School-Based Family Counseling With Refugees and Immigrants

School-Based Family Counseling with Refugees and Immigrants focuses on the practical application of School-Based Family Counseling (SBFC) with refugee and immigrant populations.

Emphasizing collaboration, mutual assistance, dialogue, and joint problem-solving, SBFC takes a systems approach that stresses the integration of school, family, and community interventions—the three most important systems that affect the lives of children. Through case studies, the book explains how to design and implement integrated SBFC interventions for refugee and immigrant populations in an explicit manner.

The book's practical, how-to approach is suitable for novice and experienced practitioners alike.

Brian A. Gerrard, PhD, is Chief Academic Officer, Western Institute for Social Research; Chair, Institute for School-Based Family Counseling; Emeritus Faculty, Counseling Psychology Department, University of San Francisco.

Erwin D. Selimos, PhD, is Professor of Sociology, West Shore Community College in Scottville, Michigan, USA.

Stephaney S. Morrison, PhD, is Associate Professor of Counselor Education and Associate Dean, School of Education and Human Development, Fairfield University, Connecticut, USA.

"If you are working with immigrant or refugee children, youth, and families, this is the research-based book that you need to read—a real hands-on practitioner's resource! It is a comprehensive book filled with descriptions of effective approaches, tools, strategies, procedures, and activities that can be used by counselors, therapists, social service providers, teachers, and administrators to build and improve the services and supports that they provide. The book includes real-life examples and case studies, often with step-by-step instructions, which make it easy for practitioners to really see how all the different strategies can be constructed and implemented. Additionally, each chapter includes insightful sections on potential challenges along with suggested solutions, multi-cultural considerations, and comprehensive lists of where to find additional resources. This book is truly a one-stop resource for those interested in not only building their knowledge and skills for providing effective interventions but also for designing programs that focus on preventing the problems that the growing number of refugees and immigrants are facing in our schools and communities."

—**Dale Fryxell, PhD,** *dean, School of Education and Behavioral Sciences; professor of Psychology, Chaminade University of Honolulu*

"Globally, refugees and immigrants form part of the daily lives of everyday citizens. Such a world-wide phenomenon is often viewed as a disruptive challenge—a challenge predicting devastating, negative outcomes for the health and well-being of families and children displaced from their familiar settings. *School-Based Family Counseling With Refugees and Immigrants* provides an alternative discourse of counseling pathways to support, heal, and enable. The text posits multiple relevant school-based family counseling models given refugee and immigrant-related challenges that are substantiated in rigorous investigation. Engaging chapters chronicle how school-based family counseling can be mobilized as resilience-enabling pathways to both buffer against the risk factors associated with being a refugee or immigrant, and promote extraordinary positive subjective health and well-being outcomes."

—**Liesel Ebersöhn, PhD,** *director, Centre for the Study of Resilience; professor, Department of Educational Psychology, University of Pretoria; secretary general, World Education Research Association*

"As a former dean, department chair, and professor of educational leadership, I highly recommend *School-Based Family Counseling With Refugees and Immigrants*. After 45 years in higher education working with public and private schools, I assumed I had the knowledge and craft to address diversity, equity, and inclusion. No time is it more important than the present to address the critical issues of refugees and immigrants in our society and schools. Reading this book gave me new insights and platforms necessary for practice. The SBFC Meta-Model provides a conceptual framework and systems approach grounded not on the refugees and immigrant families and children as problems but on opportunities for collaboration, integration, and school success. The comprehensive 19 chapters contributed by ten of the top scholars from around the world are rich with case studies, practical approaches for training, and references suitable for educational leaders and mental health practitioners alike. Our past—and our future—depends on inclusiveness of immigrant and refugee families and the integration of school, family, and community. The book, like no other, guides everyone on this critical journey."

—**Walter H. Gmelch, PhD,** *dean emeritus, professor of leadership studies, School of Education, University of San Francisco*

"*School-Based Family Counseling With Refugees and Immigrants* comprises chapters from some of the most esteemed school-based family counseling scholars, researchers, and practitioners across the globe. It fills a major void in the counseling literature, and the chapters, in the edited volume, cover a variety of topics related to refugees and immigrants. To me, this edited volume is a long-needed contribution and resource in school-based family counseling."

—**James L. Moore III, PhD,** *vice provost for Diversity and Inclusion and chief diversity officer, executive director for Todd Anthony Bell National Resource Center on the African American Male, and EHE distinguished professor of Urban Education, The Ohio State University*

School-Based Family Counseling With Refugees and Immigrants

Edited by Brian A. Gerrard, Erwin D. Selimos, and Stephaney S. Morrison

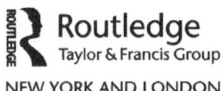
Routledge
Taylor & Francis Group

NEW YORK AND LONDON

Cover image: From Getty

First published 2023
by Routledge
605 Third Avenue, New York, NY 10158

and by Routledge
4 Park Square, Milton Park, Abingdon, Oxon, OX14 4RN

Routledge is an imprint of the Taylor & Francis Group, an informa business

© 2023 selection and editorial matter, Brian A. Gerrard, Erwin
D. Selimos, and Stephaney S. Morrison; individual chapters, the
contributors

Library of Congress Cataloging-in-Publication Data
A catalog record has been requested for this book

ISBN: 978-0-367-56469-8 (hbk)
ISBN: 978-0-367-56467-4 (pbk)
ISBN: 978-1-003-09789-1 (ebk)

DOI: 10.4324/9781003097891

Typeset in Bembo
by Apex CoVantage, LLC

Contents

Author Affiliation Table

School-Based Family Counseling with Refugees and Immigrants

Author	Affiliation
Carol E. Buchholz Holland	North Dakota State University, North Dakota, USA
Michael J. Carter	California State University, Los Angeles, USA
Claire V. Crooks	Western University, London, Ontario, Canada
Alia R. Elasmar	California State University, Los Angeles
Hans Everts	Emeritus Faculty, University of Auckland, New Zealand
Brian A. Gerrard	Western Institute for Social Research, California, USA
Kezia Gopaul-Knights	California State University, Los Angeles, USA
Emily J. Hernandez	California State University, Los Angeles, USA
Kai Yee Hon	University Malaysia Sabah, Malaysia
Sharon Hoover	University of Maryland, Baltimore, Maryland, USA
Shashank V. Joshi	Stanford University School of Medicine, Stanford, USA
Kheng Kia Khor	Universiti Tunku Abdul Rahman (UTAR), Malaysia
Otieno Kisiara	Nazareth College, New York, USA
Jin Kuan Kok	Universiti Tunku Abdul Rahman, Malaysia
Maria C. Marchetti-Mercer	University of Witwatersrand, Johannesburg, South Africa
Sudia Paloma McCaleb	Western Institute for Social Research, California, USA
Stephaney S. Morrison	Fairfield University, Connecticut, USA
Shirley Mthethwa-Sommers	Nazareth College, New York, USA
Nancy Rosenbledt	Psychologist, California, USA
Nidya Y. Ramirez Ibarra	Marriage and Family Therapist, California, USA
Natasha Robinson-Link	University of Maryland, Baltimore, Maryland, USA
Gertina J. van Schalkwyk	Emerita Faculty, University of Macau, Macao, China
Erwin D. Selimos	West Shore Community College, Michigan, USA
Maisha M. Syeda	Western University, London, Ontario, Canada
Andrea C. Tabuenca	Keck School of Medicine, University of Southern California, USA

Foreword

When my friend and colleague Brian A. Gerrard invited me to write the foreword for a book that included immigrant refugees and school-based family counseling, two of my passions and personal/professional experiences, I was delighted and yet challenged—delighted because Brian and I are two kindred souls who believe in the powerful positive benefits to children and families when the two key institutions that affect them collaborate. However, I felt challenged because of my painful recollections and experiences at the Institute for Multicultural Counseling and Education services, Inc. (IMCES), where I worked as a refugee services provider in Los Angeles and learned first-hand about refugees and their experiences both before and after their migration to the United States. One individual comes to mind. This was a bright and accomplished Bahai physician who was persecuted for his religious membership as a Bahai in Russia. Bahais were particularly threatened by the government in the then Soviet Union. After being noted for his achievements throughout Europe, this refugee had been allowed to immigrate to the United States and found himself working at a Mini Mart service station in Los Angeles. After struggling with severe depression, he committed suicide. Thus, there are many stories like this, some even more tragic, especially when it comes to children and families. For this reason I welcome this book as an excellent illustration of effective ways to reach out to this deserving group of immigrants into our society.

School-Based Family Counseling with Refugees and Immigrants is a significant compilation of the work that has been done to link schools, families, and communities for the benefit of addressing the needs of this vulnerable population. I am delighted to see how in Chapter 1 Gerrard, Selimos, and Morrison provide readers with a clear picture of this global migration of individuals and families who face enormous challenges as they dream of a better life for their children and families. I am also pleased to see this comprehensive book come together because it is my conviction that to better meet the challenge of serving refugees and immigrants, we must adopt a "system's perspective" for addressing the complex needs of diverse refugees coming from all over the world with various degrees of strengths and vulnerabilities. Moreover, it is my belief that no one institution in society, be it the schools, social service agencies, the so-called third sector of non-governmental organizations, or mental health agencies, can alone meet the complex needs of refugees.

The model of school-based family counseling has a long history in the United States and has evolved or been influenced by many theoretical and practice traditions, including family systems, the so-called one-stop shopping center model, often referred to as the school-based social services models and multicultural counseling, just to name a few of the roots informing the school-based family counseling (SBFC) model. A major strength of this book is the "applied" approach showing readers "how to" understand and apply the model in most communities, beginning with an understanding of the refugee experience, as well as their needs and practical ways to enable them to access services and resources congruent with those needs. This conceptualization is clearly outlined by Gerrard in Chapter 2, as he walks us step by step from the importance of an appropriate greeting for establishing rapport to the development of a multidisciplinary treatment plan that may involve others. Chapter 3 adds a richness to the illustration of the model by showing readers how the SBFC meta-model can successfully be applied in other countries, such as the Malaysian culture with its unique features, but whose challenges they face are similar in nature to those in the United States. In this chapter, Kok, Khor, Hon, and van Schalkwyk skillfully apply the meta-model within the context of a creative storytelling concept they describe as a collage life-story elicitation technique (CLET). The stories that emerge using this methodology add a rich and compelling picture of refugee experiences, as well as their visions and dreams of a better life.

School-Based Family Counseling With Refugees and Immigrants also addresses the myriad challenges of collaboration between immigrant families and schools, as well as the importance of working with the whole family when one hopes to make inroads for the benefit of children in a new cultural context. In Chapter 4, Gopaul-Knights, Hernandez, and Carter skillfully outline how to build collaborative relationships between schools and families in a carefully outlined step-by-step progression. Similarly, Everts helps us understand how to help migrant children by strengthening the couple's own relationship in the context of a school-based counseling model in New Zealand. In a similar manner, Ramirez Ibarra provides us with a look at the application of Narrative Therapy with undocumented immigrant families, a large population that often gets overlooked within the shadows of documented refugee migrants. This is more intensely explored in Chapter 7 where Morrison describes the challenges and opportunities to help undocumented immigrants who often have no access to public services except through the schools.

The amazing thing about *School-Based Family Counseling With Refugees and Immigrants* is its comprehensiveness. In a sense, it not only helps readers understand the strengths of the SBFC model but also explores a rich diversity of settings, situations, cultural nuances, and immigrant and refugee conditions where the model is applied and illustrated in a functional, applied manner. For example, Buchholz Holland uses a "solution-focused brief counseling" model to remind us of the meta-model and how solution-focused brief counseling once again can be an effective intervention with immigrant clients. Moreover, Morrison appropriately targets "trauma" as a major developmental challenge to refugee children and outlines a practical SBFC-informed model whose practitioners facilitate an integrated approach to provide services to children and their families. This is significant, as it has been my experience working with refugees that high levels of stress reaching traumatic elevations are common features of many refugees and immigrants.

The comprehensive and inclusive nature of this applied book on refugees and immigrants can be intimidating for its volume. However, the amazing utility and best-applied use of *School-Based Family Counseling With Refugees and Immigrants* can be found by first getting a good grasp of the SBFC model, especially the meta-model, which is outlined in Chapters 1 and 2, where the model is fully described. Each section then describes the rich application of the model by first focusing on the family, the school, and finally the community. Within each section lies the rich application of skill sets, system's formulation and applied intervention using evidence-based practice. I am proud and privileged to have the opportunity to write this preface to a book that has been part of my own professional and personal experience, both as a practitioner counselor and as an immigrant myself. It is no wonder Brian A. Gerrard and I became such close friends, for our visions are similar and our dreams for better ways to help others heal and thrive took us to the schools, families, and communities. In a way, one can say the book is encyclopedic in nature but definitive and profound in its rich contributions to the field.

Marcel Soriano, PhD

Emeritus professor

Department of Special Education & Counseling,

Charter College of Education

California State University, Los Angeles

Acknowledgments

This book began as a project of the SBFC Refugee and Immigrant Research and Intervention Team (SRIRIT), a special interest group of the Oxford Symposium in School-Based Family Counseling (SBFC). The Oxford Symposium in SBFC is an international association, sponsored by the Institute for School-Based Family Counseling. The symposium's objective is to make visible the "invisible college" of international experts in SBFC and to provide opportunity for information exchange, co-operation, and collegial networking. There are members in more than 20 countries. SBFC is an interdisciplinary, integrative, systems approach to helping children succeed academically and personally through mental health approaches that link family and school.

Firstly, we are grateful to the SBFC Refugee and Immigrant Research and Intervention Team founding members (of which we were also part): Hans Everts, Mina Fazel, Sharon Hoover, Shashank V. Joshi, and Maria Marchetti-Mercer for inspiring us to edit this book. The SRIRIT idea that lay at the heart of this book was that it would be a practical, "how to" resource for mental health practitioners and educators for collaborating with refugee and immigrant students. The support of the SRIRIT members for this book project played an important role in its completion. We are deeply grateful to Hans Everts, the founding chair of the SRIRIT, for his pioneering work in developing resilience programs for migrants, which continue to inspire us, and for his encouragement for the team to find a meaningful project. This book is the result.

Secondly, we want to thank our families for their support of our late-night vigils writing and editing.

Brian would like to thanks his wife, Olive Powell, who patiently edited his writing.

Erwin would like to thank Brian and Stephaney for being such wonderful editorial partners who made all those Zoom meetings fun and enjoyable. He would also like to thank Monique Selimos for her advice during his writing and editing.

Stephaney would like to thank God for divine strength and focus as she took on this project. She also would like to thank her husband, Rayon Morrison, and her twin girls, Victoria Grace and Sara Elizabeth, for their love and support throughout this process.

Thirdly, we would like to thank our editor Amanda Devine at Routledge for her responsiveness to our request for additional time to complete this book.

Part 1

School–Based Family Counseling Overview

1 The School-Based Family Counseling Approach to Empowering Refugees and Immigrants

Brian A. Gerrard, Erwin D. Selimos, Stephaney S. Morrison

There are increasing numbers of refugee and immigrant students present in schools worldwide. Refugee and immigrant families often experience multiple challenges in their host countries. The children and youth in those families are affected by these family, community, and school stressors in ways that can impede their learning and well-being. School-based family counseling (SBFC) is an integrative school and family approach to mental health culturally congruent with many refugees and immigrants and facilitates empowering students and families. The SBFC meta-model is presented as an organizational framework for this book.

Background

Global Increase in Refugees and Migrants

Due to wars, civil unrest, racism, and persecution, there have been an unprecedented number of persons—more than 79.5 million—displaced from home worldwide since 2018. Of this number, there are nearly 30 million refugees, and more than 15 million are under the age of 18. Over 40% of the world's displaced persons are children. Eighty percent of displaced persons live in circumstances of malnutrition and food insecurity. The top source countries for displacement are Syria, Venezuela, Afghanistan, South Sudan, and Myanmar. Out of 169 countries that have provided asylum for refugees under the UNHCR mandate, 27 countries have received more than 100,000 refugees (see Table 1.1) (UNHCR, 2020).

During 2019 there were 272 million international migrants out of a global population of 7.7 billion, amounting to 1 in every 30 persons or 3.5% of the world's population (IOM UN Migration, 2020). Figure 1.1 shows the country of origin and country of destination for migrants in 2019.

The implications are that most countries globally are experiencing increases in refugees seeking asylum and increases in immigration. This means an increased presence of refugees and immigrants in schools. While completing this book the war in the Ukraine took place and at this writing

DOI: 10.4324/9781003097891-2

Table 1.1 UNHCR 2019 Statistics for Country of Asylum Receiving More Than 100,000 Refugees

Country of Asylum	No. of Refugees Under UNHCR's Mandate
Austria	135,951
Bangladesh	854,779
Canada	101,757
China	303,379
Ecuador	104,560
Ethiopia	733,123
Democratic Republic of the Congo	523,733
France	407,915
Germany	1,146,682
Great Britain	133,083
India	195,103
Iran	979,435
Iraq	273,986
Italy	207,602
Kenya	438,899
Lebanon	916,141
Malaysia	129,107
Niger	179,997
Pakistan	1,419,596
South Sudan	289,309
Sudan	1,055,489
Sweden	253,787
Switzerland	110,162
Turkey	3,579,531
United Republic of Tanzania	242,171
United States	341,715
Yemen	268,503

there were 4 million refugees, half of them children seeking shelter in other countries and over 6 million Ukrainians displaced from their homes but seeking shelter within the Ukraine.

Challenges Experienced by Refugees and Immigrants

Migration marks a critical disjuncture in the lives of immigrants and refugees. Moving from one place to another—sometimes to areas socially and culturally much different—produces changes in one's social relationships and positions and, therefore, oneself. Through the settlement process, immigrants and refugees seek to draw coherence between their past and present lives and actively search for those things that produce a viable life in their new society of residence: safety and stability, a new home, a good job or livelihood, access to education and opportunities for self and family, and close and caring relationships with friends and loved ones. Immigrants seek to build attachments to various social institutions that make up community life, search for recognition, acceptance, respect, and avoid exclusion, misrecognition, and rejection.

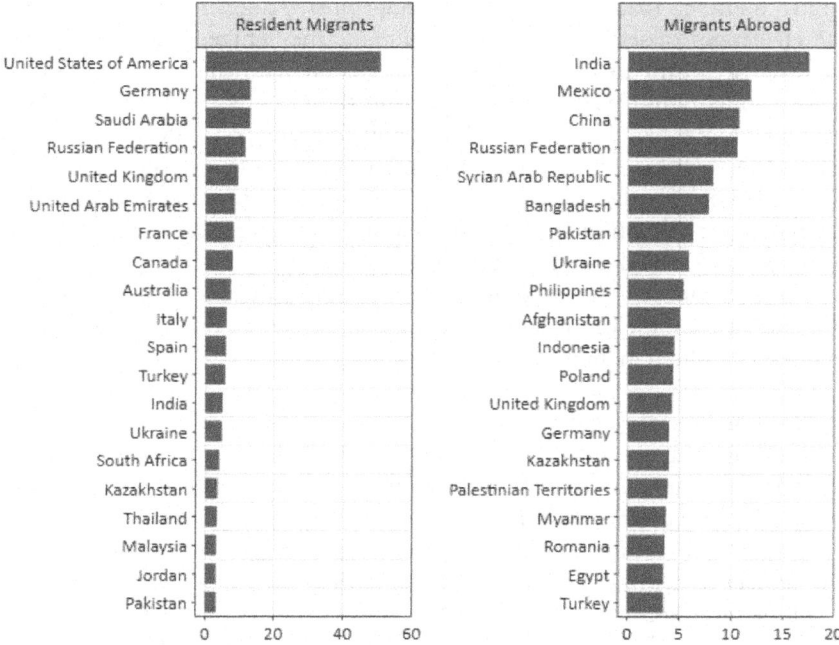

Figure 1.1 Top 20 destinations (left) and origins (right) of international migrants in 2019 (millions)

Source: UN DESA, 2019a (accessed September 18, 2019)

Research demonstrates that immigrant and refugee families face significant challenges and barriers to their settlement in new host countries. They must negotiate new cultural norms and expectations in which the degree of cultural similarity or difference between their country of origin and the receiving country may create stress that impacts their well-being (Drachman, 1992). Immigrant and refugee newcomers face barriers in finding adequate housing and accessing vital social, educational, and healthcare-related services. Many confront problems of underemployment, unemployment, poverty, and economic insecurity. Difficulty accessing social services and societal resources is often compounded by the challenges of navigating the maze of state bureaucracies—a process made more difficult when immigrants and refugees lack language proficiency or are missing necessary documentation. The challenge of building a new life is compounded by concern and worry over family members living in conflict areas and experiences of trauma. Discrimination and negative community attitudes toward newcomers further limit immigrants' access to social participation and cause injuries to their sense of worth, dignity, and belonging (Selimos, 2017).

Immigrant settlement is also an intergenerational activity. While each family member (parent, children, grandparent) struggles differently with the challenges of settlement, how immigrant and refugee families negotiate what it means to live in a new society and who they can become is worked out to and with others, especially their co-resident family members (Taylor & Krahn, 2013). Research focusing on intergenerational relationships within immigrant families demonstrates that family migration and settlement involve transformations in family relations that can produce intergenerational tensions and integration (McGovern & Devine, 2016; Selimos, 2017a; Taylor & Krahn, 2013).

The State of New South Wales Department of Education (n.d.) provides a helpful list of some of the most fundamental challenges refugees and immigrants face. These include

- finding affordable housing
- finding employment
- language and communication barriers
- racism and discrimination
- community attitudes
- impact of disrupted education on schooling
- learning English
- distance and lack of communication with families in the home country and/or countries of asylum (particularly if/where the family remains in a conflict situation)
- ongoing mental health issues due to trauma, including survivor guilt
- financial difficulties
- visa insecurity (temporary visa holders)
- separation from family members (or living in blended families)
- changes in roles and status of family members.

Of course, it is essential to note that there is incredible diversity in the social, cultural, racial, educational, and linguistic backgrounds of refugees and immigrants. These diverse backgrounds position newcomers differently in their capacity to manage and negotiate their settlement in a new host country. Furthermore, host societies and communities themselves demonstrate variation in their ability to integrate immigrants and refugees. Some societies and local communities offer many programs and services, often supported by government investments, to assist immigrants and refugees and display largely positive attitudes to immigration and newcomers. Other societies and local communities are characterized by a lack of such services, limited experience in welcoming immigrants and refugees, and, in some cases, suspicion, mistrust, and prejudice toward newcomers.

Schools are central to immigrants, refugees, and their families. As Selimos (2017) discusses, schools are often the major institution assisting in immigrant and refugee settlement and integration. They can have both positive and negative effects on how immigrant and refugee children are included in the local community. Moreover, as the proceeding section discusses, research demonstrates that immigrants and refugees typically have high educational aspirations, perceiving school success as a critical pathway to their personal/familial well-being and long-term integration in a host society. Thus, school officials and SBFC practitioners are well positioned—if not critically positioned—to be a positive force in the lives of immigrant and refugee children and their families.

Educational Aspirations of Immigrant Students and Families

The Organization for Economic Cooperation and Development (OECD) conducts periodic surveys on the performance of 15-year-olds in science, mathematics, and reading. Its Programme for International Student Assessment (PISA) survey conducted in 2006 was analyzed by Borgonovi et al. (2020) for the educational experiences of immigrant students in 30 countries. This report contains the following quotes about the aspirations of immigrant parents and students:

> What drives people from their home country is the urgent desire to make a better, safer life for themselves and, especially, their children. Immigrants are determined to make the most of any opportunity that arises from the considerable sacrifices they made by migrating. Indeed, many immigrant parents hold expectations for their children's lives that match or exceed non-immigrant families.
>
> Immigrant students themselves hold ambitious expectations for their careers. Among the countries and economies that participated in PISA 2006, immigrant students in 14 countries were more likely than non-immigrant students to expect to be working as professionals or managers when they were 30; in 26 countries, immigrant students' career expectations were similar to those held by non-immigrant students.
>
> (p. 18)

This finding highlights that immigrant families and students are highly motivated to achieve academic and career success. Teachers and mental health professionals working with immigrant and refugee students and families should regard the many obstacles these newcomers experience in schools and their host communities as only temporary roadblocks on a determined path to achieve academic and career success.

Strengths of School-Based Family Counseling

School-based family counseling (SBFC) is an integrated, systems approach to helping children and youth succeed academically and personally through mental health approaches that link family and school (Gerrard et al., 2019).

SBFC has its origins in the work of psychiatrist Alfred Adler who in the 1920s established 30 guidance clinics in Vienna, each attached to a school. Adler recognized that family and school are the two most important social institutions affecting children. By collaborating with schools and families, mental health professionals can better help children overcome problems.

SBFC has nine strengths that make it a valuable approach to helping refugee and immigrant children, youth, and families.

- School and family focus
- Systems orientation
- Educational focus
- Parent partnership
- Multicultural sensitivity
- Child advocacy
- Promotion of school transformation
- Interdisciplinary focus
- Evidence-based support

School and Family Focus

Helping children with problems by mobilizing school and family resources is the hallmark of the SBFC approach. Traditional mental health approaches to assisting children have developed in a "silo" fashion: school mental health professionals (for example) counseled children at school, and community agency mental health professionals counseled the family at community agencies. The problem with this "silo" approach to counseling and therapy is that when family problems affect students at school, the traditional approach is for the school mental health professional to refer the family to a community agency for family therapy. Unfortunately, many families do not go for family therapy because they view the problem as caused by the school or regard therapy as only for "crazy persons." As a result, minority families often do not receive the benefit of combined school and family intervention for their children. SBFC takes a different approach and combines family and school interventions in an educational framework that makes counseling and therapy more acceptable to refugee and immigrant families.

Systems Orientation

The cornerstone of the SBFC approach is that it is a systems approach to mental health that emphasizes working with a student's various primary groups: the family (parents, grandparents, siblings, and other extended family members); the school (the classroom context: students, teachers, principals, and other school personnel); the peer group (which overlaps with the school and community) and which is known to have strong influence on adolescents; and the community (in which religious, sporting, and other organizations impact children and youth). This represents a holistic approach to helping children: by mobilizing resources in multiple areas of a child's life. It is a tenet of family systems theory that one individual in a family will often exhibit behaviorally the stresses that run deep within the whole family. This individual, called the "identified" patient, is intimately linked to other family members who can remain "invisible" if the mental health professional lacks a systems view and works only with the "identified patient" (who is often a child).

The SBFC meta-model is a useful tool for the SBFC practitioner because it highlights five areas of potential systems focus (see Figure 1.2). There is an emphasis on intervention and prevention, as well as on family and school, providing four quadrants: school intervention, family intervention, school

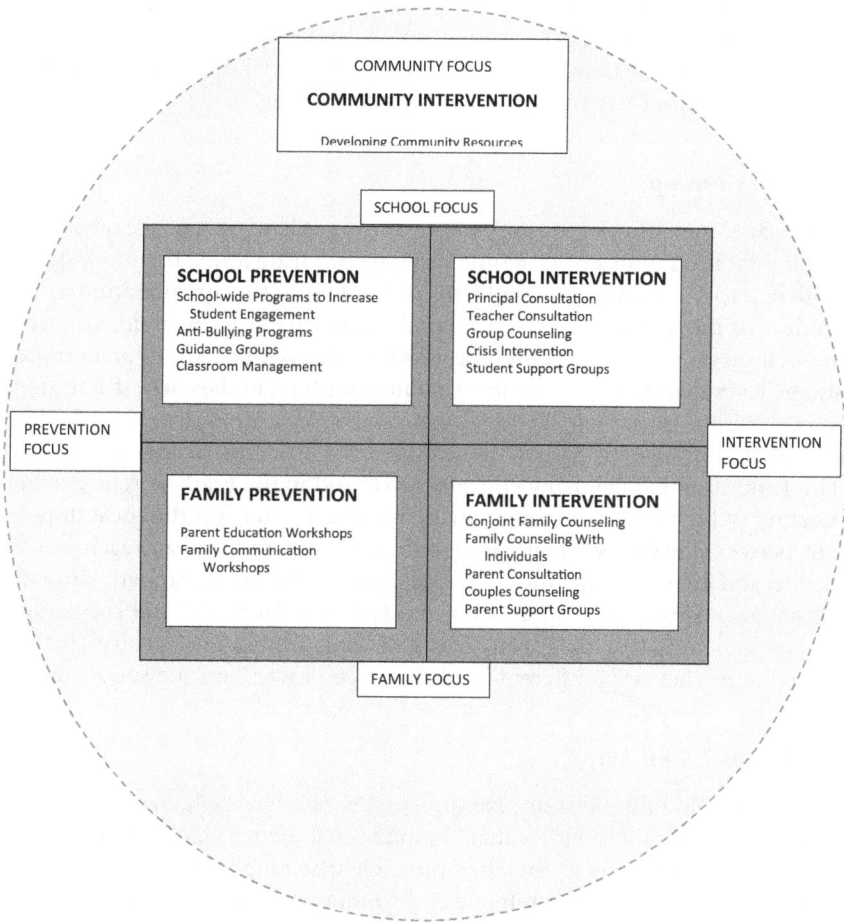

Figure 1.2 The SBFC Meta-model with Prevention and Intervention Categories

prevention, and family prevention. Both family and school intervention and prevention occur in a broader community context. When thinking systemically, SBFC practitioners pay particular attention to these five areas.

Educational Focus

The stigma of receiving mental health counseling that prevents many minority families from seeking help is avoided in SBFC because of the explicit focus taken on working with the family to promote school success for their children. Refugee and immigrant families tend to be very interested in their children doing well at school. A phone call from an SBFC practitioner inviting the parents or guardians to come to the school for a collaborative discussion on how to help their child do better at school is more likely to get a positive response from the family than if the school mental health professional phones with a recommendation that the family "seek therapy." In the context of helping parents to assist a son or daughter to do better at school, inevitably, family challenges and tensions are talked about but always in an educational, rather than a therapy, frame of reference.

Parent Partnership

The SBFC practitioner treats parents and guardians as equal partners in helping their children to overcome challenges. Historically, there is a strong tendency to view children's problems in the family therapy literature as the product of the larger dysfunctional family. Thus, to help the child, you treat the dysfunctional family. While this is often the case, the SBFC practitioner also believes that there are valuable resources within families that, if activated, bring healing. In the last 20 years, extensive research has demonstrated the critical importance of parent involvement for students' academic growth. This realization has led many educators to abandon the yearly parent-teacher meeting (which conveyed the message that the teacher was the most important person affecting student's academic behavior) and instead reach out to parents and guardians in a more inviting and collaborative manner. This collaborative, respect-based approach is fundamental for SBFC and contradicts the societal messages that many refugees and immigrants receive that, as newcomers, they are "different" and therefore "lower" on the social rung.

Multicultural Sensitivity

SBFC is a multiculturally sensitive approach because it emphasizes the importance of a family focus rather than an individual focus. That is, SBFC is not a traditional Eurocentric therapy approach that emphasizes only working with the individual. Many refugee and immigrant families come from collectivistic cultures that emphasize interdependence over independence. In addition, the SBFC practitioner assumes that cultural differences should not be viewed as challenges and obstacles but instead contain potential resources for strengthening children and families.

Child Advocacy

Because SBFC is a systems approach, the student, the family, and the school are all considered part of the client system. The SBFC practitioner has a responsibility to consider ways to empower students, families, and schools. But there is a hierarchy among these client levels, and the SBFC practitioner is a child advocate. This is because children are more vulnerable to harm and in need of greater protection. Because of this child advocacy position, the SBFC practitioner will avoid seeing only the child and doing "surrogate parent therapy" where the therapist places herself/himself in the role of the "good parent" who always listens and is rewarding. Instead, the SBFC practitioner knows that the best way to help a child is to help the parent become a more effective parent. Engaging with parents who have been treated dismissively by schools can be challenging and requires persistence on the part of the SBFC practitioner, who persists because she/he knows that ultimately this will benefit the child. Similarly, when an SBFC practitioner is dealing with a student who is being bullied and bullying is rife in a classroom or entire school, the SBFC practitioner will work to transform the bully, the classroom, and the school because it is not enough to teach a student to cope with an unjust environment. In summary, the SBFC commitment to child advocacy motivates the SBFC practitioner to engage with family and school to mobilize in these environments to benefit students.

Promotion of School Transformation

Just as families sometimes need to change to help children overcome difficulties, schools must also change to provide more positive learning environments for students. Bullying is an international problem in schools, and an important factor in bullying is the role of student bystanders who may tacitly support the bullying. In addition, teachers and principals are often unaware that the bullying is occurring. A fundamental part of the SBFC practitioner's role is to intervene in two areas of the SBFC meta-model called school intervention and school prevention. This type of intervention is an integral part of the SBFC practitioner's role with refugee and immigrant students because newcomer students can have many challenges in fitting into a new school: bullying, prejudicial attitudes of teachers, teachers lacking a background in teaching diverse students, being discriminated against because of an "accent" when speaking, and failure of the school to engage with parents. When a school is deficient in providing a constructive learning environment for refugees and immigrants, it is a core part of the SBFC practitioner's role to work with school personnel to make positive changes. This can be a challenge for the SBFC practitioner if they are an employee of the school (note:

SBFC practitioners may also be based in community agencies or in private practice). SBFC practitioners can be very helpful to refugee and immigrant students and their families by advocating for school changes that facilitate student learning.

Interdisciplinary Focus

An SBFC approach may be used by any of the mental health professions: counseling, social work, psychology, psychiatry, psychiatric nursing, and marital and family therapy. An SBFC approach is not meant to substitute for the other mental health approaches but should be viewed as a meta-model for conceptualizing family and school interventions to help students. Since the numbers of refugee and immigrant students in schools globally are increasing, the interdisciplinary focus of SBFC makes it a flexible model that can be adopted by various mental health professionals that work with schools and families.

Evidence-Based Support

There is moderate evidence-based support for the effectiveness of SBFC in nine randomized control group studies that compared combined school and family intervention with school-only intervention or no treatment and found the combined intervention superior (see Box 1.1). More than half of these randomized clinical trial (RCT) studies were done with minority clients. Gerrard (2008) reviewed more than 150 quantitative and qualitative studies on the importance of family intervention approaches being used in schools.

Box 1.1 Evidence-Based Support for SBFC

Apisitwasana, N., Perngparn, U., & Cottler, L. (2018). Effectiveness of school- and family-based interventions to prevent gaming addiction among grades 4–5 students in Bangkok, Thailand. *Psychology Research and Behavior Management, 11*, 103–115. doi:10.2147/PRBM.S145868

Conduct Problems Prevention Research Group. (2007). Fast track randomized controlled trial to prevent externalizing psychiatric disorders: Findings from grades 3 to 9. *Journal of the American Academy of Child and Adolescent Psychiatry, 46*(10), 1250–1262. doi:10.1097/chi.0b013e31813e5d39

Eddy, J., Reid, J., & Fetrow, R. (2000). An elementary school-based prevention program targeting modifiable antecedents of youth delinquency and violence: Linking the interests of families and teachers (LIFT). *Journal of Emotional and Behavioral Disorders, 8*(3), 165–176.

Flay, B., Graumlich S., Segawa, E., Burns, J., Amuwo, S., Bell, C., . . . Weisberg, R. (2004). Effects of 2 prevention programs on high-risk behaviors among African American youth: A randomized trial. *Archives of Pediatrics and Adolescent Medicine, 158*(4), 377–384. doi:10.1001/archpedi.158.4.377

Garbacz, S., McIntyre, L., Stormshak, E., & Kosty, D. (2020). The efficacy of the family check-up on children's emotional and behavior problems in early elementary school. *Journal of Emotional and Behavioral Disorders, 28*(2), 67–79.

Kratochwill, T., McDonald, L., Levin, J., Bear-Tibbetts, H., & Demaray, M. (2004). Families and schools together: An experimental analysis of a parent-mediated multi-family group program for American Indian children. *Journal of School Psychology, 42*(5), 359–383.

Kratochwill, T., McDonald, L., Levin, J., Scalia, P., & Coover, G. (2009). Families and schools together: An experimental study of multi-family support groups for children at risk. *Journal of School Psychology, 47*, 245–265. doi:10.1016/j.jsp.2009.03.001

Lochman, J., & Wells, K. (2004). The coping power program for preadolescent aggressive boys and their parents: Outcome effects at the 1-year follow-up. *Journal of Consulting and Clinical Psychology, 72*(4), 571–578.

Power, T., Mautone, J., Soffer, S., Clarke, A., Marshall, S., Sharman, J., . . . Jawad, A. (2012). A family-school intervention for children with ADHD: Results of a randomized clinical trial. *Journal of Consulting and Clinical Psychology, 80*(4), 611–623.

How to Use This Book

The first three chapters of this book present the SBFC approach to collaborating with refugee and immigrant students and their families; how to develop a culture of dialogue between schools, families, and students; and how to develop an SBFC case conceptualization to guide mental health intervention.

This book is organized around the SBFC meta-model (see Figure 1.2). For each of the four quadrants of the SBFC meta-model—*School Intervention, School Prevention, Family Intervention,* and *Family Prevention*—there are four chapters describing strategies for helping refugee and immigrant students (see Figure 1.3). *Family Intervention* deals with strategies to use when refugee and immigrant families face serious mental health challenges. These chapters deal with how to assess family strengths and challenges, how to conduct conjoint family counseling, how to strengthen couple relationships, and the use of Narrative Therapy with undocumented families. *Family Prevention* deals with strategies for strengthening families so that they become more resilient and able to handle challenges. Chapters here discuss how to promote family-school bonding, strengthen family solidarity, facilitate parent education workshops, and how to use social media to strengthen extended refugee and immigrant families. *School Intervention* deals with strategies for remediating students' problems. Chapters in this section describe ways to counsel undocumented students, use solution-focused counseling to find practical solutions, deal with student trauma, and promote school engagement. *School Prevention* presents approaches for preventing problems from

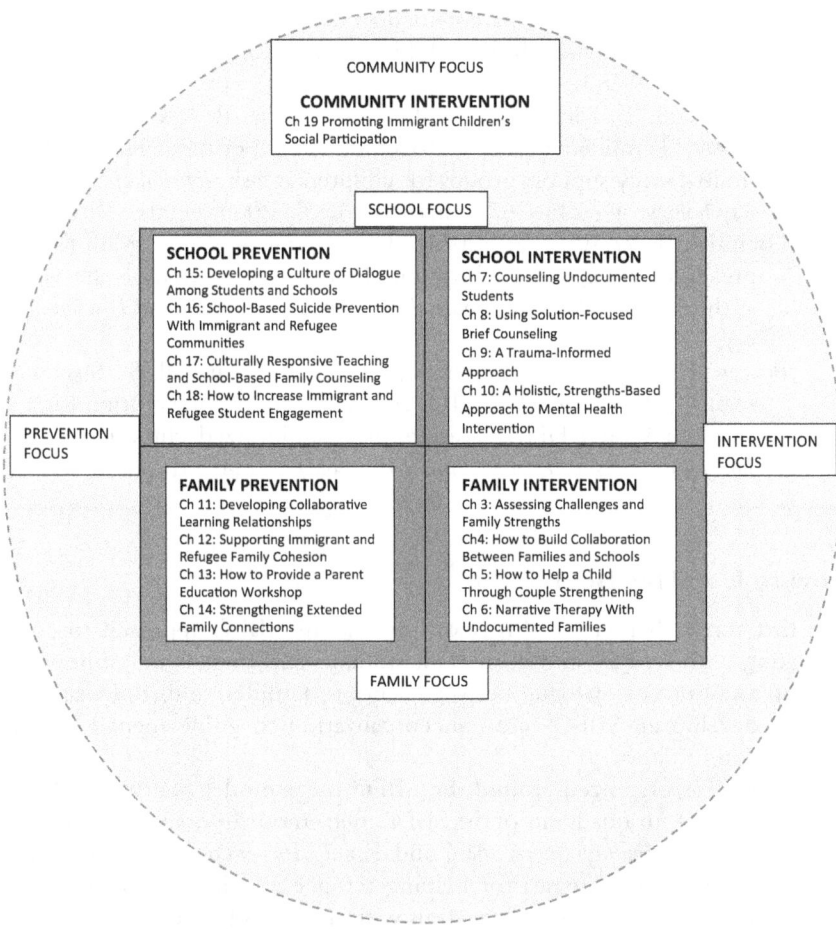

Figure 1.3 The SBFC Meta-model with Chapters

occurring in the first place. Chapters here cover suicide prevention, building on students' strengths, anti–bullying programs, and developing collaborative learning relationships between teachers and parents. A final chapter deals with mobilizing community resources to help refugees and immigrants by fostering a culture of dialogue in the community.

Resources

Books on SBFC

Boyd-Franklin, L., & Hafer Bry, B. (2000). *Reaching out in family therapy*. Guilford Press.

Fine, M. J., & Carlson, C. (Eds.). (1992). *Family-school intervention: A systems perspective*. Allyn & Bacon.

Gerrard, B., Carter, M., & Ribera, D. (2019). *School-based family counseling: An interdisciplinary practitioner's guide*. Routledge.

Gerrard, B., & Soriano, M. (Eds.). (2013). *School-based family counseling: Transforming family-school relationships. Phoenix*. Createspace.

Hinckle, J., & Wells, M. (1995). *Family counseling in the schools*. Educational Resources Information Center/Cass Publications.

Laundy, K. C. (2015). *Building school-based collaborative mental health teams: A systems approach to student achievement*. TPI Press.

Miller, L. D. (Ed.). (2002). *Integrating school and family counseling: Practical solutions*. American Counseling Association.

Palmatier, L. L. (1998). *Crisis counseling for a quality school community: A family perspective*. Taylor & Francis.

Peacock, G., & Collett, B. (2010). *Collaborative Home/school interventions: Evidence-based solutions for emotional, behavioral, and academic problems*. Guilford.

Sherman, R., Shumsky, A., & Roundtree, Y. (1994). *Enlarging the therapeutic circle*. Brunner/Mazel.

Sheridan, S., & Kratochwill, T. (2008). *Conjoint behavioral consultation: Promoting family-based connections and interventions*. Springer.

Steele, W., & Raider, M. (1991). *Working with families in crisis: School-based intervention*. Guilford.

Walsh, W., & Giblen, N. (Eds.). (1988). *Family counseling in school settings*. Charles C. Thomas.

Walsh, W., & Williams, G. (1997). *Schools and family therapy: Using systems theory and family therapy in the resolution of school problems*. Charles C. Thomas.

Internet Resources

Wikipedia.com

Wikipedia contains a concise overview of SBFC covering the following categories: The Need for SBFC, Origins, Later Developments, Strengths of SBFC, Evidence-based Support for SBFC, SBFC Challenges and Solutions in Low-Income Communities, Barriers to Entry for SBFC, Examples of Books on School-Based Family Counseling.

Oxfordsymposium-sbfc.com

This is the website for the Oxford Symposium in School-Based Family Counseling, an international organization with the mission of promoting school-based family counseling. The website hosts a 25 minute SBFC overview video with slides. The International Journal for School-based Family Counseling is also hosted on this website.

Videos on SBFC

"SBFC: An Interdisciplinary Practitioner's Guide" At this YouTube channel there are 15 role-played videos on different aspects of SBFC:

- First SBFC Interview with Parents or Guardians
- Conducting a Multimodal Assessment
- Narrative Therapy Interview
- How to Do Conjoint Family Counseling
- A CBT Approach to Family Counseling with Individuals

  Systematic Muscle Relaxation
  Cognitive Restructuring
  Systematic Desensitization
  Behavior Rehearsal

- How to Consult with Teachers
- Navigating Emotion in a Classroom Meeting
- Facilitating a Parent Support Group
- Conducting an Initial Wraparound Meeting

These videos were made to accompany the book:
Gerrard, B., Carter, M., & Ribera, D. (2019). *School-based family counseling: An interdisciplinary practitioner's guide.* Routledge.

Bibliography

Borgonovi, F., Phair, R., & Piacentini, M. (2020). Helping immigrant students to succeed at school—And beyond. *OECD Directorate for Education and Skills.* Retrieved December 1, 2020. http://www.oecd.org/education/Helping-immigrant-students-to-succeed-at-school-and-beyond.pdf.

Drachman, D. (1992). A stage-of-migration framework for services to immigrant populations. *Social Work, 37*(1), 68–72.

Gerrard, B. (2008). School-based family counseling: Overview, trends and recommendations for future research. *International Journal for School-based Family Counseling, 1*, 1–30.

Gerrard, B., Carter, M., & Ribera, D. (2019). *School-based family counseling: An interdisciplinary practitioner's guide.* Routledge.

IOM UN *migration*. (2020). World migrate on report. International Organization for Migration.

McGovern, F., & Devine, D. (2016). The care worlds of migrant children – Exploring inter-generational dynamics of love, care and solidarity across home and school. *Childhood, 23*(1), 37–52. https://doi.org/10.1177/0907568215579734

Organization for Economic Co-Operation and Development. (2007). PISA 2006: Science competencies for tomorrow's world, *1. Analysis, PISA*. OECD Publishing. https://doi.org/10.1787/9789264040014-en

Selimos, E. D. (2017). *Young immigrant lives: A study of the migration and settlement experiences of immigrant and refugee youth in Windsor, Ontario* [Dissertation]. University of Windsor.

Selimos, E. D. (2018). 'I am doing a double thing. It is for me and it is for her': Exploring the biographical agency of newcomer immigrant and refugee youth. *YOUNG, 26*(4), 332–347. https://doi.org/10.1177/1103308817715144

State of New South Wales Department of Education. (n.d.). 2020RoadstoRefuge. Retrieved December 5, 2020. http://www.roads-to-refuge.com.au/settlement/settlement-challenges.html

Taylor, A., & Krahn, H. (2013). Living through our children: Exploring the education and career 'choices' of racialized immigrant youth in Canada. *Journal of Youth Studies, 16*(8), 1000–1021. https://doi.org/10.1080/13676261.2013.772575

United Nations High Commission for Refugees. (2020). Figures at a glance. Retrieved December 5, 2020. http://www.unhcr.org/en-us/figures-at-a-glance.html

2 Developing the SBFC Case Conceptualization With Refugee and Immigrant Clients

Brian A. Gerrard

This chapter describes how to develop a school-based family counseling (SBFC) case conceptualization with refugee and immigrant clients. The case conceptualization involves assessing individual, family, school, community, and cultural factors that must be taken into consideration in planning mental health interventions. The SBFC meta-model provides an overall framework for thinking about how to help children, families, and schools. Practical suggestions are provided for assessing different system levels in a comprehensive manner.

Background

A case conceptualization is a summary of the important variables influencing a client's behavior. In using a school-based family counseling (SBFC) approach the practitioner should collect information in five areas: individual, family, school, community, and cultural. A basic assumption in SBFC is that children are profoundly affected by the interpersonal and group systems of which they are part and that family and school have a particular influence. In addition, as children age, their peer group has an increasingly important influence and, like the family, is a primary group system that should be assessed as well. It is important to note that SBFC in an approach that may be used with other mental health theoretical approaches such as behavioral, psychodynamic, cognitive-behavioral, narrative, constructivist, solution-focused, Adlerian, person-centered, and so on. However, SBFC requires a broad systems approach that is used even when only working with an individual.

Procedure

The SBFC assessment approach involves seven steps:

1. *Making Friends with the Family.* This is a critical step: if you cannot win the trust of the family you are unlikely to obtain accurate information.

DOI: 10.4324/9781003097891-3

2. *Assessing the Student's Behavior.* This involves identifying strengths and challenges in the student's relationships with family members, school personnel, peers (at school and in the community), and developing an awareness of how cultural factors influence these relationships.

3. *Assessing the Family System.* This involves collecting information on the relationships between different family members, the overall level of cohesion and flexibility in the family, the family's migrant history, and how culture affects family decisions.

4. *Assessing the School System.* This involves assessing the client's classroom and the school as systems with particular reference to what is called "social climate."

5. *Assessing Community Influences.* This involves assessing the positive and negative influences the community has on the refugee/immigrant student and his/her family.

6. *Assessing Cultural Factors.* Cultural variables must be considered in each of the preceding five assessment areas. Each of us views the world through a cultural perspective. When persons with different cultural perspectives interact, this becomes valuable information for understanding communication and miscommunication.

Assessment steps 2–6 involve taking stock of both strengths and challenges.

7. *Developing the Treatment Plan.* On the basis of assessment, the final step is formulating a treatment plan that addresses strengths and challenges affecting the student, family, school, and community.

These seven case conceptualization steps will be illustrated using a hypothetical case study involving a middle school student.

The Case of Amira

Amira Hassan is a 12-year-old girl in grade 8 in Meadow Middle School in a large urban city. Amira's teacher Ms. Ramirez has referred Amira to the SBFC practitioner, Judy, because Amira has frequently been tearful in class. Following a meeting that Judy has had with Amira and her parents Fatima and Ahmed, Judy learns that 6 months earlier the family had left Syria as refugees because of political unrest. Fatima was a physician in Syria but is not allowed to practice in the host country until she has completed additional training. Ahmed, who was a former teacher in Syria, is in a similar circumstance and has been providing income while driving a taxi. Both parents speak English. The grandparents remained behind in Syria because they were too elderly to make the arduous journey to Italy and from there to the host country.

This is the basic family background from which Judy will begin to build her SBFC case conceptualization for helping Amira. We will now examine each assessment step in detail.

Step 1: Making Friends With the Family

In order to make friends with the family it is essential to approach the parents/guardians with respect and to treat them as experts in their own right with respect to their children and family members. This can be achieved by communicating to the parents that you view them as having wisdom that will help their child succeed in school and by communicating to them that your role is to assist them as a partner in promoting their child's school success. Judy's initial phone call with Mrs. Hassan (or letter to the parents) might look something like this:

> *"Hello Mrs. Hassan, my name is Judy Riesling and I am a school mental health professional at Meadow Middle school. I am calling about your daughter Amira. Amira has been tearful a lot at school lately and her teacher is worried about her because it seems to be affecting Amira's schoolwork. I spoke with Amira briefly the other day and was impressed with how polite she was.*
>
> *I think there is a lot we can do together to help Amira, but I need your help. No one knows Amira better than you do and it would be very helpful to me if you and your husband would be willing to meet briefly with me at your convenience so that I can learn more about Amira.*

Note that the emphasis is on (a) school success (not therapy) and (b) the parents are approached as co-partners with the SBFC practitioner. If you are successful in making friends with the parents/guardians, you will more likely receive parental consent to provide counseling to the student and will likely get a first meeting with one or both parents. During the first meeting with the parents/guardians, here are some tips that may be helpful:

- Begin by thanking them for coming to meet with you.
- Explain to the parents/guardians what your role in the school is and that collaborating with parents to help children succeed at school is a core part of your role.
- Point out something positive about the child that you have noticed (or that a teacher has shared with you).
- Ask the parents/guardians what they are most proud of about their child.
- What are their hopes for their child's future?
- How do they feel about the school? Do they have any concerns?
- Be sure to involve both parents in the conversation (should both attend). Also, be aware that one parent may be regarded by the family as the "final authority" and that the consequences of your failure to detect who this is, or your ignoring them, will affect your ability to help the student. Be aware that this family member with the most influence may be in the home country (e.g., a grandparent).
- Look for things you share in common with the parents/guardians. Commenting on these helps build relationship.

- What are their thoughts about why their child is experiencing a challenge (e.g., being tearful in class)?
- Invite them to ask you questions.
- If they are willing, let them tell you their migration story. Using a person-centered counseling approach (with empathy/active listening) is generally a helpful strategy in helping clients to tell their story.
- Ask them if they have had any previous experience with a mental health professional like yourself. If so, explore what their positive/negative experience was.
- Ask them if they would be willing to work with you to find ways to help their child do better at school. Keep in mind that for various reasons they may be reluctant to work with you. For example, they may have had prior negative communication with the school (such as critical messages from a teacher or principal). If other school personnel have been abrupt or insensitive in dealing with the family, it is normal for the family to view you with suspicion. You must earn the family's trust by listening, using empathy, and avoiding being defensive. It is important to understand that it is not unusual for refugee and immigrant families to feel marginalized by school personnel. Also, keep in mind that it may take several meetings or phone conversations with the parents/guardians to build trust. It is important to be patient and not give up.

Step 2: Assessing the Student's Behavior

The assessment of the student should involve three key sources of information: an interview with the student, consultation with the teacher, and consultation with the parents/guardians. If the student has been referred to you, it is always a good idea to speak with the teacher, principal, or parent to determine the reason for the referral.

INTERVIEW WITH THE STUDENT

When meeting with the student the most important task is to make friends with the student and build trust so that the student feels comfortable sharing concerns with you. A useful way to systematically gather information about a student's concern is to use multimodal assessment (Multimodal therapy, 2019).

This involves asking the student questions that assess seven different aspects of personality and behavior:

Behavior: What did you say and do?
Affect: What emotions did you experience later?
Sensation: What sensations or tensions did you experience in your body?
Imagery: What images or pictures in your mind did you have?
Cognition: What thoughts did you have? What did what has happened mean to you?

Interpersonal: What did the other person(s) say or do?

Drugs/Biology: How was your body and health affected? Were you affected by your diet, by lack of exercise or sleep, or by taking medication or drugs?

Lazarus refers to this as multimodal assessment of the BASIC ID. When using the BASIC ID with a client, it is important to be flexible about the order in which the questions are asked. It is often helpful to begin with the "trigger" event that caused the student distress. The SBFC practitioner should also make occasional active listening (empathy) responses before proceeding to the next question.

Here is an example of what a BASIC ID would look like for the SBFC practitioner Judy during the interview with Amira when Amira revealed that another girl had bullied her.

Judy: *Please tell me more about this incident that occurred last week where you were bullied by Jane. What did she say and do to you? (Interpersonal)*

Amira: *She knocked my books off my desk when the teacher wasn't looking.*

Judy: *Did Jane say anything to you?*

Amira: *No, but she laughed.*

Judy: *Did the other students say or do anything?*

Amira: *Jane's two friends also laughed.*

Judy: *What did you say or do in response? (Behavior)*

Amira: *I picked up my books and said to Jane: "That's not nice!"*

Judy: *Did she say anything back to you? (Interpersonal)*

Amira: *She said: "Go back to Syria."*

Judy: *That must have been very upsetting (Active Listening). What feelings or emotions did you have when she said that? (Affect)*

Amira: *I felt angry.*

Judy: *Did you feel tension anywhere in your body? (Sensation)*

Amira: *My stomach felt very tense.*

Judy: *Sometimes when something like this happens, a person can feel ill later or have trouble eating or sleeping. Did anything like this happen to you?*

Amira: *Yes, I threw up my dinner that night, and I found it difficult to go to sleep.*

Judy: *Did you have any images or pictures in your head during this incident? (Imagery)*

Amira: *I thought about knocking her books to the floor.*

Judy: *You must have felt really hurt by her behavior. (Active Listening) What did this incident mean to you? (Cognition)*

Amira: *Nobody at school likes me. I hate it there.*

What Judy learned from her multimodal assessment is that this incident of bullying had a profound effect on Amira, affecting her health and sleep, and that Amira believes everyone at school dislikes her. Further, it is evident from this assessment that bystanders are supporting Jane's bullying behavior. This is valuable information that Judy can use in developing a treatment plan.

The SBFC practitioner should also ask questions about how the student gets along with fellow students at school, peers in the community, and family members at home and back in the home country. The circular relationship map (see Figure 2.1) can be used to identify significant relationships in the client's life.

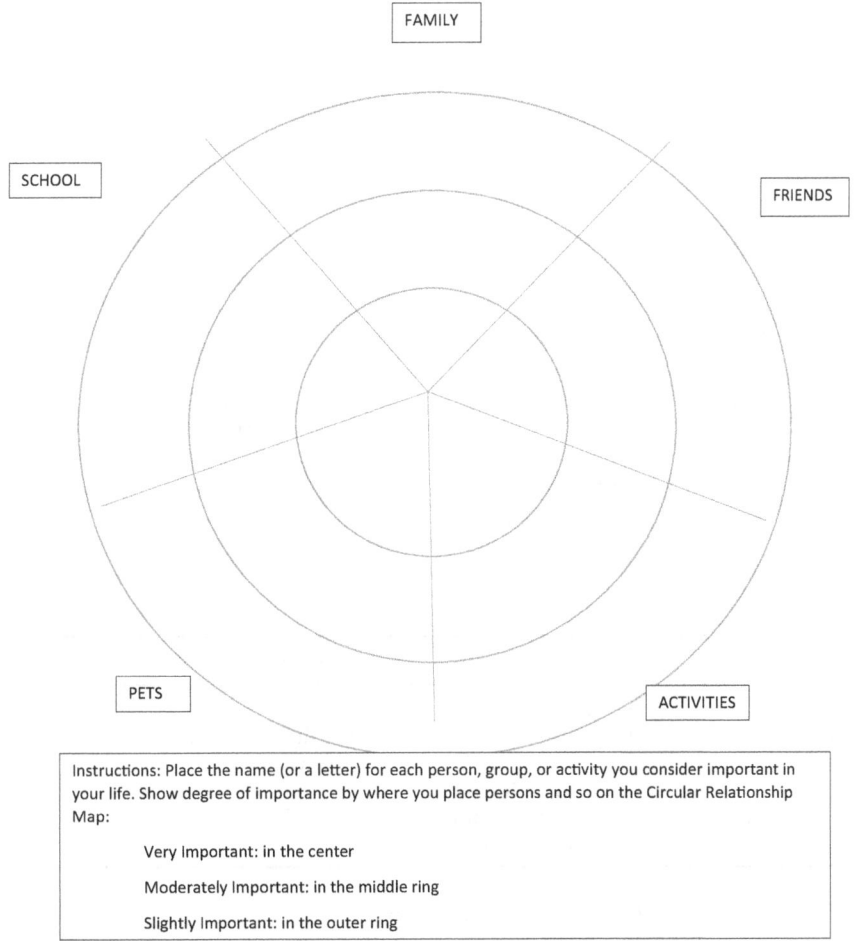

Instructions: Place the name (or a letter) for each person, group, or activity you consider important in your life. Show degree of importance by where you place persons and so on the Circular Relationship Map:

    Very Important: in the center

    Moderately Important: in the middle ring

    Slightly Important: in the outer ring

Figure 2.1 Circular Relationship Map

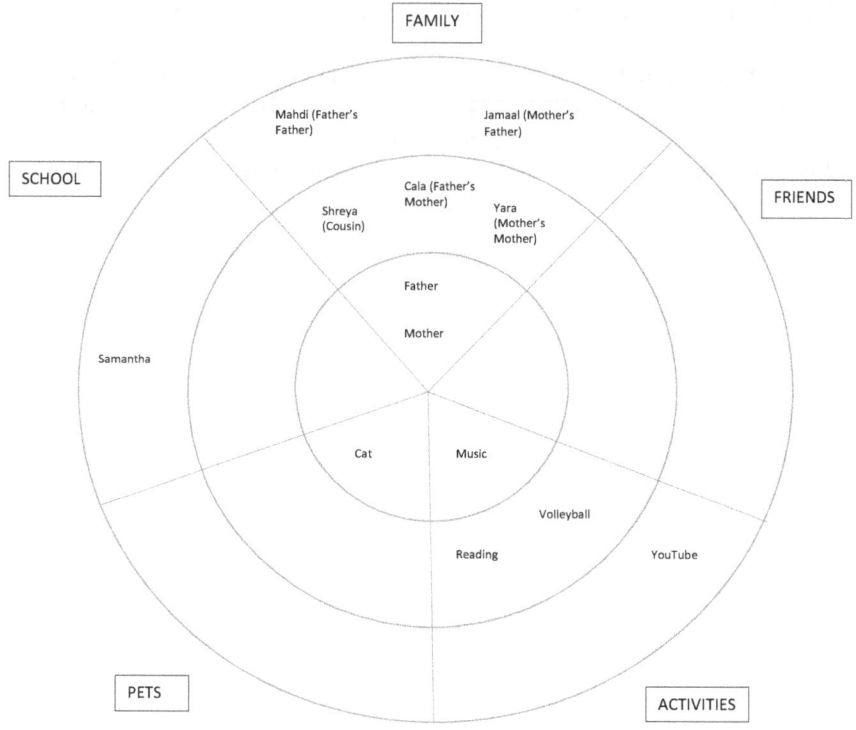

Instructions: Place the initials (or a letter) for each person, group, or activity you consider important in your life. Show degree of importance by where you place persons and so on the Circular Relationship Map:

Very Important: in the center

Moderately Important: in the middle ring

Slightly Important: in the outer ring

	Family	*Activities*	*School*	*Pets*
Inner circle	Father, Mother	Music		Cat
Middle circle	Shreya (Cousin)	Reading		
	Cala (Father's mother)	Volleyball		
	Yara (Mother's mother)			
Outer circle	Mahdi (Father's father	YouTube	Samantha	
	Jamal (Mother's father)			

Figure 2.2 Circular Relationship Map for Amira

As can be seen Amira considers her parents and her cat very important in her life. Her cousin Ali and her grandmother Yara, both of whom are back in Syria, are also important to her. However, Amira has no friends, and there is only one girl at school, Samantha, with whom she feels a moderate connection.

CONSULTING WITH THE TEACHER

In this case Ms. Ramirez, the teacher, was aware that Amira was sometimes tearful in class but was unaware of the bullying because Amira did not report it. It is often helpful for the SBFC practitioner to get permission to sit in on a class in order to observe from the back of the room how a client interacts with other students and how the teacher and students relate to the client. By doing this Judy discovered that Samantha, a girl Amira likes, but is not close to, is in the same class as Amira. However, Samantha sits on the opposite side of the classroom. Judy also noticed how Jane and two other students frequently misbehaved when the teacher's back was turned.

CONSULTING WITH THE PARENTS

The advantage of the SBFC practitioner meeting with the parents and the student together is that it allows the SBFC practitioner to directly observe how the student gets along with each parent. In addition, it allows the SBFC practitioner to get a sense of how well the parents work together and whether there is any couple difficulties (as marital discord has a profound impact on children). When meeting with Amira's parents, Judy noticed that they frequently disagreed with each other about Amira. Amira's father, Ahmed, felt it essential that Amira wear a hijab, whereas Fatima disagreed. This suggested to Judy that there was some marital discord present.

Step 3: Assessing the Family System

Constructing a family genogram is one of the most basic assessments done by family counselors. A genogram is a sort of family tree that diagrams all the family members regardless of where they are living. This is especially important with refugee and immigrant families because often the most influential family members, the ones who have the authority and power to make "final" decisions that affect the family, are in another (the home) country. Box 2.1 lists sample symbols used to develop the genogram. In addition to showing who the family members are, the genogram can also be used to show the quality of relationship between specific family members.

Box 2.1   A Basic Genogram

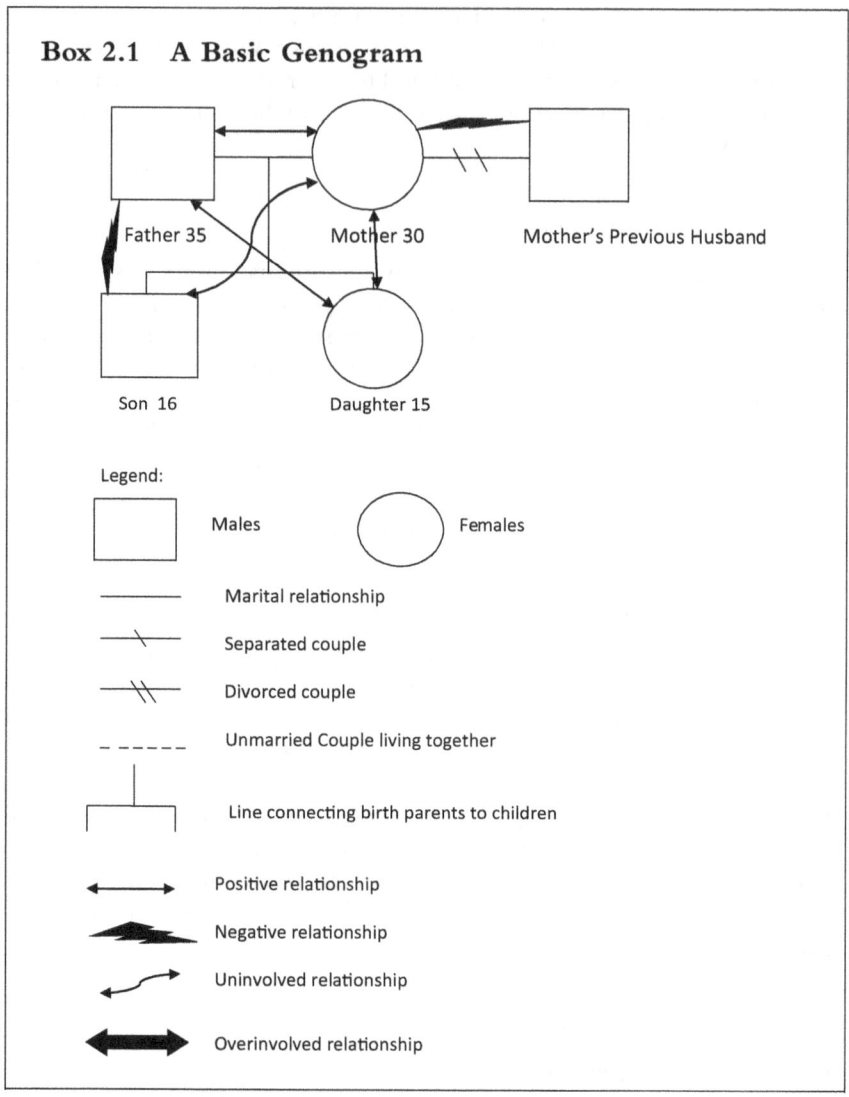

Father 35   Mother 30   Mother's Previous Husband

Son 16   Daughter 15

Legend:

☐   Males   ◯   Females

———   Marital relationship

—⧸—   Separated couple

—⧸⧸—   Divorced couple

─ ─ ─ ─   Unmarried Couple living together

⊓   Line connecting birth parents to children

◄——►   Positive relationship

◄▬▬   Negative relationship

◡——►   Uninvolved relationship

◄═══►   Overinvolved relationship

A genogram for Amira's family constructed by Judy after meeting the parents and gathering information about the family is shown as Figure 2.3.

What this genogram reveals is that there is tension between Amira's parents. The tension is related to feelings of rejection Fatima feels from her mother-in-law, Cala. Cala, who has an overly close relationship with her son, is critical of the way Amira is being raised by Fatima. Cala believes Fatima is allowing Amira to learn too many "Western" ways and that Amira needs to go to mosque more frequently. Ahmed is reluctant to ask his mother to let Fatima and him handle the parenting of Amira, and his reluctance is a source of constant friction between the parents. The frequent arguments between Ahmed and Fatima are very upsetting to Amira, causing her to frequently be

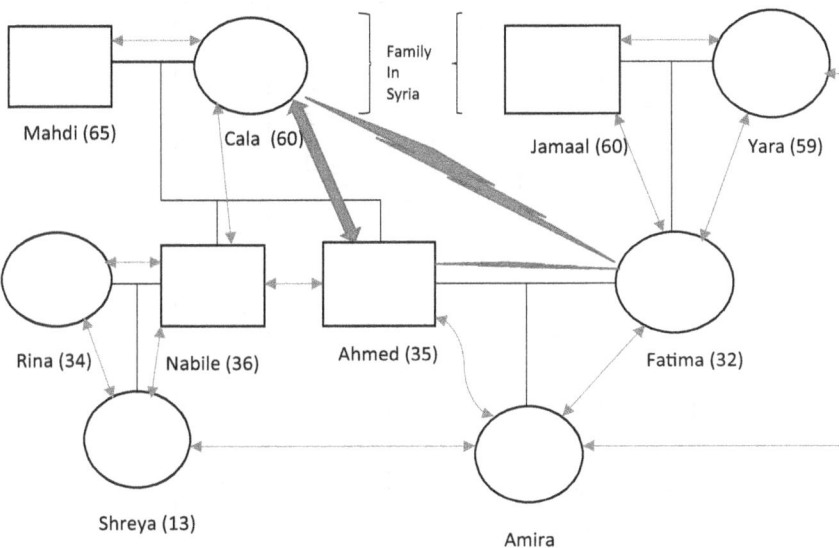

Figure 2.3 Genogram for Amira's Family

tearful at school. The genogram has helped Judy to connect Amira's tearful behavior at school with a larger family problem. In addition, the genogram reveals numerous positive relationships between family members that Judy can use to help strengthen the family and provide additional support for Amira.

There are a number of additional ways the family relationships can be assessed, but a useful one is the Circumplex Model (Olson, 1989). The Circumplex Model diagrams the family relationships on two core dimensions: Cohesion and Flexibility. Cohesion refers to the degree of closeness between family members. Generally, in a healthy family the relationship between members is Connected. If family members are too close to each other and there is little independence allowed, the family is considered Enmeshed. If there is a lack of closeness between family members, then the family is considered Disengaged. Flexibility refers to the ability of the family to adapt to change. If the family has overly strict parents, a Rigid family system is the result, and these families have great difficulty doing things differently when situations require it. If the family has parents who do not enforce any rules, a Chaotic family structure may result. This is the Chaotic family where confusion and disorder reign with no control by the parents. More constructively, families that are Flexible are able to respond to change in a flexible manner: parents are able to set limits or relax limits as the situation demands.

Each dimension (Cohesion and Flexibility) has five different levels with the extreme family types on the outside and the balanced family types in the middle (see Figure 2.4).

	DISENGAGED	SOMEWHAT CONNECTED	CONNECTED	VERY CONNECTED	ENMESHED
CHAOTIC	**Chaotically Disengaged**	**Chaotically Somewhat Connected**	**Chaotically Connected**	**Chaotically Very Connected**	**Chaotically Enmeshed**
VERY FLEXIBLE	Very Flexibly **Disengaged**	Very Flexibly Somewhat Connected	Very Flexibly Connected	Very Flexibly Very connected	Very Flexibly **Enmeshed**
FLEXIBLE	Flexibly **Disengaged**	Flexibly Somewhat Connected	Flexibly Connected	Flexibly Very Connected	Flexibly **Enmeshed**
SOMEWHAT FLEXIBLE	Somewhat Flexibly **Disengaged**	Somewhat Flexibly Somewhat Connected	Somewhat Flexibly Connected	Somewhat Flexibly Very Connected	Somewhat Flexibly **Enmeshed**
RIGID	**Rigidly Disengaged**	**Rigidly** Somewhat Connected	**Rigidly** Connected	**Rigidly** Very Connected	**Rigidly Enmeshed**

COHESION →

FLEXIBILITY

Legend: Bold type = Unbalanced family types
No bold type = Balanced family types
Bold and no bold together = Midrange family types

Figure 2.4 Circumplex Model

While generally speaking the balanced family types are considered more "healthy" or "normal" in an American Eurocentric context, there is considerable variation between different cultural groups. For example, in the traditional Syrian family, which is patriarchal, the father is the ultimate authority. Relationships between parents and children may tend to be Rigid on the Circumplex Model and yet be considered culturally appropriate. Alternatively, in a Syrian immigrant family where members are more acculturated to Western family norms, a more Flexible relationship between parents and children would be expected (Cultural Atlas, n.d.). In order to use the Circumplex Model effectively to assess families, you must take into account cultural expectations and norms.

It is important to note that the Circumplex Model is intended to measure relationships, not individuals. For example, in a relationship between a mother and daughter that is Enmeshed, the relationship is a very close one. Even though the son is a youth (e.g., aged 20) the parent will still make all the decisions, even about less important ones like what clothing to wear. The Circumplex Model may be used to classify the entire family unit or the relationship between different pairs of family members (e.g., parent-child, mother-father, grandparent-mother, and so on).

The purpose of using the Circumplex Model is to connect the family structure and relationships to the student's presenting problem. Often by modifying the family structure (e.g., helping the family to move from Rigid to Somewhat Flexible), the overall functioning of the family improves and the student benefits. Figure 2.5 shows the Circumplex Model that Judy developed for Amira's family.

As can be seen, Amira and her mother Fatima have a *Flexible, Very Connected* relationship. This is a very close relationship in which the parent exercises a more collaborative decision-making approach. Fatima insists on Amira doing well in school, checks her homework, and insists she do chores at home. However, Fatima allows Amira to go out without wearing a hijab and lets her listen to Western music and watch whatever shows on TV she wants. Amira and her father, Ahmed, have a very different relationship. They are *Rigidly Somewhat Connected*. There is some closeness between Amira and her father but not as much as Amira would like. Ahmed frequently complains to Amira that she is not behaving as a "proper daughter" because she doesn't wear a hijab and she listens to inappropriate Western music that Ahmed feels is decadent. Amira cares about her father but feels he is too strict. Fatima and her mother-in-law Cala have a *Rigidly Disengaged* relationship. They disagree sharply about how Amira should be raised. Cala believes that Fatima is permitting Amira to lose sight of traditional Syrian ways and is in danger of allowing Amira to potentially engage in immoral behaviors. Lately they have avoided speaking to each other on FaceTime. Fatima and Ahmed have a *Somewhat Flexible Disengaged* relationship. Fatima cooperates with decisions that Ahmed makes about major purchases, like where to live and buying a car, but feels that she has more responsibility for

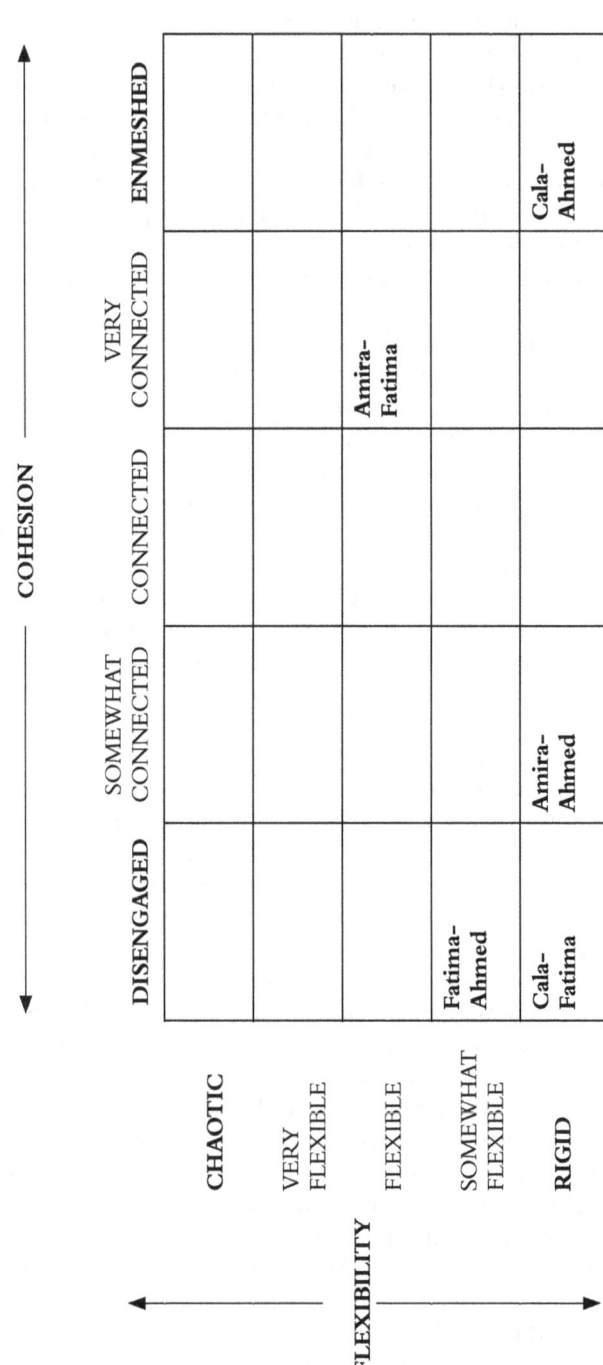

Figure 2.5 Circumplex Model for Amira's Family

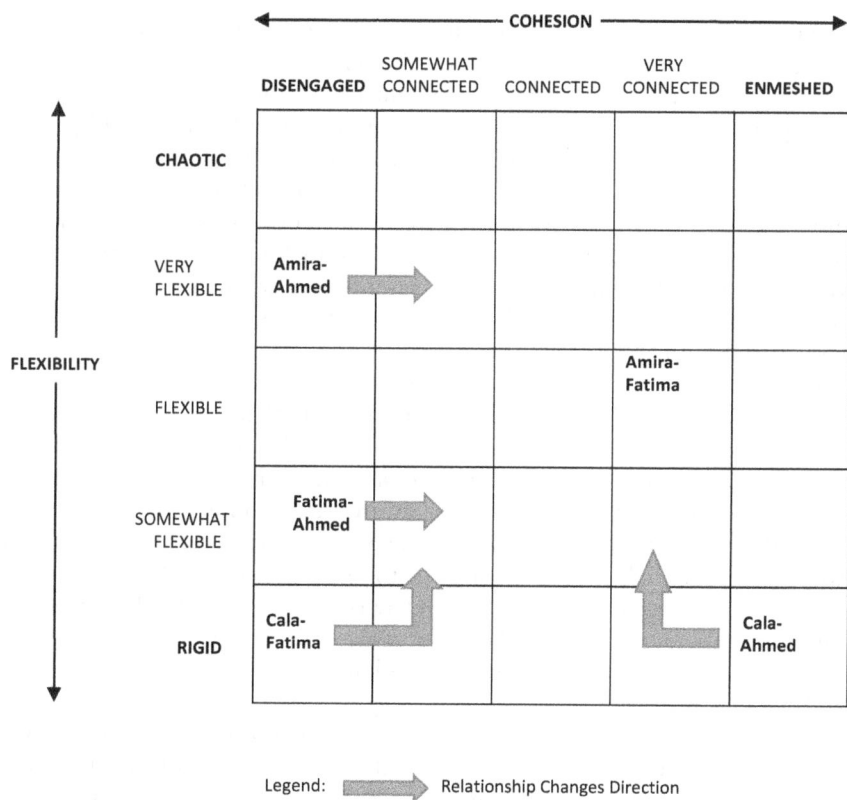

Figure 2.6 Circumplex Model for Amira's Family with Relationship Change Goals

raising Amira. Fatima especially resents the way Ahmed allows his mother Cala to interfere with how Fatima wants to raise Amira. This has caused a lot of tension between Fatima and Ahmed, and they frequently argue about who is right. Cala and Ahmed have a *Rigidly Enmeshed* relationship. Ahmed feels very close to his mother and is very reluctant to disagree with her. Cala believes she knows what is best for Ahmed and was very upset when he married Fatima. Figure 2.6 illustrates how Judy could use the Circumplex Model to identify desirable changes within Amira's family. These will be commented on later.

From the genogram and the Circumplex Model analyses it is reasonable to connect Amira's tearfulness at school with stress between her parents. In the following counseling sessions with Amira Judy was able to confirm this.

Step 4: Assessing the School System

In order to accurately assess how the school system affects a particular student, it is essential that the SBFC practitioner develop a friendship with the school personnel and be viewed as a valuable member of the school staff. This process of developing rapport can be enhanced by the SBFC practitioner having lunch with other teachers and by attending school events such as concerts and sporting events. If you are trusted by school staff, teachers are more likely to welcome you in the classroom to observe students. At many school events parents will be present, and by making friends with parents you can learn a great deal about how parents view strengths and challenges at the school. In doing this Judy learned from teachers that bullying was not widespread in the school but that it was occurring more frequently and that many teachers were concerned about it.

There are basically two school system levels that should be assessed: your student client's classroom and the entire school. At elementary and middle school levels it is easier to do classroom observations. Secondary school students are more likely to be aware that another student is seeing the SBFC practitioner, and a visit by the SBFC practitioner to a classroom would be potentially embarrassing for the student client. If a teacher has referred a student for a particular behavior (e.g., being tearful or being oppositional), by making a classroom visit you can directly observe the behavior as well as observe how the student interacts with other students and the teacher.

When Judy visited Amira's classroom, she noticed that when Amira was tearful, Jane would comment on it to other students. This facilitated Judy forming the hypothesis that Amira was sad about the stress between her parents and that Amira's tearfulness was used as an excuse by Jane to bully Amira.

The Circumplex Model can also be used to diagram relationships between your client and other students and teachers. In addition the entire classroom, as well as the school, can be classified on the Circumplex Model. Judy's Circumplex Model assessment of Amira's classroom and school is shown as Figure 2.7.

Seven sets of relationships are diagrammed in this Circumplex Model. Amira has a *Rigidly Disengaged* relationship with her bully, Jane. Jane has a *Rigidly Very Connected* relationship with three other students who give tacit support to Jane's bulling of Amira. Jane has a strong personality and exerts a leadership effect on these students. Amira has a *Somewhat Flexible Somewhat Connected* relationship with her teacher. Amira respects her teacher as the authority in the classroom and likes the teacher but would like to have a closer relationship with the teacher. The teacher has a *Chaotically Somewhat Connected* relationship with Jane, whom she regards as a "problem student." Jane alternately acts cooperative with the teacher but sometimes misbehaves to the point that the teacher has to reprimand her. The teacher confides in

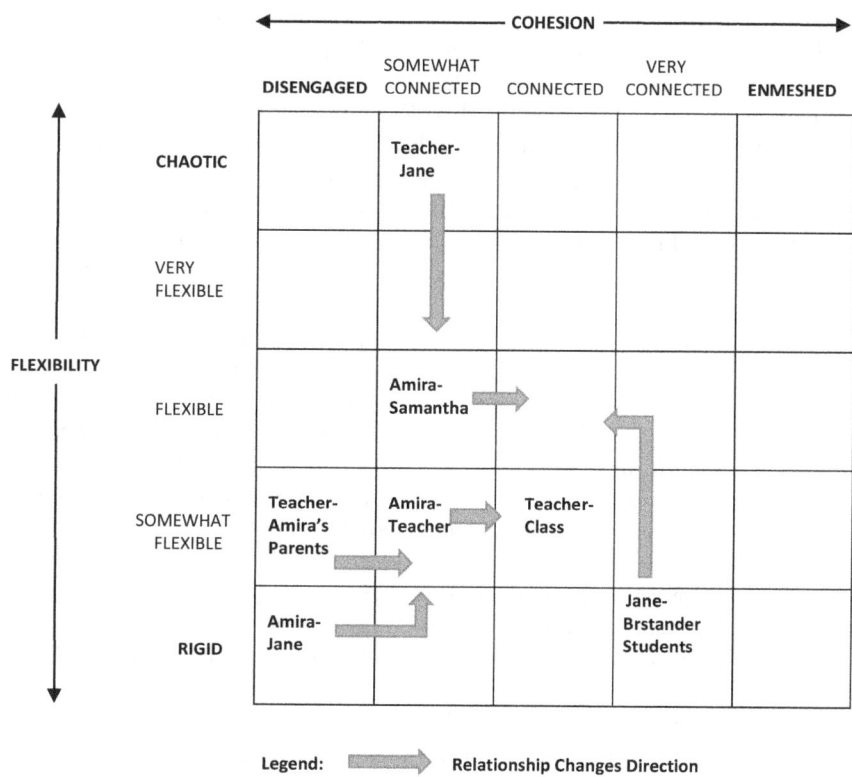

Figure 2.7 Circumplex Model for Amira's Classroom

Judy that she doesn't know what to do to handle Jane. Amira has a *Flexible Somewhat Connected* relationship with Samantha, a girl she would like to be friends with. But she is shy about making an approach. The teacher and Amira's parents have a *Somewhat Flexible Disengaged* relationship. The teacher invited Amira's parents to the school to talk about Amira's tearful behavior, but the parents did not accept because they felt the teacher only wanted to criticize them. Finally, Judy was able to observe that the teacher and her class overall had a very positive *Somewhat Flexible Connected* relationship and that students really seemed to enjoy her teaching. The arrows on this Circumplex Model show possible change directions Judy was considering for the classroom system.

Step 5: Assessing Community Influences

Assessing community influences is especially important when working with refugees and immigrants because these influences are sometimes very negative.

The majority population in a city or community may have members who are not welcoming of refugees and immigrants who seem "different" and may not speak the host language well. Being discriminated against is a common experience for many refugee and immigrant families. If you are a member of the majority group that discriminates against your client and their family, the client and family may be very reluctant to engage with you because of their past experience. It is therefore important to discuss this openly with your clients and to ask them how they feel about collaborating with you. Judy broached this topic with Fatima and Ahmed in the following way:

Judy: *I want you to know that I am very honored to be working with you to help your daughter Amira do better at school. I am working with Amira's teacher and the principal to prevent Amira from being bullied at school. Sometimes students get bullied because they come from different countries and cultures, and that is not right. I know that your family has had a long and difficult journey to leave Syria and to come to your new home in this city. While many people welcome newcomers, sometimes there are people who are not so accepting. What has it been like for you being newcomers in this community?*

Fatima: *Everyone is so friendly. We are so happy to be here.*

Ahmed: *Last week a stranger on the street told my wife, "Go back to the Middle East."*

Judy: *That must have been very hurtful.*

Fatima: *She was an ignorant woman who knows nothing of who we are.*

Ahmed: *People are generally welcoming and want to know why we left Syria. But sometimes when I am driving my taxi, there are people who won't get in when I stop for them.*

Judy: *These kinds of discriminatory behaviors can be very upsetting to deal with. How have you been able to cope when you are treated badly like this?*

Fatima: *It doesn't happen very often, but when it does we feel like we just want to stay at home. Fortunately, we have good neighbors who invite us to their homes and that makes up for it.*

Judy: *I come from the same ethnic group as some of the folks who have treated you badly. How do you feel about our working together?*

Ahmed: *We feel good about it because you don't talk down to us and you are sincerely interested in our opinions.*

In exploring community influences with Fatima and Ahmed, Judy discovered that the family's Muslim community was an important source of support. An important additional source of support for Fatima was a local university where she was taking refresher medical courses to become certified as physician in this country. Ahmed later revealed that his supervisor at the taxi company frequently made derogatory comments to him (e.g., calling him a "raghead"). Judy offered to discuss with Ahmed ways of con-structively dealing with work discrimination. This assessment of sources of support and of friction experienced by refugees and immigrants is very important because of the effect overall on family cohesion and stability and on children. SBFC practitioners are child, family, and school advocates and are willing to intervene to mobilize community resources in order to help refugee and immigrant clients.

As noted by Selimos in Chapter 19, the SBFC practitioner is a "trusted mediator between the family and the larger society." It is part of the SBFC practitioner's role to facilitate helping refugee and immigrant children, and families become successfully engaged with their community through social and leisure activities, work, and other organizational connections. Helping a child's parents to find work would have a powerful effect on promoting fam-ily independence and strengthening family resilience overall. Connecting a child struggling with language and school assignments with a community tutor can lead to significant school improvement and increased family pride. These community mediating aspects of the SBFC practitioner's role are not trivial and may achieve family strengthening as much as any traditional psychological intervention. Specific ways SBFC practitioners can perform this mediator role between family and community are described in detail in Chapter 19.

Step 6: Assessing Cultural Factors (Multicultural Considerations)

When SBFC practitioners are collaborating with refugees and immigrants, it is important to learn how culture affects the way refugees and immigrants view things. We recommend that the SBFC practitioner adopt a posture of cultural humility, defined as "ability to maintain an interpersonal stance that is other-oriented (or open to the other) in relation to aspects of cul-tural identity that are most important to the [person]" (Hook et al., 2013, p. 2). Box 2.2 contains sample questions that can be used to explore how cultural factors are important to your clients. Judy used these with Amira's family and discovered that their migration experience had been especially traumatic. While taking a boat to leave Syria, another refugee mother and her child had fallen overboard and drowned.

Judy also used the Basic Family Values Scale (see Boxes 2.3 and 2.4) to identify how Amira and her parents positioned themselves on basic cultural values expressed in the scale as opposites. Table 2.2 summarizes the cul-tural values held jointly and separately by the family members. What Judy learned from this assessment was that while the family members held many typical Syrian values in common (especially related to the importance of family), Ahmed (father) held more traditional Syrian values than Fatima (mother) and Amira. This was valuable information that helped Judy under-stand Ahmed's relationship with his mother and his conflict with Fatima.

Box 2.2 Questions for Exploring Cultural Factors

1.   **Possible Cultural Issues With the SBFC Practitioner**

"How do you feel about working with myself as someone with a different ethnicity (or different cultural background)?"

2.   **Cultural Identity Questions**

"How have the experiences you had in your native country influenced your life?"
"Please tell me about these experiences and how they affected you."
"What about your native country are you most proud of?"
"How have the experiences you have had in the host country influenced your life?"
"Please tell me about these experiences and how they affected you."
"What about your host country are you most proud of?"
"Do you think of yourself as a member of the host country or as a member of your native country or as both? (e.g. "Do you think of yourself as an American, a Mexican, or a Mexican–American?").
"Do you think of your values as being more like those of the host country or more like those of your native country?"
"Please tell me about those values and why they are important to you."

3.   **Degree of Acculturation Questions**

"How many friends do you have who speak the dominant host country language (e.g., English)?"
"What language do you speak at home?"
"What language do you speak with your friends?"
"What language do you read in at home?"
"What language do you think in?"

4.   **Migration Experience**

"What was it like migrating here? For some families migrating can be very challenging."
"What was the hardest thing for your family about leaving your native country?"
"When you (or your family) first came to this country, how did people treat you?"

5.   **Experience of Discrimination**

"Persons who belong to a minority culture sometimes are treated poorly by some members of the dominant culture. Have you had any experiences like that?"
"Please tell me about them."

6.   **Client's Cultural Explanation for Problems**

"Why do you think you are having these problems?"
"What do you think you need to do to overcome these problems?"
(Issue: Does client think of the causes and solutions for interpersonal and emotional problems in terms of mental health, counseling, scientific reasoning, rationality, or in other cultural terms?)

Box 2.3 Basic Family Values Scale

Instructions: On the following sheet please read each pair of values and indicate which one is the most important to your family (FY) or mother (M) and father (F) by placing the appropriate letter on the line joining the values. If you strongly agree that one value is important to your family, you would place the "F" closest to that value. If you feel that neither value is more important, then you would check the line in the middle. After rating the values for your family or parents, rate where you are on each value using an "S" for self.

	Very Important	Moderately Important	Slightly Important	In-between	Slightly Important	Moderately Important	Very Important	
1. Punctuality								Being flexible with time
2. Controlling the environment								Not controlling the environment
3. Sticking with tradition								Developing new traditions
4. Task-centered								Relationship-centered
5. Thoughts								Feelings
6. Expressing anger								Withholding anger
7. Family								Friends
8. Following the "letter" of the law								Following the "spirit" of the law
9. Being assertive								Being kind
10. Sitting very close while talking								Not sitting too close while talking
11. Being independent								Fitting in with the group
12. Being competitive								Being cooperative
13. Predictability								Flexibility
14. Justice								Mercy
15. Spirituality								Rationality
16. Supporting the social order								Challenging the social order

Box 2.4   Basic Family Values Scale for Amira's Family

Instructions: On the following sheet please read each pair of values and indicate which one is the most important to your family (FY) or mother (M) and father (F) by placing the appropriate letter on the line joining the values. If you strongly agree that one value is important to your family, you would place the "F" closest to that value. If you feel that neither value is more important, then you would check the line in the middle. After rating the values for your family or parents, rate where you are on each value using an "S" for self.

	Very Important	Moderately Important	Slightly Important	In-between	Slightly Important	Moderately Important	Very Important	
1. Punctuality	Father	Mother	Amira					Being flexible with time
2. Controlling the environment	Father	Mother	Amira					Not controlling the environment
3. Sticking with tradition		Father				Amira Mother		Developing new traditions
4. Task-centered	Mother	Father	Amira					Relationship-centered
5. Thoughts	Father	Mother	Amira					Feelings
6. Expressing anger					Father	Mother	Amira	Withholding anger
7. Family	Mother	Father	Amira					Friends
8. Following the "letter" of the law	Father				Amira	Mother		Following the "spirit" of the law
9. Being assertive		Father				Mother	Amira	Being kind
10. Sitting very close while talking			Mother Amira		Father			Not sitting too close while talking
11. Being independent		Mother		Amira	Father			Fitting in with the group
12. Being competitive						Mother Father Amira		Being cooperative
13. Predictability	Father Mother Amira							Flexibility
14. Justice		Father				Amira Mother		Mercy
15. Spirituality		Father				Amira Mother		Rationality
16. Supporting the social order	Father		Mother Amira					Challenging the social order

Table 2.1 Summary of Values for Amira's Family

Values for Amira	Values for Mother	Values for Father
Task-centered	Task-centered	Task-centered
Withholding anger	Withholding anger	Withholding anger
Family	Family	Family
Being cooperative	Being cooperative	Being cooperative
Predictability	Predictability	Predictability
Supporting the social order	Supporting the social order	Supporting the social order
In-between	Punctuality	Punctuality
In-between	Controlling the environment	Controlling the environment
In-between	Thoughts	Thoughts
In-between	Being independent	Fitting in with the group
Developing new traditions	Developing new traditions	Sticking with tradition
Following the spirit of the law	Following the spirit of the law	Following the letter of the law
Being kind	Being kind	Being assertive
Mercy	Mercy	Justice
Rationality	Rationality	Spirituality
In-between	In-between	Not sitting too close

7: DEVELOPING THE TREATMENT PLAN

A tentative treatment plan for Amira is shown in Table 2.2. This treatment plan is typical of SBFC treatment plans in that there is an emphasis on family intervention (e.g., teaching Amira stress reduction approaches to lower the stress that she experiences when her parents argue; parent effectiveness training to help Fatima and Ahmed handle their parenting differences more amicably); school intervention (e.g., family counseling with Jane and her parents to address her bullying behavior at school; guidance group on bullying in Amira's classroom); family prevention (e.g., school-sponsored parent workshops on bullying); school prevention (e.g., school-wide anti-bullying program); and community intervention (e.g., exploring opportunities to engage more with the non-Muslim community). This is merely a tentative treatment plan intended to illustrate how an SBFC practitioner would conduct an assessment across different systems affecting a student.

It is important to note that a wide variety of mental health approaches can be used within the SBFC case conceptualization: behavioral, solution focused, cognitive-behavioral, constructivist, narrative, psychodynamic, Adlerian, and other approaches.

Table 2.2 Proposed Treatment Plan for Amira

Treatment Level	Strengths	Challenges	Proposed Interventions
Amira	Family support	Bullied at school	Social skills training (assertion) Stress inoculation
	Good grades	Lonely, lacks friends	Social skills training Increase FaceTime with Shreya
	Enjoys music, sports	Distressed by parents arguing	Stress inoculation
Family	Parents supportive of Amira Parents have higher degrees	Parental disagreement Cala overly involved with Ahmed's parenting School parents unaware how to deal with bullying	Parent effectiveness training Discuss with parents importance of parental collaboration School-sponsored parent workshops on bullying
School	Positive classroom environment	Bullying bystanders in Amira's classroom Jane bullying Amira More widespread bullying in the school Amira lonely at school Disengaged relationship between teacher and Amira's parents	Guidance group on bullying Family counseling with Jane's family School-wide anti-bullying program Sit Amira near Samantha Facilitate meeting between Jan, teacher, and Amira's parents
Community	Supportive Muslim community Supportive university community for Fatima	Ahmed experiencing work discrimination Family feeling disengaged with the community in general	Social skills training Encouraging more activities with Muslim community Exploring opportunities to engage more with the non-Muslim community

Challenges and Solutions

The main challenge in developing an SBFC case conceptualization is that many mental health professionals are trained narrowly within their mental health discipline and are accustomed to only focusing on individual, family, or school factors separately. An SBFC approach may be used by a single mental health professional who has training and experience in individual, family and school intervention, or by two or more mental health professionals trained in intervening at different systems levels and working together as a team (e.g., professional A doing school intervention and professional B doing family intervention).

Conclusion

Conducting an SBFC case conceptualization is an essential step in practicing SBFC. In this chapter-specific approaches to gathering information about students, families, schools, and communities were described. Readers should be aware that many other assessment approaches could have been used as SBFC is a flexible systems approach meant to be integrated with different mental health approaches to collaborating with children, families, and schools.

Resources

Gerrard, B. (2019). How to develop an SBFC case conceptualization. In B. Gerrard, M. Carter & D. Ribera (Eds.), School-based family counseling: An interdisciplinary practitioner's guide. Routledge.

This chapter provides additional assessment resources for using multimodal assessment, the Circumplex Model, and assessing school climate.

References

Cultural atlas. (n.d.). https://culturalatlas.sbs.com.au/syrian-culture/syrian-culture-family

Hook, J. N., Davis, D. E., Owen, J., Worthington, Jr., E. L., & Utsey, S. O. (2013). Cultural humility: Measuring openness to culturally diverse clients. Journal of Counseling Psychology, 60(3), 353–366. https://doi.org/10.1037/a0032595

Lazarus, A. (2019, February 12). Multimodal therapy: A primer. http://www.zurinstitute. com/multimodal-therapy/. Zur. Institute.

Olson, D. H. (1989). Circumplex model of family systems VIII: Family assessment and intervention. In D. H. Olson, C. S. Russell & D. H. Sprenkle (Eds.), Circumplex model: Systemic assessment and treatment of families (pp. 7–50). Routledge.

Part 2

Family Intervention

3 Assessing the Challenges and Family

Strengths Among Refugee Children in Malaysia

J. K. Kok, Kheng Kia Khor, Kai Yee Hon, and Gertina J. van Schalkwyk

This chapter presents an exploratory case study that attempts to understand how the collage life-story elicitation technique (CLET) and a discovery-oriented narrative approach could be used as an intervention with refugee children and their families. A case study from our research has been highlighted to demonstrate how the CLET can be used to design potential interventions to assist refugee children attending a community learning center in Kuala Lumpur, Malaysia. Elaborating on the school-based family counseling meta-model, the chapter concludes with a discussion of the benefits of the CLET, where the school and the family work together to help these children to cope with their refugee status.

Background

As of October 2020, there were some 178,450 refugees and asylum-seekers registered with the UNHCR in Malaysia (UNHCR, 2021a). As Malaysia had not agreed to the 1951 Refugee Convention, there are no refugee camps in Malaysia, and the current Malaysian laws do not provide them with legal rights to remain in the country. These refugees are a marginalized group who live in overcrowded shared spaces in groups scattered in and around Kuala Lumpur in the Klang Valley (Shelter Home for Children, 2019). They do not have access to fundamental human rights. Most of them are employed on minimal wages and forced to work long hours doing dangerous work (Wake & Cheung, 2016). They are stateless migrants striving to survive and haunted by constant fears of being rounded up and repatriated to their countries of origin or even imprisoned where they are put to harsh punishment.

As of the end October 2020, the number of refugee children in Malaysia below the age of 18 was 46,730—an increase of 3,980 when compared to the figure a year before (UNHCR, 2021a). These children are deprived of their basic rights by being prohibited from gaining access to the free government education system and not being allowed to sit for the public examinations. Only 30% of the 23,823 school-aged refugee children

DOI: 10.4324/9781003097891-5

in Malaysia are enrolled in the 133 community learning centers operated by benevolent NGOs, religious organizations, and humanitarian groups (UNHCR, 2021b). However, the educational qualifications or certificates provided by these learning centers are unable/unsuitable to pave a way for them to further their studies after graduation and may not be beneficial and appropriate for their future employment. In general, most of them have become exposed and vulnerable to a wide range of adverse outcomes that span mental health problems and educational underachievement (Low et al., 2014; Shaw et al., 2018). For example, they are exposed to and at risks of suicidal behaviors, substance abuse, and criminality due to lower psychological well-being. Additionally, those children who had experienced or witnessed traumatic events (i.e., the death of their loved ones) are at higher risk of developing mental disorders or other stress-related conditions (Alemi et al., 2015). The aforementioned exposure to displacement-related stressors and being further discriminated at the hands of the local host community have cumulatively contributed to their poor mental health (Low et al., 2018).

The striving of refugee children who are motivated toward a better future needs a holistic approach as offered by the school-based family counseling (SBFC) model. The development of refugee children relies to a great extent on the enabling adults, especially the family, the school (i.e., both teachers and administrators), and the community at large. As indicated by the SBFC model, children can overcome their personal and academic challenges through mental health approaches that link family and school (Gerrard, 2008). It is hoped that with more collaboration between school and family, more appropriate interventions could be developed, delivered, and implemented for this vulnerable group of refugee children in need.

The CLET is an effective tool to work with children who are challenged in various ways (e.g., displacement through their refugee status) and those who have difficulty verbalizing their distress (Van Schalkwyk, 2010). The CLET is an arts-based approach that scaffolds autobiographical remembering and elicits both nonverbal and verbal narratives that has proven to be an effective tool to understand children's feelings that are often hidden from direct observation (Lijadi & Van Schalkwyk, 2017). Its strengths lie in allowing participants—in this case, refugee children—"free expression of their subjective and inter-subjective truths, even when [they have] difficulty recollecting their memories or the memories were about sad situations or events" (Van Schalkwyk & Lijadi, 2019, p. 9). Furthermore, the CLET is used to elicit areas of strength and weakness, coping styles, and resources that are useful when planning suitable interventions (Van Schalkwyk, 2020). This constructivist approach is also compatible with the SBFC approach, which emphasizes the conceptualization of actions and interactions within children's social and interpersonal network, and that aims to involve both family and school ensuring the child's success in life.

Using the CLET With Refugee Children to Plan an Intervention

In this section, we describe a case study from our research with refugee children attending a community learning center in Kuala Lumpur, Malaysia. The case demonstrates how the CLET could be implemented by SBFC practitioners in their own work with refugee children or any other children challenged by circumstances out of their control. The focus topic of the case study described here was "Happy Family" in an attempt to elicit strengths and coping styles from the refugee children. We conducted a two-hour group CLET workshop where step 1 of the CLET (see Box 3.2) engaged the students with making a group collage during the first hour and the fieldworkers conducting a group interview (steps 2–5 of the CLET) during the second hour. In the next section we describe the procedures for conducting the CLET workshop and analyzing the protocols in preparation of planning an intervention.

Procedure

The procedures for conducting the CLET unfolded in three phases (Van Schalkwyk, 2020):

Phase One: Planning and rapport building
Phase Two: Conducting a five-step CLET interview with a group of refugee children
Phase Three: Making sense of the CLET protocols

Box 3.1   Phase One: Planning and Rapport Building

• Before conducting the CLET workshop with the refugee children, we connected with the refugee school administrator to explore the possibility of working together, finding out the needs or possible concerns of the refugee children such as coping with challenges of transitioning to the host country. The SBFC practitioner should remain open to explore a range of domains relevant to the child's lived experiences when exploring possible challenges with the school administrators (e.g., friendship, peer relations, academic outcomes, and so forth). In our case exploration with refugee children, it was helpful to form some common objectives agreeable to the school personnel.

- A focus group format of the CLET was planned as a workshop with the refugee children on a Saturday morning when there were no formal curriculum activities. Other logistic preparations such as venue and collage-making materials (e.g., collecting local magazines for cutting images to make the collage, paper for collage-making, glue, and scissors) were also done during this initial phase.
- Parental consent was important, and the school played a role in reaching out to parents. The parents were informed about the workshop their children would participate in, and consent obtained for all children under the age of 18 years. The children were also asked for their consent to participate, and all invited participants were eager for the experience. It should be noted that, when corresponding with the parents of refugee children, it is more friendly to use the family's native language as not all parents are familiar with English even though their children might be attending an English-speaking school setup.
- Prior to the actual workshop day, the teacher asked the students to bring some photos, pictures, images, or other cuttings from magazines of their choice for the CLET workshop. These supplemented the magazines that we had collected in preparation of the workshop interviews.
- Facilitators for four focus groups, comprising psychology students at a local higher education institution in Malaysia, were trained in implementing the CLET with focus groups. The SBFC practitioner is also encouraged to familiarize themselves with the five steps of the CLET as outlined by Van Schalkwyk (2010). Whether using the CLET with an individual or a focus group, the CLET steps follow the same sequence (see Box 3.2).
- The CLET could also be implemented with the refugee family where parents and children collaborate in all the steps of the CLET (see Box 3.2). In such a setting, a flexible meeting time and multiple tools of communication might be necessary, as refugee parents often have long work-hour schedules, and they may not be allowed to take leave.

During the first contact with the refugee children included in our case study, some ice-breaking games were executed for rapport building and to allow the children to become more comfortable with the fieldworkers. We also used a color card game to organize the children in groups for implementing the five steps of the CLET (see Box 3.2).

The second phase of implementing the CLET with refugee children comprised the five steps to compile the CLET protocols (Van Schalkwyk, 2010). Our case consisted of 25 refugee students (19 boys and 6 girls, aged 10–12 years) who were recruited at a non-governmental school in Kuala Lumpur and randomly organized in five focus groups for implementing the CLET. Before conducting the CLET workshop ethical approval was obtained from the research committee at a local university where the primary investigator—who acted as the counselor in this case study—was working at the time, and parents were informed of the procedures in order to give consent for their child to participate in the workshop (see Box 3.1). The refugee children were mainly from Myanmar and Sri Lanka, most of them had arrived in Malaysia when they were 6–9 years of age and had been living in Malaysia for at least 3 years. Their parents held jobs as helpers or waiters in restaurants, construction workers, and domestic maids with monthly earnings of less than USD250 (about RM1000).

Phase Two: The five-step procedures of the CLET adapted from Van Schalkwyk and Lijadi (2019).

Box 3.2   Five-Step procedures of the CLET (Van Schalkwyk & Lijadi, 2019)

Step 1: Collage-Making

The first step required the refugee children to make a group collage by selecting images and/or cuttings from magazines, newspapers, or any printed media and pasting these on a large sheet of paper (e.g., A2). The facilitators instructed the children to create a family life-story collage using the images and cuttings to represent important and memorable experiences in the life of their family, and each child in the group was expected to paste at least 4–5 images. They could also make some drawings if they could not find an image in the magazines that fit the nonverbal "story" they wanted to tell.

Note that this step could also be carried out by the SBFC practitioner in a mental health setting or at the family home with all the family members collaborating to make a group collage (Van Schalkwyk, 2020). In the school setting, the SBFC practitioner could choose to conduct the CLET with an individual or, as in this case, with small groups in a focus group setting.

Step 2: Storytelling

Following the collage-making, each child in the focus group was given an opportunity to present one or more micro-narratives stimulated by the images on the collage. The facilitator (or SBFC practitioner) encouraged the children to tell stories about an experience/event represented in any of the pictures pasted on the collage, whether their own or an image pasted by another group member. Although the storytelling is a form of free association, the facilitator could use the following three prompts to structure the focus group (or individual) discussion: (a) Tell a story about an image on the collage, (b) what does this image mean to you, and (c) how does the image relate to an event or experience in your family life? Further prompts (except "WHY" questions) could be used to encourage participants to share their stories and narrate about their family life as refugees in Malaysia.

Step 3: Self-positioning and Missing Image

The storytelling is followed by participants having the opportunity to position themselves within the collage. Asking the participants "Where would you post a picture of yourself in the collage?" the SBFC practitioner gains an understanding of how the participants perceive of their self in the family or self in the school or everyday life, and the extent to which he/she takes ownership of the reported memories (i.e., the dialogical self and the self-other relationship patterns). Further discussion about the self-positioning could be pursued as is needed in the circumstances.

Eliciting the silent voices in narrative exploration is equally important, and in the CLET the participants were asked about any picture/image they looked for but could not find (i.e., the missing image). The silent voice—that is, a narrative expected but absent about, for example, a family member or parent—could be explored by discussing the missing image.

Note that when employing the CLET in a focus group or a family setting, the SBFC practitioner should use her/his interviewing skills to prompt as much narrating as possible asking for reasons and elaboration whenever necessary. It is also important to maintain control and ensure that all participants have an equal opportunity to express themselves, which might mean silencing the bold ones (in some family cases a very vocal parent) and encouraging the silent ones with more prompts. Rules of engagement should be established at the outset.

Step 4: Juxtaposition (Comparing Similarities and Differences)

In this step, the participants (e.g., groups of refugee children or family groups) are then asked to juxtapose negative events with positive events or to reflect on two pictures whose meanings were related in terms of either similarities or differences.

Step 5: Reflection and Closure

The final step of the CLET focuses on reflection and debriefing prior to the participants leaving the focus group setting. On the one hand, the participants are given a chance to elaborate on their stories told during Step 2 and/or adding details to their stories that had been previously overlooked. They could also reflect upon how they experienced participating in the CLET and, if able to (e.g., a parent in a family setting), elaborate on what they have learned from their participation (see Van Schalkwyk, 2020). On the other hand, a participant who feels saddened or confused about something that happened and/or a story told by him-/herself or another party, would have time to reflect on their feelings and could be assisted by the SBFC practitioner to regroup and leave the session less distressed.

Following the five steps of the CLET, the SBFC practitioner now has to make sense of the stories following an analytical phase that allow for exploring the autobiographical memories of participants before planning an effective intervention. In Phase Three (see Box 3.3) the CLET protocols of the refugee children were prepared, transcribed, and then analyzed following an in-depth thematic analysis in the interpretative phenomenological tradition (Smith & Osborn, 2008). It is important to label the protocols anonymously with pseudonyms when the analysis is done in a group in order to protect the child and/or family's privacy.

Box 3.3   Making Sense of the CLET Protocols

- To make sense of the CLET protocols, we first analyzed the non-verbal texts (i.e., the collages, Step 1 of the CLET) without reference to the micro-narratives (Steps 2–5 of the CLET). Reading the collages, we established the denotative or concrete meanings of the images as well as, and most importantly, the connotative or symbolic meanings embedded in each image. This means that we independently (as a team collaborating on this project) read the collages for the nature of the images (denotation), the symbolism and/or metaphors expressing possible tensions embedded in the participants' memories, and the narrative tone to examine potential meanings that could not be verbalized (see also Van Schalkwyk, 2013; Van Schalkwyk & Lijadi, 2019, p. 4).

Note that each image denotes a memory about people or objects or events and related or embedded symbolic actions and interactions. Each image also represents alternative meanings expressed as metaphors concerning possible tensions embedded in the participant's memories and potentially an area to focus on for the intervention.

- Following the collage analysis, we explored the micro-narratives (Steps 2–5 of the CLET) for further clues or themes regarding the strengths and weaknesses, the coping styles, and resources that the refugee children talked about in their storytelling. The collage images served as stimulus for the storytelling and allowed the children to give voice to their experiences and feelings without talking directly about these feelings that could be disturbing. We also checked for unexpected themes and meanings relevant to the context of being a refugee family in Malaysia, as well as cultural-specific meanings that could be utilized when planning an intervention. Reading through all of the micro-narratives and comparing these with the denotations/connotations embedded in the collages helped us identify several themes that could be further explored in developing an intervention to strengthen the children's prospects for a better future.

Note that making sense of the CLET protocols could be done by the individual SBFC practitioner or by a team including also the parents, the school counselor, teachers, and other stakeholders (e.g., community members). Being designed for cross-cultural research and practice, the CLET expects that the SBFC practitioner be sensitive to sociocultural cues through the use of locally relevant magazines for collage-making and by interpreting narratives within context rather than in accordance with predisposed labels and categories. Working as a team that involves the parents when analyzing the CLET protocols of refugee children could therefore assist the SBFC practitioner to test their assumptions and hypotheses prior to conceptualizing an intervention with the child independently (see also Van Schalkwyk, 2020). Furthermore, the CLET is a strength-based approach that aims to conceptualize cases through the lens appropriate to SBFC and hypothesizing the participants' problems and strengths in accordance with their available resources and coping styles (Van Schalkwyk, 2013, 2020).

- In the final part of Phase Three, the SBFC practitioner conceptualizes an intervention that can be offered either within the school context or directly in consultation with the parents. In our case study with the refugee children in Malaysia, the aim of the intervention was to strengthen the children's mental health, assist with their goal-setting and overall helping them to achieve the "better life" they wanted with their families in the host country. Further exposition of the intervention follows the presentation of the case in the next section.

A Case Study in Malaysia

In this section, the analysis of a case study demonstrated how the CLET served as a discovery-oriented approach allowing the voice of refugee children in Malaysia to be heard regarding their perceptions of family life and their coping strategies. We conducted the CLET procedures (see Box 3.2) in a group setting and collected collages and narratives from five groups. After conducting both in-case and across-case analyses of the CLET protocols (Yin, 2009), we summarized and integrated the repeated occurrence of themes from the nonverbal (pictures) and verbal storytelling that could give a deeper understanding of the participants' lived experiences in the family and as refugee children in Malaysia (Lijadi & Van Schalkwyk, 2017; Van Schalkwyk & Lijadi, 2019). For the purpose of our case study exploration, the five collages were collected and numbered for easy reference (Figure 4.1). In a further presentation of the evidence given, reference to these were made as "Fig. 1, Col1:3" for collage 1, picture 3 or "Fig. 1, Col3:8 & 9" for collage 3, pictures 8 and 9.

In the analysis of the CLET protocols, it was assumed that the children will paste many images of people representing their perspectives of the family and family lives of refugees in Malaysia (Step 1 of the CLET). Although human-related images dominated the five group collages (64% of all images), only a few images directly portrayed family life as such (see Figure 4.1). Many were of individual persons (i.e., 23 of 48) or persons who stirred up memories of the past or visions for the future. In their storytelling (Step 2 of the CLET), the children did, however, make connections to their family lives through identifying the symbolic meanings of the pictures and linking them to their experiences as refugees living in Malaysia. They could also use the human-related images as metaphors in their group collages to narrate stories about their families and the impact of their refugee status on their lives generally as well as more specifically.

Following through with the narrative style of the CLET and conducting both within-case and across-case analyses of the five groups (Yin, 2009),

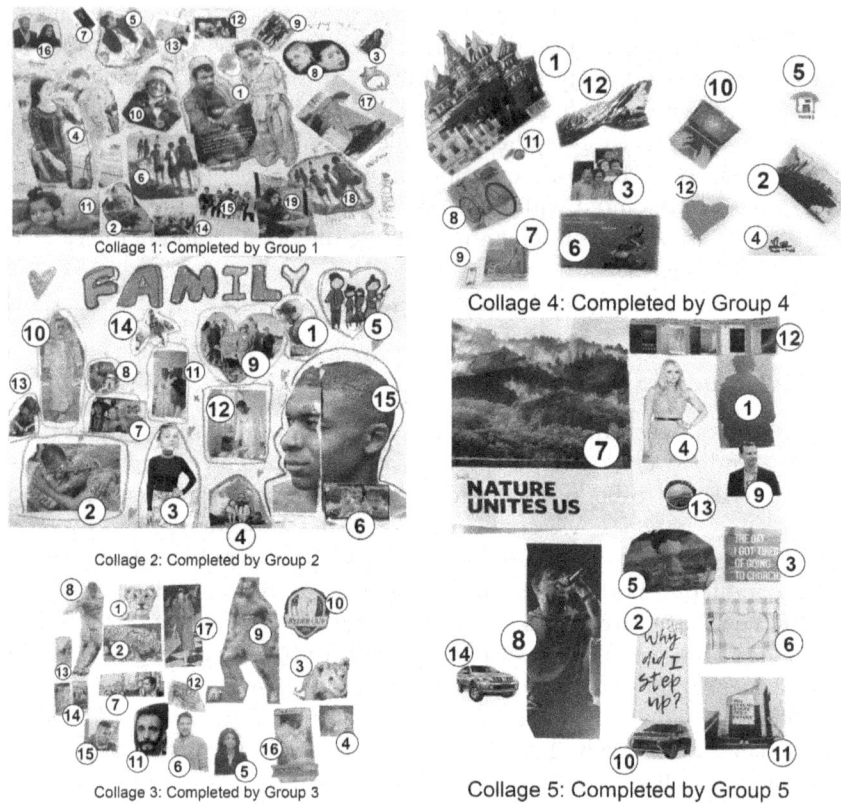

Figure 3.1 Five Collages Made by Refugee Children

the themes emerging from the CLET protocols are presented in Tables 3.1, 3.2, 3.3, and 3.4, both visual (nonverbal) stories as embedded in the collages (Figure 4.1) and the verbal storytelling with direct quotes in the children's own voices (in italics). Overall, the themes pertained to (a) separation and disruption, and for the children we interviewed, leading to feelings of isolation and loneliness; (b) vulnerability regarding the children's perceptions of the family being refugees living in Malaysia. The themes continue to express how the family is also perceived as a (c) source of strength, while other (d) enabling adults empower them to overcome the adversities they face as refugee children in Malaysia. In presenting the themes emerged from the case study, we used pseudonames to protect the child and/or family's privacy.

From this case study, the first two themes revealed the internal landscape and emotions of these refugee children, while the other two themes related to their coping strategies. In the next section we discuss the development of a potential intervention plan with the refugee children in Malaysia and how

Table 3.1 Summary of Micro-narratives for Theme 1: Separation and Disruption of Family Life

Theme	Analysis and Interpretation
Separation and disruption	1. This theme regarding family life was narrated by many of the refugee children in relation to war and other abuses that had caused separation and disruption in their lives. Many refugee families had been forced to leave behind family members or a parent might leave the family behind in the home country in search of a safe haven and/or a better future. Examples: • "*I miss my grandma and I also miss the snow at grandma's house*," said a girl named Cynthia, in Group 4 when talking about a picture of a snow-capped mountain (Fig. 1, Col4:12). Her grandmother lives in the northern parts of Pakistan, and she had not seen her since they came to Malaysia 4 years ago. • A boy in Group 1, Koko, had pasted two pictures, one of a mother and daughter together and one of a man sitting alone to the side. He narrated a story about the mother and daughter being reunited after the initial separation (Fig. 1, Col1:4), and the father as still being alone and separated from his loved ones (Fig. 1, Col1:5). While Koko was apparently happy when talking about the reunion between mother and child, his tone changed, and he became visibly sad when talking about the lonely father. Another boy in the group said: "*The father is feeling sad for being faraway.*" • Moe Chit, a girl in Group 1 pointed to a picture of a man holding a frightened little girl in his arms and a little boy standing close by (Fig. 1, Col1:1). Moe Chit did not say anything but showed an emotional face before changing the topic of discussion away from the sadness expressed in the picture. • Other expressions of separation, loss, and vulnerability emerged in several group narratives such as "*giving away the child,*" "*leaving behind,*" "*losing life,*" and "*without a family you are nothing.*" Minh, a boy in Group 2, presented some insights when narrating about his group's collage (Fig. 1, Col2: 1 & 2) saying that picture 1 represented "war" and the loss of life, while picture 2 showed the contrast of "*gaining of lives*" where "*two individuals hugged each other.*" 2. Living in Malaysia also meant a sense of isolation and loneliness represented in the refugee children's visual and verbal storytelling about single persons on the collages (e.g., Fig. 1, Col1:3; Col2:3 & 13; Col3:6 & 15) as well as lone objects (e.g., Fig. 1, Col4:7 (empty chair); Col5:6 (empty plate)). Many parents of refugee children in Malaysia worked as construction workers or as helpers in restaurants, where they worked long hours and seldom had time to spend with their children, specifically not when the children were awake (i.e., during the day). The children were therefore left behind to take care of themselves and their younger siblings.

(Continued)

Table 3.1 (Continued)

Theme	Analysis and Interpretation
	Example:

- Maung, a boy from Group 5, pointed to one of the single female images who reminded him of his mother (Fig. 1, Col5:4)—he did not know the existence or the whereabouts of his father. Pointing to an empty plate on the collage (Fig. 1, Col5:6) he said, "*I wish I could have meals with my family.*" His mother worked as a domestic helper, was always busy, and did not have much time to spend with him, although he described her as always smiling and never sad.
- Maung also commented on missing his extended family, his "*uncle and aunty*" with whom he went swimming and kayaking during the summer (Fig. 1, Col5:5) before they came to Malaysia. Apparently, Maung did not care much about his father's whereabouts and did not talk at all about his father or the missing father figure in his life, although he tended to divert attention away from negative emotions by doing other things such as coloring and doodling.

Table 3.2 Summary of Micro-narratives for Theme 2: Vulnerabilities

Vulnerabilities	The refugee children's emotional narratives expressed the challenges and difficulties they faced. While some would narrate stories related to war atrocities, others talked about "being bullied" by older siblings or family members or about feeling "powerless" in the face of difficulties living in the host country, Malaysia. Bullying could be interpreted as yet another form of disrupting a child's life, particularly when sibling rivalry emerges.
	Examples:

- Thakin, a boy in Group 3, initiated his storytelling by choosing two images of seemingly powerful people, a politician and two football players on the group collage (Fig. 1, Col3:7, 8 & 9). He described the football player as "*a show-off*" and the politician as "*a bully*" without any further elaboration. During a more relaxed phase of the interview (Step 5), Thakin added that his two older siblings have been bullying him and that they were always rough with him or made fun of him or getting him to do things he would rather not do. He also admitted to defacing another image by adding a beard to the face (Fig, 1, Col3:11) indicating his disgust with someone who, in his view, represented a bully.
- In Group 3 the children echoed the theme of being powerless. Wanting to be powerful to overcome the adversities they were facing, Ken talked about a footballer (Fig.1, Col3:9) and a trophy (Fig.1, Col3:10), all of which represented the wish or the desire to be powerful and strong—the footballer had power and authority and would enable Ken to tell others what to do instead of always being told: "*If I am like him, I can tell everybody what to do, and they have to obey me.*" He also liked to win, and thus the trophy signified winning.

- The refugee children talked about being bullied by older siblings or by peers. This concept is further reinforced in all five group collages, which had images of figures with authority, such as politicians (Fig.1, Col3:7), the military or police (Fig.1, Col1:1, Col2:1), businesspersons (Fig.1, Col5:9; Col3:5; Col5:4), or sports persons (Fig. 1, Col2:14; Col3: 8 & 9) who might have represented unverbalized stories of power, harassment, or abuse. There were also images of fierce, powerful, and threatening animals (e.g., tiger, lion) and an image of a faceless person holding up a sign of hope (Fig.1, Col5:11). The inclusion of the images of authority figures as well as threatening animals was interpreted as visual stories of bullying—that the children and perhaps their parents and other family members had experienced but were unable to verbalize in their storytelling. The faceless person (Fig. 1, Col5:11), however, was puzzling. The researchers interpreted this as the refugee children hiding their stateless identity in a host country that was not particularly welcoming of their presence.

Table 3.3 Summary of Micro-narratives for Theme 3: Family as Source of Strength

Family as source of strength	In contrast to perceiving the family as being disrupted, and having other vulnerabilities, the refugee children in this study also perceived the family as a source of strength in the face of adversity. In three of the group discussions the children (i.e., Groups 1, 2, and 4) voiced their feelings of "happiness" when talking about the reunion of family members (Fig. 1, Col1:4; Col2:2) while being with both parents and extended family members (Fig. 1, Col4:3) and when doing things together collectively. Examples: • Jia (a girl from Group 2) drew nine heart shapes on Collage 2 as indicative of family love, and she said, *"It's a happy family."* There seems to be an apparent longing for the times when the family could do things together whether reflecting on the past (e.g., visiting family in the country of origin) or imagining the future (e.g., going on a holiday or supporting one another through difficulties). • *"Without a family you are nothing,"* said Amid from Group 4 who came from Pakistan via Sri Lanka. Pointing to a huge mosque (Fig. 1, Col4:1) and a giant cruise liner (Fig. 1, Col 4:2) he continued to narrate: *"Family needs to have love, leisure time, and playing time and going for holidays"*; explaining that being together as a family will be a great strength when faced with adversities. • *"I enjoyed the happy moments where all family members get together, all the mums and aunties would be busy cooking and all our cousins would play together,"* said a girl, Shinh, pointing to a picture (Fig. 1, Col2:7). • Sai, a boy, pointing to (Fig. 1, Col4:7), *"It was my brother's birthday, and my father gave him a bicycle as a present. We were so happy as a family."* • Anjana, a girl in Group 1, happily showed a red heart shape she drew (Fig. 1, Col4:12) and positioned herself between the heart shape and the picture of grandma together with grandchildren (Fig. 1, Col4:3): *"This is a happy family."*

Table 3.4 Summary of Micro-narratives for Theme 4: Enabling Others

Enabling others	Another coping strategy emerging from the narratives of the refugee children interviewed involved the support from compassionate teachers and other community leaders. This theme particularly coincides with the SBFC model proposing collaboration between the two main institutions in the child's life when planning an intervention—that is, the school and the family.
	Examples:
	• Betsy, a girl in Group 1 expressed positive emotions of home and happiness with colorful drawings on the group collage stating that she had a teacher who was very supportive and helpful to her: *"Teachers give us hope and lead us. They help bringing my hopes and dreams to reality. I am very grateful to my teachers"* (Fig. 1, Col1:17). Other members in Group 1 agreed that their teachers were *"like an angel"* who would guide them to fulfill their dreams *"of becoming a successful person in the future."* It was also observed that Betsy tried to bring happiness into the group conversation by starting to sing and talking about her teacher.
	• Rico, a boy, and Ruth, a girl, in Group 2 respectively pasted images of a man in white clothes and turban (Fig. 1, Col2:10) and of religious people wearing robes and a doctor attending to a woman on a bed (Fig. 1, Col2:11 & 12). In their storytelling, Rico and Ruth elaborated that these people represented persons of influence and power who could resolve certain issues in their country (of origin). They were important people and could effect change. Knowing such community leaders, either in their country of origin or in the host country, seemingly gave the children a sense of well-being and empowerment for coping with the adversities they were facing as refugees.

it fits in with the SBFC model of holistic support for children's well-being on all levels.

Developing an Intervention

Following the execution of the five-step CLET procedures (Phase Two) and analyzing the CLET protocols (Phase Three), the SBFC practitioners in collaboration with the school and family (parents) develop an intervention either with individual children or with a group of refugee children to explore enabling properties of living and thriving in the host country, Malaysia. In Tables 3.5 and 3.6, we explicate possible intervention strategies for this group. For this purpose, only some of the more pertinent cases (individual children) who expressed specific narratives related to the four themes were identified in the analysis.

School and family are two important systems that could advocate for the betterment of children's lives (Gerrard, 2008). Therefore, we propose a close working relationship between the school and family. Isolation, loneliness, and disruption were constant themes emerging from the Malaysian case study. We propose providing after-school arrangements for refugee children

Table 3.5 Strategy for Proposed Intervention for Refugee Children

Theme	Difficulties revealed	Goals	Proposed intervention
Separation and disruption	Koko reunited with his mother after the initial separation while the father is still alone and separated from his loved ones.	Strengthen Koko's adapting skills.	Family intervention: Meet with Koko's mother and use the CLET methods to help Koko express his emotions to his mother and help him further to adapt in Malaysia.
	Maung did not know the existence or the whereabouts of his father and did not talk at all about his father; negative emotions observed during CLET process.	Enhance emotion expression and increase cohesion in family.	Family intervention: Meet with Maung's mother and use the CLET to explore Maung's emotions and help his mother to better understand his sense of separation from the father figure.
Vulnerability	Thakin complained about sibling bullying.	Eliminate bullying and improve sibling relationships.	Family intervention: Meet with Thakin together with his two older siblings and parents and use the CLET to help the family express reasons for the bullying and discuss possible solutions.

Table 3.6 Strategy to Strengthen the Relationship Between School and Family

Theme	Strengths discovered	Goals	Proposed intervention
Source of strength	Most of the refugee children indicated family as their source of strength.	Help parents to find ways to nurture their children better.	Family intervention: Meet with family members and follow up the positive vibes in the family; discuss with the family the importance of understanding the needs of the individual family members and source out possible community programs that could further support the family.

(Continued)

Table 3.6 (Continued)

Theme	Strengths discovered	Goals	Proposed intervention
Enabling adults	Most of the refugee children mentioned teachers are angels in their lives.	Give support to teachers so that they could play this important role in the lives of the refugee children.	School intervention: Meet with teachers to explore more possible support structures for them, such as their training needs and the provision of teaching resources; recruit more volunteer teachers to meet the serious shortage of English teachers within the refugee community; liaise with NGOs to advocate for the educational needs of refugee children.

so that they are not left unattended when their parents are at work. With the children perceiving their schoolteachers as "angels," these educators could play a greater role through providing the necessary support when other systems had failed this vulnerable group of children. Since the family (even for the vulnerable refugee family in Malaysia) is perceived by the children as a source of strength, we need to empower refugee families to support their children better, despite the challenges they face in their daily lives. This could be achieved by advocating for greater collaboration in the relationship between the school, the family, and the community. The local community in the host country should engage more actively with the refugee families to assist with care, taking and integrating within the local context. For example, a local family could team up with a refugee family advising them about child care, the legal system, and the health care system, to name but a few.

Overall, to improve the lives of refugee children in Malaysia we need to go beyond the family and school settings to advocate for more humanitarian assistance from local NGOs, faith-based communities, and local charity organizations and perhaps even have close collaboration with UNHCR to provide affordable medical assistance and quality training for volunteer teachers and SBFC practitioners who could plan for appropriate and effective interventions for these vulnerable families and their children. By helping the family, we help their children. One such opportunity exists in the Picha Project (Low, 2017), a social enterprise that aims to create a sustainable source of income for refugees through food-catering and delivery services as a means to provide a friendly living environment to assist refugee families in Malaysia.

Multicultural Considerations

When using the CLET to gain an understanding of the vulnerabilities and needs of refugee children and to plan for interventions, the SBFC practitioner needs to take note of the characteristics of "family functioning" in an Asian context (Kok & Low, 2017; Van Schalkwyk, 2017). Being in a patriarchal society where the norms of interpersonal relationships are positioned in a hierarchical order, children are expected to submit to authority, including that of their parents and their teachers. Most Asian children are afraid to openly discuss their negative experiences with their parents, and they may not be willing to disclose their perspectives about their family lives with outsiders, as this would be regarded as disclosing family shame. In the case study, it was discovered that the children did not openly discuss the atrocities of authority and the adverse effects on their family lives. As noted by Kitano and Chinn (1986) as is typical of Asian culture, there is a general inability to voice such negative experiences involving those in a vertical social hierarchy.

The CLET is, however, sensitive to such multicultural considerations and cultural diversity. In their protocols, the children who participated in the collage-making and storytelling used contrasting images and narratives as well as images with negative meanings or connotations as metaphors for the difficulties and challenges they experienced within their family lives (Van Schalkwyk, 2010). They used these images to express that which is difficult to talk about while presenting supposedly socially acceptable narratives to voice their feelings and experiences. Being in a minority position and possibly being warned by their parents to maintain low profiles when talking to others (strangers), the children were cautious and did not elaborate on instances of bullying except for revealing sibling conflicts and showing feelings of anger and resentment. Similarly, while attempting to solicit and to draw out collaboration from the parents of refugee children, there is a need to apply cultural sensitivity to avoid labeling their child as having problems or blaming them for the negative emotions expressed by their children, which may result in shame and embarrassment or even imply that they had not been taking good care of their children.

Challenges and Solutions

The CLET is not a psychological test aimed at diagnosing specific disorders, and the SBFC practitioner using this approach should not attempt to arrive at such a diagnosis based solely on his/her analysis of the CLET protocols. Rather, the CLET is a visual arts-based tool to draw out autobiographical remembering narratives from clients who otherwise have difficulties verbalizing their distresses or curtailed by cultural constraints of what is socially acceptable. The CLET serves to elicit the voices of refugee children and their families who may not be able to sufficiently articulate either their strengths or weaknesses using the host country's language (Van Schalkwyk &

Lijadi, 2019). In this regard, the CLET as a tool for engaging refugee children in telling their stories links well with the SBFC model that wants to provide children around the globe to express that which concerns them most and help them succeed in life.

Furthermore, the CLET also provides a channel into the internal landscape of deeper meanings that children make from their lived experience. Understanding how meanings are constructed in a social context is important to develop coherent interventions that could support vulnerable populations such as refugee children. In addition, using symbolic and projective skills working with children enables participants to construct new meanings (Lijadi & Van Schalkwyk, 2014) and solve problems that they did not yet know they had. In the case study presented earlier, the children identified "trophy" as "winning" and "tiger" as "powerful," while an "empty plate" was used to project their dream of having the parent's company.

Conclusion

Our case study reveals that the CLET is a useful tool for the SBFC practitioner who wishes to give a voice to the refugee children. By eliciting stories stimulated by the images pasted on a collage, the CLET is a strength-based approach that allows for changing intervention planning from problem-solving to empowering clients to be resilient and utilize whatever resources they have in story. Using externalizing language and symbolic objects during the collage-making process furthermore avoids children feeling threatened into exposing family secrets (or shame) and labeling the refugee family as problematic or even as abnormal. Such labeling will only exacerbate the social injustices to the family that is already encountering difficulties due to the socioeconomic system and environment of the host country. This is consistent with SBFC approach, which identifies child's issues in a broader context. By advocating the needs of refugee children, implementing programs to improve their well-being, utilizing a collaborative approach with a framework of school-child-family interconnectedness, SBFC can maintain a social justice approach that is strength-based.

Acknowledgment

The authors would like to record our gratitude for the case study mentioned in this chapter that was funded by Lao Hooi Kee Research Fund, UTAR.

Resources

Van Schalkwyk, G. J. (2010). Collage life story elicitation technique: A representational technique for scaffolding autobiographical memories. Qualitative Report, 15(3), 675–695. https://nsuworks.nova.edu/tqr/vol15/iss3/11/. https://doi.org/10.46743/2160-3715/2010.1170

Van Schalkwyk, G. J. (2020) (Chapter 14. Case study: A family in distress. In B. A. Gerrard, M. J. Carter & D. Ribera (Eds.), School-based family counseling: An interdisciplinary practitioner's guide (pp. 361–377). Routledge.

Van Schalkwyk, G. J., & Lijadi, A. A. (2019). Creating space for children's voices: Utility of the collage life-story elicitation technique. Journal of Psychological Research, 1(3), 1–11. https://doi.org/10.30564/jpr.v1i3.592

Bibliography

Alemi, Q., James, S., Siddiq, H., & Montgomery, S. (2015). Correlates and predictors of psychological distress among Afghan refugees in San Diego county. International Journal of Culture and Mental Health, 8(3), 274–288. https://doi.org/10.1080/175 42863.2015.1006647

Gerrard, B. (2008). School-based family counselling: Overview, trends, and recommendations for future research. International Journal for School-Based Family Counselling, 1(1), 1–30. http://www.instituteschoolbasedfamilycounseling.com/docs/ IJSBFC20-%20Volume%20I(1)%20-%20Gerrard.pdf

Kitano, M. K., & Chinn, P. C. (1986). Exceptional Asian children and youth (An ERIC exceptional child education report). Council for Exceptional Children.

Kok, J. K., & Low, S. K. (2017). Proposing a collaborative approach for school counseling. International Journal of School and Educational Psychology, 5(4), 281–289. https://doi.org/10.1080/21683603.2016.1234986

Lijadi, A. A., & Van Schalkwyk, G. J. (2014). Narratives of third culture kids: Commitment and reticence in social relationships. Qualitative Report, 19, 1–18. http://www.nova.edu/ssss/QR/QR19/lijadi49.pdf, (article 49). https://doi.org/10.46743/2160-3715/2014.1213

Lijadi, A. A., & Van Schalkwyk, G. J. (2017). Place identity construction of third culture kids: Eliciting voices of children with high mobility lifestyle. Geoforum, 81, 120–128. https://doi.org/10.1016/j.geoforum.2017.02.015

Low, S. K., Kok, J. K., & Lee, W. Y. (2014). Perceived discrimination and psychological distress of Myanmar refugees in Malaysia. International Journal of Social Science and Humanity, 4(3), 201–205. https://doi.org/10.7763/IJSSH.2014.V4.346

Kim Low, S., Aun Tan, S., Kuan Kok, J., Nainee, S., & Viapude, G. N. (2018). The mental health of adolescent refugees in Malaysia. PEOPLE: International Journal of Social Sciences, 4(2), 428–439. https://doi.org/10.20319/pijss.2018.42.428439

Low, X. E. (2017). Rohingya curries and Syrian sweets from refugees are making start-up a hit. CNBC. http://www.cnbc.com/2017/12/10/the-picha-project-rohingya-and-syrian-refugees-cook-for-start-up.html. SHAW, S. A., Pillai, V., & Ward, K. P. (2018). Assessing mental health and service needs among refugees in Malaysia. International Journal of Social Welfare, 28, 44–52.

Shelter home for children. (2019). Refugees and their children in Malaysia. http://www.shelterhome.org/index.cfm?&menuid=13

Smith, J. A., & Osborn, M. (2008). Interpretative phenomenological analysis. In J. A. Smith (Ed.), Qualitative psychology: A practical guide to research methods (pp. 53–80). SAGE.

United Nations High Commission for Refugees. (2021a). Figures at a glance in Malaysia. http://www.unhcr.org/en-my/figures-at-a-glance-in-malaysia.html

United Nations High Commission for Refugees. (2021b). Education in Malaysia. http://www.unhcr.org/education-in-malaysia.html

Van Schalkwyk, G. J. (2013). Assessing individual or family dynamics through the Collage Life0Story Elicitation Technique (CLET). In B. Gerrard & M. Soriano (Eds.), School-based family counseling: Transforming family-school relationships. Createspace.

Van Schalkwyk, G. J. (2017). Socio-cultural barriers to entry for school-based family counseling. International Journal of School-Based Family Counseling, Special Topic Issue, 2017, 1–10.

Wake, C., & Cheung, T. (2016). Livelihood strategies of Rohingya refugees in Malaysia: We want to live in dignity. Humanitarian Policy Group.

Yin, R. K. (2009). Case study research: Design and methods. SAGE, Inc.

4 How to Build Collaboration Between Immigrant Families and Schools Using Conjoint Family Counseling

Kezia Gopaul-Knights, Emily J. Hernandez, and Michael J. Carter

This chapter can be used by school-based family counseling (SBFC) practitioners who are interested in collaborating with immigrant families in conjoint family counseling processes within a school context. Understanding the importance of conjoint family counseling and being able to incorporate it into one's counseling practice is an essential part of being a culturally competent SBFC practitioner. The procedures described will assist trained mental health practitioners with experience in family therapy with the challenging task of working with immigrant families and in applying conjoint family counseling to a school setting.

Background

School-Based Family Counseling

The skills of conjoint family counseling are a critical component of school-based family counseling (SBFC). SBFC is a specific conceptualization of how conjoint family counseling processes can be applied directly to student problems in schools. SBFC can be implemented by mental health professionals in school settings, such as school counselors, school social workers, and school psychologists, so long as those professionals are trained in its core processes. These professionals should have education and training in addressing the complex problems that can arise in a family system (Carter & Evans, 2008). School personnel may be in the best position to implement SBFC because the focus in a school setting is on improving student functioning for success as opposed to addressing mental health issues.

Conjoint Family Counseling

Conjoint family therapy applied in SBFC can also be useful for schools because of its collaborative and open processes. The SBFC practitioner is

DOI: 10.4324/9781003097891-6

trained to work with the whole family to create a more consistent and stable environment in the student's home by addressing the needs of the parents, siblings, and other relatives as well. Family counseling is very different from individual or group counseling because it typically involves dealing with a high degree of interpersonal conflict and requires a more active and directive approach. At its core, effective family counseling often requires mental health practitioners to help a family to address the unresolved conflicts that create so much anxiety for family members, especially children. Skill in family counseling requires knowledge of individual cognitive and emotional development and understanding of what these look like in natural settings from infant to grandparent. It also requires familiarity with the stages of the family life cycle and normal and abnormal responses to stage transitions for a family from the birth of a child to the aging and death of parents. Family counseling involves the willingness to bring out conflict and the skills to resolve it in ways that help each member develop greater awareness and compassion for each other. These skills enable a mental health practitioner to feel prepared to handle a lot of what happens in assisting parents to help their children develop, especially in the emotional and behavior areas that can greatly affect school progress.

Working With Immigrant Families

Immigrant families face a multitude of challenges in the United States and stand to benefit greatly from the conjoint family counseling process. The term "immigrant" is often used to describe all persons leaving one country to enter another country permanently. The literature has made a distinction between economic immigrants and refugee immigrants in which the former group relocates to a country in search of better economic prospects while the latter group relocates due to persecution (Cortes, 2004). The move for economic immigrants is voluntary, and, depending on their immigration status, they are often able to return to their homeland to visit friends and family left behind. However, for refugee immigrants, the move is involuntary and returning home can be threatening to one's life. Factors in the home country and new host country impinge on the family system and will influence whether the immigrant family thrives or struggles to adjust to their new life. The SBFC practitioner is in a pivotal role to work with immigrant families since the school is usually the first point of contact. However, the process of school-based conjoint family counseling may not be appropriate for refugee immigrants or those immigrants initially settling in the United States due to their focus on survival and adjustment. In these situations, the SBFC practitioner would prioritize assisting the family in accessing basic resources such as housing, food, medical needs, and the like.

The challenges that immigrant families encounter in the United States are numerous. There is often a language barrier that immigrants encounter when attempting to assimilate into the United States. Many immigrants speak a language other than English, and within each of these languages are dialects. Dialects are also common even among English-speaking immigrants. For instance, in the English-speaking Caribbean, variants of English are spoken called "Patois" or "Creole." Immigrant children often take English as a second language (ESL) when they first enter school, but there is still a language difference between families and the schools that threatens effective communication. The historical and cultural context of the education system in the immigrant's host country should also be considered as it is often neglected when interpreting the concerns immigrant children present. Many countries have a two-tiered education system (i.e., elementary and secondary school), while the United States has a three-tiered system (i.e., elementary, middle, and high school). This fundamental difference, added to the fact that many immigrant children do not receive formal education or have interrupted schooling in their home country, makes the adjustment to the United States' education system difficult. Immigrant children are often diagnosed with learning disabilities, attention disorders, and emotional disorders although the symptoms they exhibit may be more accurately explained by the school factors or trauma mentioned earlier. Many immigrants may experience trauma in their home country, during the migration process, or while living in the United States. These experiences must be prioritized when working with the student and family because the experiencing of trauma symptoms can interfere greatly with availability and access to learning.

In attempting to work with immigrant populations, SBFC practitioners may identify unwillingness on the part of immigrants to engage in the helping process. There are many reasons for this, which will need to be explored and addressed. Immigrants often have a distrust for government systems through their own experience or from observing the experiences of those similar to them. The undocumented status of many immigrants also contributes to the lack of willingness to accept help because of fear of deportation. Additionally, immigrants often fall into minority groups and experience racial and social injustices. The current political and social climate can lead to a greater sense of insecurity that may further limit immigrants' trust and acceptance of help from others. Economic challenges are also common among immigrants. Although there are immigrants who prosper economically, there are many who are homeless or live in cramped housing or apartments and who live below the poverty line. They may also work multiple jobs or long hours, and accepting help may mean that it is taking away time that can be used to gain financial resources. Accepting help from others may be further obstructed by cultural differences and clashes that exist between the home and the school. In many cultures, family concerns are not spoken of outside the family, there are taboos or stigmas regarding receiving help in any form from others, and the spiritual or village leader is considered the healer. Many Latinx families and immigrants firmly believe the reality of negative energy, spirits, and curses due to their own experiences and cultural and historical backgrounds.

Despite these challenges, immigrants possess a significant number of strengths that can be mobilized during the SBFC conjoint family counseling process. Berger Cardoso et al. (2019) categorized immigrant strengths into four categories: pre-migration ecological (external) strengths, pre-migration individual strengths, post-migration ecological strengths, and post-migration individual strengths. Pre-migration strengths are those that existed prior to migration, and post-migration strengths refer to those that exist in the host country. Pre-migration ecological strengths include extended family network, community and neighborhood support, and churches. Individual-level pre-migration strengths include resiliency, grit and determination, survival skills, cultural values, spirituality, and ability to travel long distances. Post-migration ecological strengths include pro-bono legal services that may exist to help with undocumented status, community-based organizations, churches, and extended kin family support. On the individual level, post-migration strengths include the psychological flexibility, future orientation, desire to learn and work, motivation to achieve goals, and multilingual development. SBFC practitioners must consider how past and present strengths interact with each other and influence the resiliency of immigrants.

Procedure

This proposed model can be used by practitioners who are interested in integrating conjoint family counseling processes in their work with immigrants within a school context. The procedure consists of eight steps, with six of the steps being in direct contact with the family. The first step is crucial to establishing the foundation for the work with the family. This eight-step procedure follows a framework that was first described in detail in chapter 3 of the School-Based Family Counseling: An Interdisciplinary Guide (2019, Gerrard, Carter & Ribera (Eds.).

Step 1: Initial Referral/Information Gathering

The first step in the process is the initial referral. The initial referral usually comes from the school or community agency after many interventions have been completed including meetings with the student, classroom observations, conferences with the counselor, teacher, and/or parent. There are times when the referral for therapy services comes from an outside agency, such as Child Protective Services, after the family has encountered problems with mode of discipline or neglect due to economic circumstances. Families may be less willing to participate in the counseling process as a result. Resistance may also originate from fear or stigma attached to therapy due to cultural beliefs and traditions. SBFC practitioners must anticipate possible resistance from families and spend additional time in the rapport-building process and simultaneously display sensitivity to immigrants and their concerns.

Another important aspect of this first step is information gathering to get a comprehensive view of the student's academic history and better understanding of the presenting problem. Reviewing previous academic history allows a holistic view of the student and may shed light on the current presenting problem and provide a guide to be able to pinpoint when difficulties may have started. Having an understanding of the academic history will help the SBFC professional have a more in-depth understanding of the root of the presenting problem and provide for a more accurate plan and intervention for working with the student and family. SBFC practitioners must anticipate the lack of availability of school records for immigrant students. Cumulative academic records typically do not follow the children when they migrate to another country. The SBFC practitioner and the school team may need to do a thorough interview with the family to gain as much insight into schooling history, especially given the variations in education systems across countries and incomplete or lack of schooling for some children. The next step focuses on how to make the first contact with the family.

Step 2: First Contact—How to Get the Family In

The establishment of rapport begins in the initial phone call by communicating to the parent(s) the need for the family to be involved in order to assist the student, who may be the primary reason why the family is seeking help. It is important to remember that many parents do not truly understand what mental health intervention is about and may feel very defensive about a request for their child or themselves to be involved in counseling. They may feel that counseling, or therapy, is for "crazy people" or that personal information should never be shared outside the family. In these cases, it's critical for the SBFC practitioner to explain that this intervention is part of the educational process that helps children learn. In many cases involving a referral for school-related problems, parents may feel that only the child needs to be involved in counseling. Helping parents to understand why their involvement is required is an important first step in establishing rapport. Some parents may ask: "If my child is having the problem why do I need to be involved?" Great care should be taken in answering this question because parents may become defensive if it is implied that they need to be involved because they are the *source* of the problem. This "source-solution attribution" (Compas et al., 1982) occurs when parents assume that if the *solution* to a problem is their involvement, then the *source* of the problem must be themselves. It is important to interrupt this attribution by explaining to parents that "while many things may cause a child's difficulties, parents know and love their child, so they can be of great help in addressing the problem."

Additional consideration to have when working with immigrant students and families is that a phone call may not be the best way to make initial contact with immigrant parents. Immigrant families may not have a phone or, if they do, are unwilling to agree to the counseling process over the phone.

Rapport may be better established through a home visit or by setting up a meeting at the school. SBFC practitioners may find that rapport is also more easily established with the family through collaboration with community leaders and advocates such as a spiritual leader. Importantly, the primary language spoken by the immigrant family, and the need for translation during the entire process, must be strongly considered. As a word of caution, the student should never be used as a translator during the counseling process, even if the language is uncommon and there is difficulty with locating a translator. This would give the child another role in the counseling process that will inhibit their participation as a student and a family member. The next step in the procedure is establishing the first family meeting.

Step 3: First Meeting With Family—Learning More About Strengths and Challenges

The first family session is the most important because it sets the stage for subsequent sessions and the main accomplishment is *making strong connections with the parents and family* so that they return and continue in the process. This rapport is more important than anything that is discussed and should always be the *utmost priority*. It is worth mentioning again in this step that school-based conjoint family counseling may be inappropriate for economic and refugee immigrants who are very new in the United States, are adjusting to trauma related to the migration process, and are operating in mere "survival" mode with the struggle to meet foundational basic needs. This stage requires that immigrants and refugees are somewhat settled in having their basic needs of food, shelter, and safety met. Given this, the first family session will focus on what family counseling is about and how it might help the child to earn more money and experience less anxiety (i.e., due to unemployment) when they become adults (see Figure 4.1). In addition, it will include a discussion of family counseling and the focus on communication and learning about our strengths and challenges.

Expectations and Ground Rules

At the first meeting, expectations and ground rules are discussed with the family. This involves committing to attending all sessions and reviewing communication and confidentiality. Communication and confidentiality focus on (a) the family's openness about what is going on in their lives and their thoughts and feelings about it and their thoughts about our views, (b) freedom for every member to share without fear of punishment, and (c) ensuring safety and protection for everyone.

Identifying Strengths and Challenges Including the Presenting Problem

The assessment begins by interviewing the parents with the *SBFC Interview Procedure* (Carter & Evans, 2008), which involves interviewing the parents, children, and teacher(s) with a focus on strengths, challenges, and what has been tried to address these challenges (see Resources at the end of this chapter). The SBFC practitioner may also find it useful to consider the student and family's strengths and challenges from an ecological perspective, while examining pre- and post-migration experiences, to gain a deeper insight into their overall functioning. For instance, an SBFC practitioner may highlight that the immigrant family had a large family network to rely on pre-migration. However, in post-migration this wider family network may not be available. The lack of kinship network may contribute to feelings of isolation and consequently impact the family's functioning. These and other considerations may reveal critical needs that must be addressed in order to improve the student and family's functioning.

When interviewing the parents in this session, include an exploration of the following:

1. The parents' viewpoint of the history of the problem
2. Anything they would like you to know in order to help the family
3. Their viewpoint of how well they operate together as a team
4. The general level of marital satisfaction and any unresolved conflicts
5. Family genogram.

Exploration of Family Challenges and the Presenting Problem

The family challenges and presenting problems will then be explored with the family. While some of this information may be known from the initial referral, it is still important to explore this with the family. Explain that it is normal for each family member to have different views of what the family needs to work on. In general, start by asking the *student* what they think the family needs to work on and then move up, finishing with the parent(s). This allows the children to have some input before the parents give more detailed descriptions. As the family talks, be sure to explore EACH person's perspective and SUMMARIZE what they say and how they feel. As you listen, think about how the problem may be related to normal stressors that occur during each of the family life cycles that the family may be in at this time.

Additional Family Counseling Techniques to Facilitate in the First Session

Exploring the family challenges and presenting problem is likely to bring about some tension or conflict in the session. The SBFC practitioner may need to use reframing, interrupting, and interventions to address the family conflict as needed. If family members interrupt and disagree with each other, reiterate that it's natural for every person to have their own viewpoint and that each person will get a chance to give their view. If the parents start to discuss marital issues or other issues that violate healthy subsystem boundaries, then immediately interrupt the discussion with a brief explanation of the types of issues that are best discussed together as a family (e.g., expectations of parents and children, family rules, consequences, and so on) and the types of issues that are best talked about in private (issues that the parents have with each other, issues that the parents have with a child that might embarrass the child if discussed with siblings, and the like). Then ask the parents to save that discussion for later when you will talk with them separately from the kids.

Summarizing the First Session

Depending on what arises in the session, it may be possible that the SBFC practitioner does not complete all aspects of this first meeting, but it is very important to save time to summarize what has happened in the first session before it ends. After each person has given their view, tell the family that the plan is to address *each* of the problems that they have talked about but that the family will have to work on one at a time in order to make progress so that everyone will feel better.

As you summarize what the family has done to deal with the problem, remember to do as follows:

> *Acknowledge* the family and individual strengths and specifically *praise* the family *for their effort* in trying to make things better, even if it didn't seem to solve the problem. Remind them that if they *continue to try*, things will get better.
>
> Assure the family that, while it will take time for things to get better, today is a great start because everyone knows more about the situation and we can now start to help the family to work together to improve the situation a little each day.
>
> Get a consent for counseling form signed and, if necessary, get a consent to release information form signed in order to talk with other important parties (e.g., school, outside service provider, other professionals, other family, or community members).
>
> Remind the family of the next session date and time, give them an appointment card with this information and your phone number, and then say goodbye.

Step 4: Second Meeting With Parents—Psycho-education

The second parent meeting consists of psycho-education, a process of providing information, education, and support to assist the family to understand their situation and cope. This stage of the conjoint family counseling process requires the SBFC practitioner to be familiar with the cultural and historical background of the immigrant family. This is because the SBFC practitioner takes on the responsibility for prioritizing the problems to be addressed in the session, which can only competently be done if there is a thorough understanding of the family's background and problems that are presented. Additionally, another important consideration for SBFC practitioners is the role present and past traumas place in the family's functioning. The immigrant family may not recognize how the trauma that they have experienced has impacted the problems they now encounter. Making this connection during the counseling process may be beneficial in understanding the nature of the crisis and developing solutions. As the SBFC practitioner moves toward the psycho-education phase, there will likely be some resistance from immigrant parents due to differences in child-rearing practices in the immigrants' home country versus the United States. Demonstrating sensitivity to these differences and acknowledgement of how difficult this must be for families will be important in getting buy-in from parents.

Psycho-education topics may vary, but in general psycho-education when working in a school setting should consist of the following.

4a The Most Important Issues and Current Crises

The SBFC practitioner provides a summary of the first session to remind the family of what was done and the reasons for working together. Following this narrative discussion, the parents are then presented with the SBFC practitioner's view of the family's most important issues and current crises, the latter being the initial focus of treatment. The most important issues usually are related to the presenting problem, although the SBFC practitioner's view of the presenting problem is typically different from the family's because the counselor is objectively considering many more aspects of the family from the dimensional analysis. After speaking with the parents, the counselor then gives feedback to the whole family with an emphasis on strengths and family life cycle stressors that normally challenge all families, while safeguarding any information that would increase anxiety. Feedback from the parents is actively solicited throughout this process.

Throughout the evaluation process, the SBFC practitioner is looking for any crises that need immediate attention before continuing with further treatment. These require the SBFC practitioner to engage in crisis counseling, which typically involves the following:

1. Identifying the possible harm that may occur and helping the family to understand that immediate action must be taken to *prevent harm to anyone.*
2. Developing a specific behavioral plan to assist the family in helping each other to cope constructively with the crisis.
3. Assisting the family to recognize what the crisis reveals about their family dynamics and what they can do to prevent further occurrence of the crisis.

If crisis counseling is involved, this becomes the priority. An additional session may be required in this procedure after the crisis is stabilized to review psycho-educational information with the family.

4b General Psycho-educational Topics to Introduce

A general introduction to these topics is provided in this session. Since this procedure is an abbreviated form of a longer-term conjoint family therapy intervention, these psycho-educational topics may be applied as needed or as appropriate. These topics will be reviewed again during additional sessions and integrated into the treatment plan.

The psycho-educational topics include the following:

- The three rules of kindergarten
- The three high-risk behaviors of adolescence
- The main protective factors to prevent these high-risk behaviors
- The three outcomes of young adulthood
- Introduction and review of basic academic school counseling information
- The ten positive methods of discipline and redirection techniques

It is important to note that many parents may not be consciously aware of their role and influence in teaching their children appropriate behavior. Most rely upon their own cultural and familial experiences to make decisions regarding how best to deal with their children and may not be aware of the specific expectations of the school and classroom environment. Many parents may feel uncomfortable discussing their own discipline techniques that may include yelling or spanking, which may have been experienced in their own upbringing. Children learn best when discipline methods are consistent across all environments, especially in school. That's why it's important to explore the specific techniques that have been used in the past so that any necessary modifications can be made in the present in order to maximize the child's academic and personal development.

The psycho-educational topics listed earlier are described in more detail here.

> The Three Rules of Kindergarten: The three rules of kindergarten provide a discussion of the following teachable behaviors: (a) keep hands and feet to self, (b) follow directions, and (c) respect others and their property.
>
> High-Risk Behaviors of Adolescence: Another aspect to explore in the parental subsystem with adolescent children concerns the high-risk behaviors of adolescence: (a) substance and alcohol abuse; (b) romantic relationships, sexual behavior, pregnancy, and sexually transmitted disease; and (c) negative influence of peers. The main protective factor to prevent these behaviors is an open and trusting relationship with a credible adult such as a parent (Fraser, 2004). Many parents, however, are not aware of this protective factor that can help to prevent significant problems regarding these high-risk behaviors.

The Three Outcomes of Young Adulthood: Another focus is typically centered on three areas of competence (usually in their early 20s), which are (a) to be self-maintaining, (b) to have one good friend, and (c) to stay out of jail. These outcomes may seem minimal, but if a child is able to accomplish these, they'll have a good chance of being happy and successful as an adult.

Being self-maintaining requires satisfying all physical, financial, and psychological needs including health, cooking and cleaning, work skills to provide and live within one's means, and other skills required to live independently. Having one good friend (which safeguards one's mental health) requires the ability to identify and manage one's own emotions; express thoughts and feelings adequately; listen carefully to others; be flexible enough to accommodate the needs of others while also advocating for one's own needs; and other interpersonal skills. Staying out of jail requires the ability to understand and follow rules, respect authority, and understand the social consequences of human behavior. These "three outcomes of young adulthood" often become the basis for the development of family rules within the household as children grow older. It's also necessary to acknowledge the increased ability of the adolescent to participate and give input into family discussions regarding decisions that affect them and to also take more responsibility for their part in implementing these. This enables parents to move from "managers" to "consultants" as adolescents become adults.

4c Introduction and Review of Basic Academic School Counseling
Information With the Student and Family (Secondary-Level Students)

This part of the session includes an individual review of the student's academic history with the family, including grades, test scores, credits, college course requirements, and progress toward graduation (or promotion for younger students). Many immigrant children attended school in their home country but may not have any records or documentation so it's important to discuss this with the family and explore schooling prior to the current school. It is critical to include the parents in this conversation because children may not be able to articulate their academic histories or the reasons for academic transitions in their lives.

While this general academic information may appear to be general knowledge, it's very common for students to move through high school and not have an understanding of what is needed to graduate and what options are available to them. This information is often provided in large group settings such as assemblies, classroom presentations, or workshops, where students may not be fully attending and "fall through the cracks." Particularly for immigrant students, this information should be delivered in their primary language in small group settings and be relevant to their experiences. Collaborating with a primary counselor who can develop a more personal relationship with the immigrant students is critical to the connection necessary to gain trust.

"Teaching" the basics of academic counseling to students is an important aspect for SBFC practitioners. Providing this information within a family counseling context allows for an assessment of their current level of knowledge, improved understanding of the concepts, and individualized assistance and support. The SBFC practitioner should also assess nonverbal reactions and use that information in the counseling process.

Reviewing academic information with the family provides a basic common knowledge of academic information and helps them be on the same page to establish family expectations, rules, and goals. Understanding the family's goals is important in working with immigrant students. Some may feel like higher educational pathways are not a good fit for them or may never have thought it was an available option. This is a good opportunity to personalize the information, advocate for available post-graduation opportunities, and use the "Education Pays" chart (see Figure 4.1) to make the connection between education and improved financial power and less unemployment. The SBFC practitioner should conduct a basic review of grades, how grades are converted into points, which become a grade point average (GPA). There should also be a review of school credits, how they are earned, and how many credits are needed to graduate (this information varies by school, district, and state). Families must understand that an "F" grade equals 0 credits, and, while a "D" in a class may allow them to graduate, it will disqualify them from applying to a 4-year university unless they retake the class. Also, to provide educational equity, many state graduation requirements now involve students completing an A-G course curriculum (courses required for college acceptance to a 4-year university).

4d Positive Methods of Discipline and Redirection Techniques

It's important to help parents to see the connection between early childhood experiences of parental discipline and the quality of the parent-child relationship during adolescence. This is a good time to reiterate that this relationship constitutes the primary protective factor against the three high-risk behaviors of adolescence.

This discussion typically leads to explanation and training of positive discipline techniques that acknowledge the child's feelings and give two structured choices of how to deal with their feelings. This also includes a specific, detailed procedure that uses "Breaks," which are modified "time-outs" that allow the child a chance to think about their behavior and more constructive ways of getting what they want. Let the family know that this use of "time-out" or "Breaks" will come in the next session because kids need to have consistent attention to positive behaviors before time-outs or Breaks will work.

The positive methods of discipline and redirection techniques are reviewed with the parents only. The student can be excused to return to class or work on an independent assignment if the parents are seen after regular school hours. This information is adopted from Kay Manning: Positive Methods of Discipline and Redirection (2018) (see Resources at the end of this chapter). Essentially, this is: understanding and acknowledging the feelings behind child behavior, positive redirection, and giving two structured behavioral choices. It also involves positive reinforcement, using "I" messages, being positive versus saying "No," avoiding labels, modeling feelings in a positive way, explaining, and trusting in the child's developing competence.

As the psycho-educational meeting with the family is summarized, the parents are encouraged to implement these positive discipline techniques until the next session.

Step 5: Third Meeting With Family—Co-constructing Rules, Expectations, and Consequences

The third family session helps the family to co-construct a positively oriented system of behavior management based on what is consistent with societal and school system requirements in order to be successful. Again, it is emphasized that this work at home can help the child to develop the skills necessary to be successful in the school/work environment, which leads to earning more money with less unemployment in adulthood. The session covers checking the implementation of positive discipline; co-constructing expectations and co-constructing rules; and consequences with the use of the objective discipline procedure (ODP), "Break" system, and behavior chart, a method of recording what happens whenever inappropriate behavior such as noncompliance or aggression occurs (Carter, 2013). Including children in the development of rules and expectations may be uncomfortable in some immigrant households based on how children are raised in their culture. Some cultures will view this practice of including children in the development of rules and expectations as giving a child "too much say" in how things are run in the family. SBFC practitioners should be aware of this hierarchical structure in the way communication occurs in the family and be sensitive to the discomfort that parents experience. This discomfort may be addressed by allowing parents to share their honest opinions about the methods being suggested, which is then followed by the SBFC practitioner providing a rationale for each method and how it will benefit the family.

5a Checking the Implementation of Positive Discipline

The third family meeting begins with a check-in regarding the implementation of the positive discipline techniques reviewed in the last session. What you're hoping to get from the children is a description of the parents providing positive attention whenever the children are behaving positively and providing an acknowledgment of their feelings and two structured choices whenever they are behaving inappropriately. If not, then ask the parents if they remember how they responded to the children when they were behaving positively or inappropriately. If necessary, review the basic concepts of positive discipline (Carter, 2013).

5b Co-constructing Expectations

After assessing the implementation of the positive discipline techniques, the next step is to work with the family to "co-construct" the expectations, rules, and consequences of how things will operate in the home. This process of "co-constructing" is critical in order for the children to understand and "buy-in" to this family plan. This process begins with a review of the three outcomes of young adulthood and the skills that are necessary in order to achieve each of these.

5c Co-constructing Rules and Consequences With the ODP "Break" System

The next important process of this session is to co-construct with the children and parents the specific rules and consequences and specific procedures that the family will use to implement these. While parents retain authority for final approval, this co-construction process is critical in order to incorporate the child's input into the development of the behavior management system. This typically results in less resistance on the part of the children to participating in the system because of their ownership over how it was developed. This involves exploring the *current* behavior management situation in the family and then co-developing new ways of dealing with noncompliance with parental directions.

Using the ODP given in the later section can help the family in dealing with noncompliance and following parental directions. This procedure can be used for children aged 5 and older, while a general time-out break can be utilized for children aged 2–4. This procedure may be a source of discomfort if the parents interpret that privileges are rewards given for good behavior. Some cultures believe that children should do what they are told without compensation for this obedience, and a reward can be deemed as a "bribe." This concept must be reframed by explaining that appropriate behavior is the requirement for maintaining access to privileges versus a "reward." It should be discussed and understood that child privileges are not entitlements but rather must be earned through appropriate behavior. Most parents withdraw privileges from children as an immediate consequence for inappropriate behavior, often for long periods of time without the child having any input. This prevents the child from the opportunity to slow down and make an informed choice about complying with the rules before being "grounded" from privileges. One effective technique to address this is the ODP (Carter, 2013) with the use of a 5-minute "Break" where the child sits for 5 minutes without any attention so that both parent and child can reflect on how to improve the situation before grounding. If the child refuses to take the Break, then the child is "grounded" from all electronics and favorite activities until the child chooses to take the Break. The child does not necessarily have to sit in one place during grounding. After the child takes the Break and complies with the original direction, they are then grounded for an additional 30 minutes and then all privileges are returned as long as the child continues to comply with the rules. These inappropriate behaviors, Breaks, and groundings should be charted with the ODP chart to give the counselor a detailed description of implementation information (see Resources at the end of this chapter).

Step 6: Fourth Meeting With Family—Checking on Progress and Focus on Family Fun

The fourth family meeting begins with a reminder that these counseling sessions will help children be more successful and happy in their lives now and in the future. This meeting provides an opportunity to check on the progress of the implementation of the positive discipline and ODP including troubleshooting, problem-solving, and effective communication through "dyad" work. Once these are accomplished, the focus then turns to how the family experiences fun together.

6a Discussion of Strengths and Positive Behavior and Challenges During the Past Week

The counselor facilitates a family discussion of the positive aspects of the past week, particularly those that are related to appropriate child behavior such as following directions immediately. It's important to ask the children if they can recall how they and the parents felt during these positive experiences and to remind everyone that the ability to follow directions is highly correlated with competence and future success in life. Competence is what makes us feel good about ourselves and allows us to praise ourselves, which leads to more confidence and optimism about the future.

6b Checking on the Progress of Implementation of the ODP

After this, the counselor reviews the behavior chart to better understand what has happened during the previous week. The counselor notes any behavioral trends related to the day of the week and the time of the day (e.g., Mondays, mornings, afternoons, and so on) as well as which child and parent is most noted and if any of the breaks might be related to lack of established morning, afternoon, or evening routines. Parental errors might include giving breaks at bedtime or in the morning when children are less available for learning and the Breaks might be ineffective due to time constraints such as needing to get sleep or getting to school. Until the Break system is firmly established and understood, these times and tasks need to have pre-established routines and incentives for completion in a timely manner. These might include earning some extra screen time if the child is ready for school on time or story time with parents if the child is ready for bed on time. Often, an older child may be more successful in adapting to the system and have fewer incidents, which is natural given the expectation of more maturity. It's also important to remind everyone that, even if there were lots of incidents during the week, this constitutes family progress because these important learning experiences lead to improvement.

During the discussion, the SBFC practitioner reframes the behavior that has resulted in the most "Break" incidents as an opportunity for everyone to learn rather than feel bad. It's best to first ask the child involved in these incidents to try to remember what happened and what they were thinking and feeling at each step of the inappropriate behavior. The child can then be encouraged to ask other family members to add to the narrative. It's also important to ask the child whether the initial direction seemed reasonable in terms of the child's ability to comply.

Finally, the child is asked to comment on how the parent seemed during the incident. Was the parent calm or upset, did the parent speak clearly or with a raised voice? Then, check to see if the parent agrees with the child's perception or views it differently. Regardless, it's important to point out that progress happens when parents are role models for children in learning to remain calm and positive, even when upset. It's also useful to teach the family mindfulness of emotions and ways of calming down including relaxed breathing. It may also be necessary to review the ODP, including further role-play of the process.

6c Improving Family Communication Through Active Listening Skills and
Practice in "Dyads"

Communication styles can be quite different across cultures. Communication in some immigrant families may be hierarchical in nature with greater value placed on what adults say than what children say. Furthermore, children may be spoken to and not allowed to voice their opinions in the family. The shift to children and parents having an equal voice in the counseling session may be uncomfortable for family members and should be addressed in the session. As the communication increases between parents and the child, the SBFC practitioner may recognize there are differences in the worldview of the immigrant parent and the child. This may be because the assimilation stage may be different for the child and parent. Some parents may hold strong to their cultural values while the children may more easily assimilate into the host culture. Highlighting this within the session may bring more clarity to the family and allow a greater level of perspective taking from each party. Facilitating "dyad" work can assist with psycho-education about this process, increasing awareness and decreasing the tension in the family.

Dyad work is an important process to address differences of opinion between family members by practicing active listening skills with two family members. While it may seem simple, many family disagreements are caused by ineffective communication where neither person is really listening to what the other is saying. Active listening skills are often the most important thing for families to learn. Briefly, active listening involves asking one person (i.e., Person 1) to express one positive thing about the other (Person 2), who is directed to listen carefully with the expectation that Person 2 will be asked to reflect back to Person 1 what they said and how they felt. Then, Person 1 is asked if Person 2's reflection was accurate, and if not, then Person 1 corrects misperceptions of content or feeling with Person 2 again reflecting back what Person 1 said. Then, Person 2 gives a reaction to what Person 1 said, with Person 1 reflecting back the content and feelings of Person 2's reaction. Then, Person 2 expresses one positive thing about Person 1, and the whole process is repeated.

An example of this discussion could be as follows:

> *"Mom, I'd like you to begin by telling Julie one positive thing about her, either something she's done or perhaps something you feel good about her. Julie, after your Mom finishes, I'm going to ask you to reflect back to her what she said and how she felt about it."*
>
> *"Julie, please tell your mom the basics of what she told you. Please tell her how she seemed to feel about what she said."*
>
> *"Mom, how accurate was Julie in her perceptions about what you said and how you felt?"*
>
> *"Julie, now that your Mom feels that you understood her, could you please give your reaction to what she said. Mom, be sure to listen carefully because when Julie is finished, I'll ask you to reflect back to her what she said and how she feels about it."*

Once both persons are successful in actively listening to positive comments with this process, then they are each asked to tell the other person one thing that they would like the other person to improve on, using the same process. During this phase, it is critically important for the counselor to help each person to focus on the content and feelings involved in what is being said, before responding to what the other person said. While this may seem slow at times, it's an important building block in improving patience and the effectiveness of family communications.

6d Assessing Existing Family Fun and Exploring New Activities

While it's important to address specific problems within families, it's also important to improve the quality of family functioning by focusing on how they experience *fun* together. "Fun" may seem unimportant to some families, especially those with challenges in their own families of origin, but fun is an important ingredient in experiencing happiness. Happiness often involves positive, meaningful relationships with others, and enjoyable interactions lead to these. As discussed earlier, one of the primary protective factors against the high-risk behaviors of adolescence involves a strong, open and trusting relationship with a credible adult, preferably a parent. Experiences of fun with parents and family help to promote this type of relationship and create positive family memories that help maintain interpersonal connections between siblings as they grow older. Begin by asking each person about what family activities are most fun for them, including fun between smaller groups of family members as well as the whole family.

After assessing current family fun, explore other family activities that might be fun, especially low-cost activities such as taking a walk or cooking a family meal together. Interactive board games such as "Apples and Oranges" or "UNO" card games can focus on enjoying experiences together, whether you win or lose. Larger scale family fun trips such as camping can be an inexpensive way to spend quality family time together in an outdoor environment.

One of the greatest challenges to family fun is technology such as smartphones, which distract family members from being fully present while together. At home and during family outings to restaurants, it's more commonplace to see families together, but attending to their smartphones rather than to each other. Accordingly, it's important to facilitate family discussion about specific boundaries needed around time spent with the family to create positive, lasting memories. This also requires that parents focus on activities that are fun for everyone, not just for themselves.

The fourth family meeting concludes with a summarization of the session, highlighting the positive progress and continuing challenges in using the behavior management system and communicating effectively as well as renewed focus on increasing family fun together.

Step 7: Fifth Meeting With Family—Termination, Generalization, and Transfer

The fifth family meeting is focused on assessing progress, troubleshooting and problem-solving, and beginning the process of termination by introducing the concept of "family meetings." Explanation and practicing these important family functions help the family to generalize and transfer the knowledge and skills learned and to monitor progress and address future challenges. At the end of this session, a 1-month follow-up appointment is made.

7a Termination of Conjoint Family Counseling

As the family learns to deal with crises, improve family structure and functioning, and to address and resolve specific family problems, the process of termination begins with the introduction of "family meetings." In these, the family takes more responsibility for facilitating the family counseling sessions, which enables the counselor to measure how well the family can work together without assistance.

7b Family Meetings

Family meetings are an opportunity to get together to discuss the positive and negative things that are happening. Family members rotate the facilitator role, helping to run the meeting and monitor the communication rules. The SBFC directs this initial "family meeting" to ensure maximum participation and success and chooses a family member to assist them. The meeting begins with *each* family member commenting on something *positive* that has happened in the family during the past week, and after summarizing these, *each* family member shares one thing they would like to see *improved* during the next week, with discussion of how the whole family can help make this happen. During discussion, the counselor focuses on reminding the family to use their "active listening" and other effective communication skills to attend to each other and to reflect back the content and feelings of their statements. When necessary, the counselor points out mutual points of agreement and areas of difference and creating ways of compromise to resolve these. This discussion also allows the counselor to assess to what degree the family is consistently using the tools of positive discipline and the "Break" system.

7c Crisis Prevention Through Family Life Cycle Preparation and Problem-Solving

Resilience is enhanced when a family anticipates problems that may come up in the future and learn to deal with them through proactive family problem-solving processes. Transitions into new stages of the family life cycle often create great stress and conflict in families. Specific explanations of these stages, especially those in the near future, help a family understand what adaptations are needed to maintain success as their family develops and provide opportunity to explore the family's problem-solving process. It's often useful to use the most recent family life cycle stage to explore how the family dealt with previous problems. Family resilience can be enhanced by integrating the concepts given earlier into the conjoint family counseling processes of family evaluation, treatment, and termination. These can help the family recognize and use their own resources to maintain healthy structure and communication and to solve family problems now and in the future.

In moving beyond the family counseling session, the SBFC practitioner must recognize the challenges that immigrant families face in attempting to generalize and transfer the skills learned in the sessions and provide ways to address them. Many immigrant families will continue to face external and internal challenges that threaten their resiliency. Some of these external challenges include poverty, racism, and lack of familial support. Internal challenges include learning disorders and other disabilities, mental health challenges, and physical/health challenges. SBFC practitioners should anticipate these challenges and mobilize both internal and external protective factors and resources to address concerns. For some families this may mean connecting them with local food pantries, helping them complete paperwork to receive monetary support from social services or referral to community agencies for mental health services.

Step 8 Follow-Up Session and Identifying Need for Additional Sessions

Lastly, a follow-up session is scheduled within a month's time to check in with the family regarding progress, updates about the presenting problem and implemented interventions, and anticipating possible future obstacles or crises. Psycho-educational concepts will also be revisited and reinforced as needed and additional resources and referrals may be provided. In scheduling this session, the SBFC practitioner should plan to be flexible due to immigrant families' work and other time constraints.

Another important process is helping the family to identify when they might need continued family counseling and to understand and identify individual and family symptoms that indicate problems. Individual symptoms may include reduced functioning in any of the main life functioning areas (school, work, financial, self, and so on) as well as maladaptive responses to specific situations. Family symptoms may include reduction in the frequency of family fun and time together or an increase in family conflict or negative mood. When these occur, the family should reactivate the processes of family meetings and problem-solving. If the family does not improve significantly following these strategies, then the family should contact the counselor sooner than later to prevent crises.

It's also important to remind the family that teachers, administrators, and staff will continue to monitor the student's performance in the school environment and report back to the family if any challenging situations occur. If the parents become concerned about the child's school functioning, they should contact the counselor for a phone call or in-person booster session if necessary. Another important part of this process is to help the family gather the necessary referral information just in case these are necessary later.

Multicultural Considerations

This chapter has addressed ways to apply conjoint family counseling with immigrant children and families in the school by integrating multicultural considerations in each stage of the process. However, there are some general cultural considerations for working with immigrant families that warrant mentioning separately. Getting immigrants to accept the counseling process for their children may take multiple attempts, patience, and understanding from the SBFC practitioner. SBFC practitioners should gently show the benefits of counseling for the child and family but also recognize that parents should have autonomy to make decisions that they deem are best for their family. If parents decide to reject the opportunity for counseling services, or need additional time to ponder the idea of accepting services, the SBFC practitioner should work with other school personnel to provide resources needed for the family that can help alleviate some of the current concerns. Additionally, the SBFC practitioner should recognize the unique experiences of each child and family with whom they work and allow them to be the "experts" in providing information about their functioning and their background. This means using active listening skills, additive empathy, and other micro counseling skills to help draw out the clients' stories (Ivey et al., 2017).

A critically important aspect of effective conjoint family counseling is specific consideration of the cultural and historical backgrounds of the family. These must be included in the evaluation of the family in order to improve understanding and reduce resistance. It's critical to focus on family history as well as cultural background to avoid making faulty generalizations that can adversely affect conjoint family therapy success. Counselors often make assumptions regarding cultural background, particularly regarding variations within the same ethnic group. It's important for the counselor to create a narrative that involves exploration of the family's specific cultural beliefs and family history and how these affect individual family members' development and the presenting problem. In this sense, the cultural and historical story of the family becomes the context for present-day problems. Presenting this narrative in a compassionate way creates new connections and increases awareness for the family of the systemic issues that the family has faced and continues to face due to race, ethnicity, religion, class, immigration status, and any other cultural factor. Any family intervention must consider not only the individual and systemic functioning of the family itself then but also the way in which systemic factors in society interact with and affect the family's ability to function.

Challenges and Solutions

There can be many challenges to applying the "8-Step SBFC Procedure for Conjoint Family Counseling in Schools." This process can be difficult, time-consuming and requires knowledge, training, and experience in working with family systems. A review of some of the other challenges and corresponding solutions is here.

Obtaining buy-in from administration to integrate more work with families in schools may take time. Align with administration by developing strong rapport and working relationships with them. Provide regular updates regarding your work and outcomes to administration and demonstrate skills in working with families by volunteering to intervene in situations involving parents/families and be visible in your interactions fostering family engagement in school.

School focus is on the student versus including the family in intervention. Provide research and studies on the importance of family engagement in the school setting. Provide information about how frequently the problems that are affecting students in the classroom are related to issues outside of school.

SBFC practitioner gaining access to school campus. The school/district can hire counselors with training and experience in working with families and school counseling. School/district can contract or partner with local agencies that can work collaboratively with the school staff and support team.

Time management and other assigned non-counseling job responsibilities. This is where the importance of administrator buy-in comes in so that administration and staff understand the positions, roles, and responsibilities in advocating for working with families and explanation of the time investment. Be visible on campus in your work with families.

Billable services. This process doesn't usually involve the billing for remuneration of services, so administration may feel it's not incurring a visible profit and may believe that counselor time is better spent in other areas. Working with families usually increases attendance and decreases behavioral incidents, providing an added value to the school that is directly observable and measurable. Provide a cost-benefit analysis related to assigned tasks and how increasing attendance increases revenue for the school/district through average daily attendance (ADA) monies.

Appropriate education and training level in multicultural counseling and understanding of family systems are needed. School/district can hire counselors with training and experience in working with families and school counseling. More school counseling programs are integrating work with families and multicultural counseling into their degree offerings. Provide professional development at the school site.

Administrators may also worry about complicated family issues (child abuse, marital conflict, domestic violence, or underlying psychiatric issues). But these issues cause trauma in children, which directly hinders academic functioning. Focus on trauma-informed practices in the schools and how counseling in the schools addresses this need. Focus on having an expert on campus that can intervene with complicated family dynamics and provide appropriate screening, treatment, and referrals for more intensive services as needed.

Negative school climate. "Hurt people, hurt people." Focus on interventions that include trauma-informed practices, positive school climate, student engagement, and implementing tier 1–level interventions to build morale within the school, faculty, and staff.

Logistical issues (time, space, confidentiality, work hours, working parents' inability to attend daytime meetings, and so on). Allow for flexible counselor schedules that may include Saturday shifts, later start times to accommodate evening hours for seeing families, and so on. This also addresses space and confidentiality issues with more private space available and accommodates parent work schedules.

Conclusion

Immigrant children present significant behavioral and emotional needs in the school setting that can be addressed through SBFC. The challenges that immigrant children exhibit in the schools must be conceptualized within the context of the trauma they have experienced, economic depravity, documented status, and their historical and sociocultural background. This chapter has outlined an eight-step procedure that SBFC practitioners can engage in when working with immigrant children and their families. Each step of the process is fully outlined and includes specific multicultural considerations and practical strategies for executing the procedure with immigrant families. Toward the end of the chapter, more general cultural considerations are highlighted along with challenges and solutions to executing the conjoint family counseling process in the schools. As SBFC practitioners engage in the counseling process with the immigrant family, they must involve themselves in a self-reflective process of addressing their own biases and assumptions and understand the historical and cultural context of the immigrant family. SBFC practitioners must also seek out consultation with others, including community leaders and professionals, who are knowledgeable about the specific immigrant group from which the immigrant family comes. These are critical steps that must be taken by the SBFC practitioner to continue to evolve as a multicultural competent practitioner. Overall, the SBFC practitioner is charged with the responsibility of forming a partnership that includes and attends to the immigrant family's worldview and uses their assets to help them move through the change process.

Resources

SBFC Interview Procedure (Carter & Evans, 2008) (pp. 9–10, Appendix A). This procedure involves interviewing the parents, children, and teacher with a focus on learning more about strengths, challenges, and what has been tried to address these challenges.

Positive Methods of Discipline and Redirection (Kay Manning, 2018) (pp. 89–93). These positive methods of discipline and redirection techniques are reviewed with the parents.

The Objective Discipline Procedure. This procedure uses a 5-minute "Break" where the child sits for 5 minutes without any attention so that both parent and child can reflect on how to improve the situation before grounding. The full description is in chapter 3 in Gerrard, Carter & Ribera (Eds.) (2019) School-Based Family Counseling: An Interdisciplinary Practitioner's Guide, chapter 3, Appendix B, Routledge.

Bibliography

Cardoso, J. B., Brabeck, K., Stinchcomb, D., Heidbrink, L., Price, O. A., Gil-García, ÓF., Crea, T. M., & Zayas, L. H., . . . Zayas. (2019). Integration of unaccompanied migrant youth in the United States: A call for research. Journal of Ethnic and Migration Studies, 45(2), 273–292. https://doi.org/10.1080/1369183X.2017.1404261

Burr, W. R. (1970). Satisfaction for the various aspects of marriage over the life cycle: A random middle class sample. Journal of Marriage and Family, 32(1), 29–37.

Carter, M. (2013). Objective discipline procedure for noncompliance (with grounding). In B. Gerrard & M. Soriano (Eds.), School-based family counseling: Transforming family school relationships. creates pace. Appendix B.

Carter, M. J., & Evans, W. P. (2008). Implementing school-based family counseling: Strategies, activities, and process considerations. International Journal for School-Based Family Counseling, 1(1), 9–10, Appendix A.

Compas, B. E., Adelman, H. S., Freundl, P. C., Nelson, P., & Taylor, L. (1982). Parent and child causal attributions during clinical interviews. Journal of Abnormal Child Psychology, 10(1), 77–84. https://doi.org/10.1007/BF00915952

Cortes, K. E. (2004). Are refugees different from economic immigrants? Some Empirical Evidence on the Heterogeneity of Immigrant Groups in the United States. Review of Economics and Statistics, 86(2), 465–480. https://doi.org/10.1162/003465304323031058

Fraser, M. W. (2004). Risk and resilience in childhood: An ecological perspective. NASW Press.

Glied, S., & Cuellar, A. E. (2003). Trends and issues in child and adolescent mental health. Health Affairs, 22(5), 39–50. https://doi.org/10.1377/hlthaff.22.5.39

Hernandez, E. J., Ribera, D., & Carter, M. J. (2019). Family intervention: How to build collaboration between the family and the school using conjoint family counseling. In B. Gerrard, M. Carter & D. Ribera (Eds.), School-based family counseling: An interdisciplinary practitioner's guide. Routledge.

Ivey, I. E., Ivey, M. B., & Zalaquett, C. P. (2017). Intentional interviewing and counseling: Facilitating client development in a multicultural society (9th ed). Cengage Learning.

Karpel, M., & Strauss, E. (1983). Family evaluation. Gardner Publications.

Manning, K. (2018. (2019). Positive methods of discipline and redirection. [Class Handout]. California State University – Los Angeles, & COUN. Introduction to family evaluation and counseling. In B. Gerrard, M. Carter & D. Ribera (Eds.), School-based family counseling: An interdisciplinary practitioner's guide, 5200 (pp. 89–93). Routledge.

McGoldrick, M., & Gerson, R. (1988). Genograms and the family life cycle. In E. A. Carter & M. McGoldrick (Eds.), The expanded family life cycle: Individual, family, and social perspectives (3rd ed., pp. 164–189). Allyn & Bacon.

Minuchin, S., & Fishman, H. (1981). Family therapy techniques. Harvard University Press.

Whitaker, C. A., & Keith, D. V. (1981). Symbolic-experiential family therapy. In A. S. Gurman & D. P. Kniskern (Eds.), Handbook of family therapy. Brunner and Mazel.

5 How to Help a Child Through Couple Relationship Strengthening

Hans Everts

This chapter describes how strengthening a couple's relationship makes an important contribution to their ability to provide effective parenting for troubled children in the context of school-based family counseling (Gerrard, 2008; Gerrard & Soriano, 2013). The evidence-based concept of couple resilience is a core element in the New Zealand–based Migrant Family Resilience project (Everts, 2013), which comprises a variety of psycho-educational programs designed to prevent the development of serious problems in families facing major challenges such as immigration or having refugee status.

Background

The Family and the Parenting Couple in the Settlement of Immigrants and Refugees

Chapter 1 in this book makes important points on how the school-based family counseling (SBFC) approach helps empower immigrant and refugee families. This includes SBFC's emphasis on a systems orientation to the family, on the importance of partnership between parents and professional helpers, on multicultural sensitivity, on an interdisciplinary focus, and on evidence-based support. While these core points are by necessity limited in detail and specificity, some illustrative examples are provided—a child's role as identified patient in a dysfunctional family system, parent involvement in decision-making about student academic development, and sensitivity to cultural differences between Western individualism and Eastern collectivism. These examples illustrate issues, which will be elaborated in the current chapter.

At the present chapter's core lie three paradigms, all developed in New Zealand. The first comprises a model of functioning (MOF) for the family as it seeks to attend to its three core tasks—meeting the needs of its members, meeting the requirements of society, and maintaining itself as a functioning unit—all this while struggling to adapt to life in a new country (Everts, 2003). All core aspects of the family system are affected—personal

DOI: 10.4324/9781003097891-7

functioning, couple relationships, child-rearing practices, gender roles, communication, and decision-making (Everts, 2003, 2013). The second paradigm comprises the concept of Migrant Family Resilience (MFR) as developed by New Zealand's MFR project (Everts, 2004b, 2011a, 2013). Resilience refers to the ability to cope successfully with challenge and maintain, if not enhance, one's resourcefulness. Many families develop resilience, or new strength, through the very fact of having to face the challenges of transition. As Froma Walsh notes "family resilience is forged through adversity, not despite it" (Walsh, 2006). The challenge of immigration can be a time of positive crisis, and judicious intervention can facilitate the development of family system strengths as well as prevent the development of more serious problems (Everts & Wu, 2004).

The third paradigm is that of the couple resilience (CR), central to this chapter, which refers to the resilience or strength, which the couple as a team draws on to deal with challenge. Where present, it is primarily responsible for the family's success in adapting to life in a new country. In the same way that the family is a social system, the parenting couple is a social system that exists to meet the personal needs of each partner, to take responsibility for meeting society's requirements, and to maintain itself as a functioning unit (Everts, 2003). Its ability to deal with a child's problems at school is very much a function of its integrity as a team. During migration and settlement, however, that integrity is challenged. Partners may struggle with depression or personal doubts (Wong & Everts, 2002). Unemployment or discrimination may undercut an immigrant couple's self-image and self-esteem. Diminished earning power can challenge the family's hierarchy and create tension in the marriage system, made worse by changes in gender role when women sometimes acculturate faster than men. Couple relationships may become overloaded through lack of social support. Communication and decision-making may deteriorate. As Gerrard and Soriano (2013) note, SBFC counselors often work with the parenting couple as principal allies in helping the troubled child. To do so effectively the SBFC counselor must have a conceptual framework that explains how couples function—for better or worse. The SBFC counselor must then translate this rationale into purposeful and effective action strategies that enable counselor and couple to collaborate in dealing with family-related challenges like the child's ability to cope with problems at school. That will hopefully help a couple maintain or strengthen its integrity as a functional team. The New Zealand–based MFR project is based on the MOF and includes the development of the CR model and its associated intervention processes. These tightly integrated paradigms form the crucial underpinning for all intervention programs and activities alluded to in this chapter.

The New Zealand–Based MFR Project

The influx of migrants from East Asia into New Zealand during the last 35 years created a perfect opportunity for the development of the MFR project, the CR paradigm of this chapter, and their integration with SBFC

(Everts, 2004a, 2004b, 2007, 2008; Vong, 2002; Wong & Everts, 2002). This work was extended to include the refugee community as one whose needs are even greater and more complex. While aspects of this work are unique to New Zealand, the underlying themes are universal, and it is our hope that the New Zealand experience has relevance for SBFC in other countries. The project team comprises a small group of multicultural helping professionals, both migrants and refugees, with qualifications in psychology, counseling, social work, medicine, and religious ministry. All are in leadership positions in their own communities. This team took responsibility for the development of the evidence-based programs described in this chapter, their adaptation to and translation into the language of the recipients, the training of group leaders and community resource personnel, the actual running of programs, the conduct of evaluation and follow-up, and liaison with recipient organizations. The nature and quality of the team have been essential to the success of the MFR project to date. In the last 3 years, much of the project's community work has been carried out by the New Settlers Family and Community Trust in Auckland, whose current focus includes providing professional services "by refugees for refugees."

Psycho-educational Prevention versus Therapeutic Counseling

Both MFR and CR activities address themselves primarily to the issue of family prevention—where problems are apparent in children, schools, families, and parenting couples and where a briefer process of preventive intervention may stop the development of more serious problems demanding more intensive treatment. Such preventive intervention often involves the use of a more structured psycho-educational program. Intervention that is seen as educational and strength-based is frequently more familiar and acceptable to immigrant and refugee families. It falls more into the family preventive quadrant of the SBFC paradigm, as outlined in this book's first chapter. At the same time, MFR leaders are both educator and counselor in their facilitation of a psycho-educational program, which deals with couple or family issues. Participants in such a program may well raise issues (sometimes indirectly), which are too complex, too serious, or too personal to be able to be handled within the limitations of a structured program. The group leader must recognize that, respond appropriately, and guide the participant toward a situation in which a counseling/therapeutic intervention can take place. This process must move smoothly from family prevention to family invention, as described in the SBFC meta-model. This eventuality is incorporated in the CR activities listed in the following section, where circumstance helps determine the best activity to be undertaken.

The Couple Resilience Model: Evidence-Based Development

The author has been involved in exploring the concept of CR since the 1990s, as an outgrowth of his work in family systems and family therapy

(Everts, 1999). This coincided with the development of the multicultural MFR project team, providing a springboard for the conceptual and clinical initiatives outlined in this chapter. The concept of CR was originally developed using a field-based, qualitative model, based on a questionnaire given to more than 600 subjects in six countries (Everts, 1999). Using a modified grounded theory approach, 17 categories of response were identified and grouped into 4 themes (see Appendix A). Of these, a couple's emotional bonds constitute the most prominent resource that contributes toward a couple's resilience, accounting for 43% of the total responses recorded. This is followed by its action skills (26%) and the personal resources of individual partners (22%). Lastly, but still worthy of note, is the couple's community support (9%). The 17 specific qualities and skills can also be ranked in terms of frequency of citation. When divided into three levels, the top level (★★★) includes love, commitment, and tolerance (all aspects of emotional bonds), communication as an action skill, the personal quality of optimism, and the presence of a support network in the wider community. The second level of prominence (★★) includes similarity of values, the couple's ability to collaborate, its past history, and people's personal awareness, religious or spiritual faith, and strength. The third level of categories (★) includes intimacy time, self-sacrifice, physical resources, self-protection, and the presence of role models. This framework or model has a measure of consistency across different nationality samples and indicates that couples draw on a range of qualities and skills in coping with challenge and in maintaining or enhancing the quality of their relationship. While indicative, these research findings cannot be taken as prescriptive for individual couples. Any one couple will develop its own set of resources that determine success in coping with life challenges. However, our findings indicate that some such resources are more likely to be of help than others and that a couple is well advised to develop as many qualities and skills as possible. These research findings have been used by the CR project team to underpin and justify the development of a range of couple strengthening programs and activities for use within a variety of new settler communities in New Zealand and elsewhere. A number of these are outlined in the next section.

Procedure

Activity 1—The Successful Families Program, Used With Newly Arrived Refugees

This two-session program is distinctive by being used right at the outset of the settlement process of newly arrived refugees in New Zealand. It covers similar content themes as the generic parenting program but in highly condensed form. It also includes a significant segment on problems of anger and family violence, which feature in many refugee families—illustrative of the corrosive effects that trauma and long-term displacement have on family systems and family members. Running this program posed several significant challenges to the author as its developer and deliverer over 2 years. Each group comprised freshly arrived families from different refugee communities and included teenage children (sometimes younger), unattached young adults, single parents, parent couples, and grandparents. Multiple, simultaneous translations addressed often-bewildered participants in the context of an overwhelmingly busy 6-week induction program in Auckland's refugee reception center.

Ten out of 24 programs delivered over a period of 2 years were evaluated and indicate that in this context there was consistent acknowledgement of core universal values, interaction strategies, and patterns of family relationship that were held in common by respondents regardless of nationality, religion, gender, or age. These results also affirm the relevance of the essential elements of the CR model, as noted in the handout material for session 1 (Appendix B).

Over the 24 programs run, the author developed several strategies that proved helpful. Strong, direct, personal but culturally appropriate rapport establishment was necessary. Being older, male, a migrant himself, long married, a grandparent, and a professional teacher, all inspired respect. Constant affirmation fostered confidence and enthusiasm. Humor bonded the group and lightened the session's mood. Inviting questions and comments helped bring out content that could be woven back into the process. Finding and articulating underlying universal values provided necessary validation (or reframing) of nonnegotiable attitudes, at the same time as establishing a willingness in participants to consider new learnings that would enhance successful family adaptation in a new society. The author's use of personal illustrative examples, both positive and negative, lent credibility to teaching points. Running this program validated core values about personal and family integrity held by the author. It also tested every one of his professional skills as counselor and educator. Within the limited scope of its brief, the relative success of this preventive crisis-intervention program for family systems may connect with the work of other SBFC counselors in a conceptual and practical way that warrants further exploration.

Activity 2—Couple Strengthening in the MFR Parenting Program

Somewhat further through the settlement process we have incorporated the CR theme into the context of the wider parenting program for immigrant and refugee families (Migrant Family Resilience, 2007a, 2007b; Everts, 2013). This is in line with the project's emphasis on relating couple functioning to parenting effectiveness and thus to SBFC. Specifically, we have a session on strong couples, responsible parents early in the standard parenting program. Its rationale is based not on the notion that couples want to look at their relationship for its own sake (which, in our situation, they avoid doing in public) but that being effective as parents requires them to work together as a functional and resilient team. As a couple they face a parenting crisis that contains both opportunity and danger—both yin and yang as in the Chinese definition of crisis. With appropriate help, both their child and their relationship may benefit; without it, both may suffer further. How this session is handled as part of the MFR parenting program is described in detail (Everts, 2013), and the interrelationship between CR and effective parenting is referred to repeatedly in other sessions of that program. Where further help with family discord is needed, a parent or parenting couple in our New Zealand project may be referred to the Protecting Family Happiness program, described later.

Evaluation data from 344 participants in 31 parenting programs for immigrants and refugees, conducted over 9 years, indicates that parents (and grandparents) rate the session on couple functioning as highly or fairly useful. Even allowing for a culture-based tendency for respondents to be polite and say the "right thing," it indicates the perceived relevance of this topic to a couple's task of effective parenting in a society that is new and challenging for their families and to the school system that receives their children.

Activity 3—Protecting Family Happiness Program—for Preventing Family Violence

The generic parenting program (Migrant Family Resilience, 2007a, 2007b) is pre-structured to cover a series of inter-related topics. That may be sufficient to meet the needs of parents who are in an at-risk situation and thus prevent the escalation of their children's problems at home or school. However, it is unlikely to meet the needs of parents whose problems are more severe. They need something more personalized and flexible. The Protecting Family Happiness Program was developed for such parents and couples (Migrant Family Resilience, 2009). Going through the generic parenting program would have (hopefully) given them a background framework of understanding, a degree of trust in process and leadership, and motivation to be openly and honestly engaged. The Protecting Family Happiness Program can be used as follow-up from either the generic parenting or the successful families program—though the latter has not yet occurred in our project.

While broadly educational in orientation (thus more culturally acceptable), the actual session process is relatively flexible and allows for more personalized interaction than its precursor. The evaluation feedback from the few groups run to date indicates that, while generally successful, the selection and preparation of participants are important if they are to be fully engaged in and benefit from the process. Even then, families typically drift back to homeostasis, and the complex nature of systemic change means that one of two follow-up activities is normally required. For one, the consolidation of change processes started in a preventive program typically requires ongoing monitoring and support in the community—by professional or semi-professional resource personnel. Alternatively, more time and intensive individualized intervention may be necessary—in the form of family counseling rather than family prevention in Gerrard's typology. In summary, the Protecting Family Happiness Program constitutes an appropriate follow-through for some couples or parents who have completed a generic parenting program but is likely to require either consolidation in the community or more intensive therapeutic intervention—neither of which has been systematically explored in the present project. Comparison with the work done by others in this field from an SBFC perspective would be invaluable.

Activity 4—Making Strong Couples Program

While not directly related to the task of parenting, the MFR project has also developed the Making Strong Couples Program, a six-session couple strengthening program based on the CR model (Migrant Family Resilience, 2012a, 2012b). Its session topics include personal well-being or integrity, the couple's emotional relationship, effective communication, teamwork, and effective action. A program like this fits couples who wish to enhance a satisfactory relationship or ones who want to improve an at-risk one. While such programs are popular in the wider community, we have found little appetite for them among immigrant and refugee families. There is, however, some interest in this program among younger immigrants who are preparing for marriage. The Making Strong Couples Program has been run for such a group in the Chinese community, where we found among its members two cross-cultural couples (Chinese woman, New Zealand man) and one couple who were already married but experiencing difficulties. The feedback from this trial group indicates that they found it relevant, supportive, and challenging. A similar program was run for Chinese couples and helping professionals in Shanghai.

Activity 5—Empowering Community Organizations

The MFR project team is also responsible for the training of group leaders, community resource personnel, and organizational leaders. *Group leaders* are qualified helping professionals who are inducted into leadership via an apprentice training process and, once certified, are required to continue receiving supervision.

The training of community resource personnel is essential for the generalization of learning from the time-limited MRF programs in the community. Such people may have a professional or semi-professional background, be in a paid or voluntary role, and are typically members of the community they serve. They have not usually trained to run MFR programs themselves. To help support, follow up on, and consolidate client learnings, they must know what the programs contain, personally accept the basic premises involved, and have the ability (under supervision) to generalize the outcomes of MFR programs. Two 7-hour Train the Trainers programs of this kind have been conducted, informal training has taken place for others, and two half-day workshops on this issue were conducted in Hong Kong and Indonesia. Evaluation results strongly indicate the importance of taking community resource personnel through the generic parenting program and discussing their role in following through on that program with clients who have completed it, as well as others in the wider community.

Where the MFR project has worked with existing community organizations, it has deliberately engaged their executive teams to ensure that MFR programs are appropriate to their needs and that they in turn will support and foster the continued use of the resources that are provided. This has worked well with a range of such community organizations, some of whose working brief spans both family and school, as reflective of SBFC thinking.

Challenges and Solutions

Some challenges pertain directly to the theme of this chapter, including the following:

- The long stretch from couple functioning to a child's school adjustment—this requires helping professionals to have a conceptual framework and collegial network that stretches across that gap, whether they work at the family end or the school end of the continuum alluded to in the SBFC literature (Gerrard, 2008).
- Working across very different or incompatible belief systems—one can compromise in a conflict of needs, but not in a conflict of values, so one has to work from within the value system of the clients to find core beliefs that are sufficiently universal to apply in both cultures (see Appendix B). This is augmented by the argument that couples, if they wish to be successful as couples and parents in New Zealand, have to adapt. This is a challenge for us as representatives of the recipient community as well as for the new immigrants. While we have been able to make a successful start in this process within the context of our programs, such adaptation takes years and requires further preventive intervention as well as the support of within-community resource personnel—an example of the collegial network in action, as referred earlier.
- The possible presence of trauma—as noted in the chapter on MFR (Everts, 2013), the presence of post-traumatic stress in the history of couples, especially refugees, remains an issue that program leaders must be constantly aware of and able to have addressed. Individual trauma intervention may well be required before couples can be expected to develop a resilient relationship that allows them to collaborate in effective parenting in a new country. This is one of the reasons why a couple focus is relevant to SBFC work.

- The many configurations of couple/parenting relationships—in our programs we have worked with informal as well as married couples, single parents with or without support from other family members, separated couples, one spouse whose partner is unable or unwilling to attend (e.g., Lim, 2010), and grandparents with major parenting responsibilities. We have found that the principles of CR hold true in any intimate relationship between two, or even more, partners. Even when such a relationship is in the process of formation (e.g., the pre-marriage program) or has broken down, reflection on what it consists of and how it can be created or recreated is valuable in a situation where people are reflecting on the challenges of parenthood in a new context.
- The limited scope of the present project—this chapter deals only with the unique but limited nature of our research and our research-based clinical activities. The reader needs to be cautious in evaluating what has taken place in New Zealand but hopefully be able to relate this to what is being done elsewhere and work with us to enhance SBFC internationally.

Conclusion

This chapter explores how preventive couple strengthening provides a necessary foundation for effective parenting of children under stress and for ultimately aiding the collaboration between home and school—though that issue is not addressed directly here. The work described here is part of the overall MFR project designed to help immigrant and refugee families adapt to life in a new country and culture. The choice of a preventive approach to couple strengthening is made in part because, where possible, prevention is better than cure and in part because the communities involved have a cultural preference for education rather than therapy. The concept of CR provides the conceptual core of the project, with its emphasis on identifying the qualities and skills that enable a couple to have a close relationship, as well as deal effectively with life challenges. This CR framework connects very well with SBFC, insofar as its emphasis on effective parenting leads into the enhancement of home-school collaboration.

The couple strengthening project has focused its applied work on the settlement of immigrant and refugee families into the New Zealand community for a variety of reasons—the need to maintain family integrity in a new environment, couples struggling with alternative parenting models, children entering a strange school environment, community leaders seeking help, and helping professionals in need of training. The MFR project was initiated to take on that challenge. The project's programs that address the parenting couple's needs include the Successful Families Program, the Couples Session in the Parenting Program, the Protecting Family Happiness Program, the Making Strong Couples Program, and a range of activities designed to develop the skills of community resource personnel. The entire project is multicultural in its applications and, while still in the process of developing its scope fully, is demonstrably relevant to the family prevention and intervention aspects of the SBFC paradigm. We hope that this chapter will encourage readers to relate aspects of the project to their own work and to liaise with the author, so that our collective experience may enhance international applications of SBFC. For further communication regarding any aspect of this chapter, please contact the author.

Resources

Everts, H. (2013). Developing migrant family resilience. In B. Gerrard & M. Soriano (Eds.), School-based family counseling: Transforming family-school relationships (pp. 211–233). San Francisco: Institute of School-Based Family Counseling.

Everts, J. F. (2003). An integrated model of functioning for use in counselling and reaction pattern research: Occasional paper. Auckland University of Auckland.

Lim, G. (2010). Parenting programme for Korean Fathers [Program manual]. Auckland University of Auckland.

Migrant Family Resilience Project. (2007a). Parenting programme [Program manual]. Auckland University of Auckland. Faculty of Education.

Migrant family resilience project. (2007b). Parenting programme. Session 2: Strong couples make good parents, Session, M. Auckland: University of Auckland. Faculty of Education.

Migrant family resilience project. (2009). Protecting family happiness programme [Program manual]. Auckland: University of Auckland. Faculty of Education.

Migrant family resilience project. (2012a). Making strong couples programme [Program manual]. Auckland: University of Auckland. Faculty of Education.

Migrant family resilience project. (2012b). Making strong couples programme. Nine suggestions for making a family successful. Class Handout. Auckland University of Auckland, Faculty of Education.

These are programme descriptions and handouts used in the Migrant Family Resilience project.

Bibliography

Everts, H. (2004a). Vision and challenge in school-based family counselling. Paper presented at the Second Annual Oxfords Symposium in SBFC. Brasenose College, Oxford.

Everts, H. (2004b). Migrant family resilience. Paper presented at the Inaugural International Asian Health Conference. Auckland, New Zealand, November.

Everts, H., & Wu, P. (2004). Identity and resilience in families facing cultural transition through migration—with illustrative reference to Chinese families in New Zealand and Taiwan. Paper presented at the Third Biennial International Conference on Intercultural Research, National Taiwan Normal University, Taipei, May.

Everts, J. F. (1999). Couple resilience: A definition and analysis of the concept. New Zealand Journal of Counselling, 20, 47–65.

Everts, J. F. (2007). Applying principles of school-based family counselling to preventive intervention with migrant and refugee families. Paper presented at the Fifth Oxford

Symposium in School-Based Family Counselling. University of Hong Kong, Hong Kong, June.

Everts, J. F. (2008). Integrating supportive care in schools with the enhancement of family resilience—A New Zealand project for immigrant families. International Journal for School-Based Family Counseling, 1, 57–64.

Everts, J. F. (2011). Building resilience in migrant families—An illustration of school-based family counseling in action. Paper presented at the Symposium on School-Based Family Counseling. Hong Kong Institute of Education, Hong Kong, June 25.

Gerrard, B. (2008). School-based family counseling: Overview, trends, and recommendations for future research. International Journal for School-Based Family Counseling, 1, 6–24.

Gerrard, B., & Soriano, M. (Eds.). (2013). School-based family counseling: Transforming family-school relationships. San Francisco: Institute for School-Based Family Counseling.

Vong, C. (2002). The impact of migration on the Chinese family. New Zealand Journal of Counselling, 23, 21–24.

Walsh, F. (2006). Strengthening family resilience. New York: Guilford.

Wong, J., & Everts, H. (2002). How Chinese families develop resilience. New Zealand Journal of Counselling, 23, 25–32.

Appendix A

Couple Resilience—Outline of the Model

PERSONAL RESOURCES (22% of total resources mentioned)

Optimism—hope and faith in the future, even in the middle of problems; having a sense of humor.★★★

Awareness—having an awareness or understanding of self and others.★★

Religious or spiritual faith—having a religious or spiritual faith.★★

Personal strength—being tough, courageous, or determined in the face of stress.★★

EMOTIONAL BONDS (43% of total resources mentioned)

Love, affection—having love, trust, care, or respect for each other.★★★

Commitment—being committed or faithful to each other; being determined to see things through together, for better or worse.★★★

Tolerance—being tolerant, patient, forgiving and flexible toward each other; able to give and take.★★★

Similar values—having similar values, goals, and beliefs to each other.★★

ACTION SKILLS (26% of total resources mentioned)

Communication skills—being able to listen, discuss, make decisions, or solve problems together; able to express oneself; able to find solutions, which leave both parties happy; able to not lose one's temper or panic.★★★

Collaboration—being able to work together as a team to solve problems or cope with stress.★★

Past history—having a long or good past history with each other; having coped with or learned from past problems.★★

Intimacy time—having time together in recreation, fun/rest that makes that relationship a better one.★

Self-sacrifice—making personal sacrifices for the sake of the other.★

Physical resources—having money or possessions to help cope with difficulties.★

COMMUNITY SUPPORT (9% of total resources mentioned)

Support network—having other family members, friends, professionals, or even pets, available to support and help the couple.★★★

Self-protection—being able to protect oneself as a couple against the bad influence of others in the wider community.★

Role models—having role models (good or bad) that are available to the couple.★

★★★—very helpful resources;   ★★—helpful resources;   ★—resources that are of some help

Appendix B

Nine Suggestions for Making a Family Successful

1. Make Couples Successful—Happy and Strong

A couple is successful when each partner is happy, when both love and respect each other, when they talk and work together as a team, and when they get support from others. A successful couple (if there is a couple) lies at the heart of a successful family.

2. Parents Work as a Team to Get Things Done

The parent team is strong when they agree on how to run the family and set a good example.

3. Parents Teach Children How to Be Responsible by Showing Them

Parents teach children to be responsible by inviting them to join in family decision-making as soon as they are old enough.

4. Doing the Right Thing Is Rewarded

Reward and praise are more powerful than punishment—so reward and praise each other whenever people do the right thing.

5. Doing the Wrong Thing Is Punished

If someone breaks a rule, the agreed punishment is given. Losing out on reward or praise is often the best punishment.

6. Be Disciplined Where It Is Important

It is important for the whole family to agree on basic rules, rewards, and punishments that are necessary in making it run well. Discipline means sticking to making them work.

7. Punish in a Fair Way

Ignore smaller issues; make some allowance for the situation. Give warning, then don't argue, don't give in, but punish as agreed.

8. Punish With Love and Respect

Show love and respect for the other person, even while you punish someone's behavior. Don't lose your temper. Don't overdo the punishment.

9. Talk About Things That Have Gone Wrong

When people are calm, talk about what has happened and what was learned. If something needs to be changed in how the family works, do it.

© Migrant Family Resilience Program (2011)

6 Narrative Therapy With Undocumented Families

Nidya Y. Ramirez Ibarra

This chapter will review the application of Narrative Therapy with families who have an undocumented status and seek support from school-based family counseling practitioners (SBFC) in their community. The focus will be on reviewing the use of Narrative Therapy practice called externalization as a strategy for SBFC practitioners to engage with undocumented children, adolescents, and families. Conversations with undocumented families regarding the resources and referrals that they request and necessitate for their life will be presented as an avenue toward the use of externalization. The SBFC model aims to frame the child's challenges in all of their socialization context or networks such as family, peer group, classroom, school (teacher, principal, other students), and community. The SBFC model is a used as a guide when implementing Narrative Therapy's externalization. Explorations with families of their experiences and responses to an undocumented status through conversations about resources and referrals will be illustrated.

Background

Undocumented parents, children, and adolescents may enter psychotherapy with requests for community resources and referrals to alleviate a myriad of issues and problems, from feelings of hopelessness to concerns with familial relationships. The lived experiences of undocumented families are impacted by the political landscape and discourses in communities about immigrants (Cross et al., 2020, p. 1459). Undocumented families move within familial, societal, community, and school cultures with limited access to rights, benefits, and resources, limiting access to educational and economic mobility. In 2017 it was estimated that 16.7 million people in the United States have at least one family member residing in their household with undocumented status (Mathema, 2017). Using externalization in conversations about a family's need for resources and referrals can explore the effects of undocumented status on different aspects of family life. Therapists and family members can also witness the family's collective and individual skills, abilities, resistance, knowledge, and values.

DOI: 10.4324/9781003097891-8

An undocumented status can impact a family in many ways. For each family member, the influence of an undocumented status expands, similarly and differently, to every aspect of daily life. Families navigate the effects of undocumented status on relationships, health, employment, finances, mental health, education, housing, and rights. Undocumented families may often initiate mental health services and family therapy without directly identifying a connection between the presenting problem and their undocumented status (Cha et al., 2019). Research by Balderas et al. (2016) with undocumented families revealed three themes regarding the extent and depth of conversations in undocumented households about living with undocumented immigration status. Notably, many parents initiate conversations with their children regarding their undocumented status because of external factors such as the deportation of a parent or a child's greater awareness of the benefits of documentation. Some parents felt the need to instill feelings of pride and worth in their children and prepare them for experiences of discrimination through direct conversations about their undocumented status. Other parents chose to guard their children's emotional well-being by refraining from those conversations for as long as necessary. Discourses within a family about navigating an undocumented status are not homogenous. Disclosing an undocumented status outside of the household to a professional or mental health provider entails a deliberate and calculated assessment for many families and individuals. Alejandra, a 22-year-old undocumented Latina interviewed for the Raza et al. (2019) study, explains that a critical consideration in that process is the potential responses to the disclosure.

> If I do not know what a person's political stance on immigration is . . . I get a little bit uneasy and I withhold that information until that person either says something, hints at it, or you know, I can somehow collect that information from them. Otherwise, if I know that people are supportive or sometimes even neutral to the issue, I do not mind sharing.
>
> (p. 198–199)

An SBFC practitioner's political awareness and position matter determining the level of trust undocumented people can place on the therapeutic process and disclosure of their status. In my work with families, disclosures about undocumented status usually emerge in conversations about a family's necessity for resources and referrals that address challenges posed by a lack of legal status. I am aware that as a service provider, I am in a position of power and situated as an institutional agent that can choose to embody the characteristics of an empowerment agent. An institutional agent is described by Stanton-Salazar (2011) as an individual holding a role in which they "directly transmit, or negotiate the transmission of, highly valued resources" to others in a similar social group (p. 1067). An empowerment agent recognizes how "social structures" can limit people's access to resources. They actively advocate for people to benefit from awareness and access to institutional support and distribute their knowledge about information and resources (Stanton-Salazar, 2011). It is in practicing as an empowerment agent that trust can be built with undocumented families.

Although there is a standard view of clinical work and case management as existing separately from one another, Narrative Therapy's externalization encourages a consciousness in the potential of these conversations to elicit opportunities for change, exploration, and enactment of life stories. Many undocumented people choose the risk of disclosing their immigration status when it could lead to much-needed resources. Madsen proposes the metaphor of "walking and talking" to represent journeying with people in work that comprises "practical assistance with purposeful conversation" (2014). During a session, an adolescent described having difficulty sleeping for fear that their mother would be detained by Immigration and Customs Enforcement (ICE). She had recently learned that her aunt had been arrested by ICE at her home. She and her mother inquired about any no-cost or low-cost legal support for the aunt, and know-your-rights information for the mother had to be prepared should ICE also look for her. A mother I worked with mentioned becoming increasingly concerned about a medical issue she had been enduring for a long time. She feared her health was getting worse without medical treatment. She wondered if there was any resource that could guide her toward medical assistance for undocumented adults. Her children also expressed worry for their mother's health and hoped that a community resource could lead her to the help she needed.

Introductory Practice of Narrative Therapy's Externalization

Narrative Therapy, founded by Michael White and David Epson, adopts a narrative metaphor regarding a person's lived experience. Instead of organizing families within "systems" or "patterns," it considers dominant and "taken for granted" stories in cultures and societies. Attention is drawn to the dominant and alternative stories that people are living and how these are all shaping each other (1990). White (2007) explains that many people initially enter therapy with the belief that the problems of their lives are a direct reflection of "truths" about their or other's identity, character, or nature. This, in turn, causes someone to delve further into the problem they are attempting to change. One may examine how anti-immigrant messages that criminalize undocumented families influence the stories that shape a family's life and the meaning they ascribe to their individual and collective experiences. Narrative Therapy works with families to understand their preferred meanings, identities, knowledge, and values.

Externalizing questions and conversations are a core practice of Narrative Therapy that entails examining the problem and people's relationship to the problem as the problem itself. This contrasts with a typical diagnosis in which a person's fixed internal qualities are established as the problem. Michael White (2007) states:

> When the problem becomes an entity separate from the person, and when people are not tied to restricting "truths" about their identities and negative "certainties" about their lives, new options for taking action to address the predicaments of their lives become available . . . if a person's relationship to the problem becomes clearly defined, as it does in externalizing conversations, a range of possibilities becomes available to revise this relationship.
>
> (p. 26)

Externalizing supports families and children to define the problem using their language and definitions. The SBFC practitioner privileges the child or family's language to name the problem and organizes questions that objectify the problem itself. The questions used in this process focus more on the problems impacting the children and families rather than them beingproblem (Jill & Combs, 1996, p. 31). For example, a practitioner may inquire into when worry surprises a child during their day rather than positing questions about "being" an anxious child. An SBFC practitioner will need to listen for the language that the family and child use when describing and labeling the problem. It is through this intentional listening that SBFC practitioners can intervene with questions and techniques that stay close to the family's descriptions and definitions of their experiences. For examples, depending on a family's culture an experience, typically labeled as anxiety, may be uniquely described as worry, heartache, nervousness, and more. Definitions of the identified problem in externalized conversations can stay constant throughout therapy or evolve in the process.

Problems can develop from an issue someone is grappling with or from feeling disempowered; therefore, there may be practices an undocumented family enacts as reminders to hold pride in their immigrant story. This relationship to an undocumented status can also be essential to expand on with a child and family. By deepening alternative stories and different instances in which people are taking a stand against the problem, new insight on possibilities for life, relationships, and well-being arise.

Facilitating externalizing conversations necessitates a particular stance from the therapist. For the problem to be named and exposed, White and Epston (1990) suggest an "investigative reporter-like position" in which a therapist works with a family or person to unveil the actions, intentions, roles, and characteristics of the problem (p. 27–28). Directly confronting the problem or being on a quest for solutions is not the goal at this point in the conversation. By avoiding a dichotomous construction of the problem where it is either positive or negative, good, or bad a family can gain greater perspective on the context of the problem and what it is upholding and giving value to.

Utilizing externalization in conversations about resources and referrals with undocumented families can have the following therapeutic benefits:

- Unity among family members in responses to the effects and influences of living with undocumented status.
- Honors abilities, skills, and actions and opens more possibilities to acknowledge a family's responsibility, hope, aspirations, and agency.
- Diminishes blame, failure, and shame about living with undocumented status and recognizes the influence of culture, politics, and power.
- Positions the mental health provider as a partner concerning the problem.
- Undocumented families are centered as experts of their own lives.

In the practice of externalizing conversations with children and families with undocumented status, the strengths identified by Soriano and Gerrard (2019) of school-based family counseling are adopted as guiding values. Specifically, SBFC practitioners can benefit from maintaining a systems-focused lens and an approach that reinforces a partnership with the parents and caregivers. SBFC affirms that children are connected to systems made up of their family, school, peers, and community. Since families living with an undocumented status navigate and are impacted by multiple systems and institutions, the SBFC practitioners' role is to acknowledge and frame the complexities of a child's experience and interconnection between school and home from a systems perspective. Aligning with the parents or caregivers as a partner in the cultivation of family changes and accomplishing goals, the SBFC practitioner can model to the family practices, like externalization, for interacting with each other in ways that the family prefers and believes will support their well-being.

Procedures

After many years working with undocumented families, I have developed a skillful ear for expressions from family members that identify a need for potential resources, information, or referrals. Conversations with undocumented families about resources or referrals that address a specific area of need can emerge throughout different points and sometimes multiple times in our work together. An undocumented family's needs can include legal consultation, food, medical treatment, psychiatric evaluations, transportation support, and financial assistance. Listening and responding as an SBFC practitioner to these expressions of the need for referrals and resources can construct an opening into explicit conversations about the impact of undocumented status on the children, parents, and family. The practice of externalizing objectifies the undocumented status as the problem and separates it from attributions to internal characteristics of a child or a family. It shifts from questions like these: How is it to be an undocumented child?

Table 6.1 Examples of Externalizing Questions About Referrals and Resources

---

What are some of the situations in which the need for this resource has become more
noticeable for you and your family?
What conclusions about your life or relationship have led you to identifying this
resource as something that could be helpful for you?
What do you imagine might be possible for you if you were to obtain this resource?
How long have you and your family been noticing the need for this resource?

How has living with an undocumented status shaped your relationship with
your parents? This can be particularly significant for families living with an
undocumented status who are constantly a focus of hostile messages about
their existence (i.e., illegal alien, lazy, criminals, thieves, invaders, and so on)
that they may come to internalize or be affected by. Therefore, externalizing
is more than a use of a technique. Externalizing establishes a foundation for
all the work with an undocumented family to unfold. Externalizing avoids
generalizations about families with undocumented status and remains open
to the meanings and possibilities that can arise from these conversations
for each undocumented family and their experience. Families can build on
metaphors that represent their experiences while also being supported by
their therapist to identify metaphors that fit. Tables 6.1–6.3 are examples of
past sessions with undocumented families presented and externalizing questions and conversations.

The Case of a Single Mother

A single mother and her 13-year-old son both hold an undocumented status. The mother sought family therapy to address the constant anger her
son has been expressing toward her. During the intake process, the mother
mentions that she wants to know of any legal resources available in the community that could help her evaluate whether she and her son may qualify
for an immigration visa.

Example of Externalizing Questions and Conversation

SBFC Practitioner:	How might the need for this resource relate to some of the challenges you and your son have been experiencing in your relationship?
Mother:	I am always so tired by the time I get home. My schedule changes every week, and most of the time I only have one day off to do everything else that I need to do at home.

SBFC Practitioner:	What about for you (son)?
Son:	Yeah, it is true, she is hardly ever home and when she is, she is on my case about everything I do or do not do. It is annoying.
Mother:	Even though I work almost every day of the week, I am always aware that it was difficult for me to get this job having an undocumented status. I must be careful not to lose it because it is all we have. It frustrates me that I get home and there is so much that needs to get done, which he could be helping with. Instead, I put up with his anger and disrespect toward me when I tell him what he needs to do.
SBFC Practitioner:	What do you hope could be more possible for your relationship if you did attain the immigration visa?
Son:	I hope that she can be less stressed when she is home and maybe we can spend more time together.
Mother:	If I have my papers (permanent legal status), then hopefully I will be able to get a job that is less stressful where I can earn more and have at least one more day off. I just want to be able to spend more time with my son and pay more attention to what he does.
SBFC Practitioner:	What do you all think your search for support and legal assistance shows about the position you are taking on the effects of living with an undocumented status?
Mother:	I think for me I know that I need and want to spend more time with my son, so I am trying to find a solution and have some courage to investigate something that we are not sure will happen.
Son:	I am still trying to figure it out, but I do think it would be nice if my mom did not have to work so much and we could do things together more often. I think us having an immigration visa would really make a difference with that.

Table 6.2 Possible Follow-Up Externalizing Questions

How do you see the anger and effects of an undocumented status relating with each other?

How has the anger's recent presence in your relationship influenced the actions you are taking toward obtaining support?

How does living with an undocumented status impact your relationship?

How does living with an undocumented status impact you individually?

Are there ways in which you are already not allowing the impact of an undocumented status to sneak into how you interact with each other?

The Case of a High School Student

Some families and children may enter therapy or counseling with a clearer idea of how an undocumented status is affecting their well-being, as is the case of the following family who reached out for counseling services. The parents noticed that since their daughter had begun her last year of high school and was coming to understand the challenges of living with undocumented status, she was crying all the time, blaming her parents for bringing her to the United States, and expressing hopelessness for the future. During an initial session, they mentioned that the daughter had applied to several scholarships already. They all wondered if the practitioner was aware of any more scholarships for high school students dealing with undocumented status. The daughter also asked if the practitioner knew a local organization that could aid with the assessment and cost of the Deferred Action for Childhood Arrivals (DACA) program. DACA grants temporary administrative relief from deportation and a work permit to youth who have been living with undocumented status in the United States and meet other specific requirements set forth by the United States Citizenship and Immigration Services (USCIS, 2021).

Example of Externalizing Questions and Conversation

SBFC Practitioner:	How long have you all been noticing the sadness show up in relationship to living with an undocumented status?
Daughter:	I noticed it come up more and more when I started applying to colleges and universities. I realized that I would not qualify for any financial aid to attend the different schools, not even the waiver to apply.
Mother:	This year has been hard for her since she is noticing that there is a lot, she may not be able to do compared to her friends. She sometimes cries for hours after getting home from school.
Daughter:	I also cannot get a driver's license or get a job.
SBFC Practitioner:	You mentioned that the sadness has come up more and more recently and your mom said that you spend a lot of time crying after school. I am curious what happens to the sadness when you research scholarships and financial assistance that may be available for students with an undocumented student?
Daughter:	I think the sadness is still there in some way, but I am also trying, at the same time, to have some hope that I will find scholarships and find a way. There are so many goals that I want to accomplish and ways that I wish I could help my parents.

Table 6.3 Possible Follow-Up Externalizing Questions

Along with the real challenges that you are facing, what else does the sadness tell you about your life and your future with an undocumented status?

When in the past have you also held on to some hope in the face of sadness?

What kind of relationship does each of you want to have with the sadness when it shows up?

What is the sadness letting you know about the impact that an undocumented status is having on your life currently?

What type of things occur during a particular day that may invite the sadness or hopelessness?

Father:	I do not know how she does it, but even with all the sadness and frustration I do see her putting so much effort into finding scholarships and immigration information like DACA.
Practitioner:	Are there other moments when the sadness about living with an undocumented status does not fully team up with hopelessness?
Daughter:	Probably when I am with the teachers who help me to complete my college applications. They are the only ones I have talked to so far about having an undocumented status. Also, my friends because even though they do not know what I am going through, spending time with them is fun and motivating.

Multicultural Considerations

Language can be a different experience among members of immigrant families, including within undocumented households. A mental health provider may find it helpful to maintain awareness that each family member can experience varying levels of fluency and comfort in English and their native language. During family sessions, I will typically notice a child speaking in Spanish and English while their parents only express themselves in Spanish. At this point, I usually share this observation with the family. In the research of Babino and Stewart (2017), elementary-age children have nuanced experiences navigating two languages. They indicate that when they are in an environment with bilingual individuals, such as in school or with siblings, they choose to speak only English or a combination of English and Spanish, while mostly favoring English. This coincides with students choosing to speak to one another in English during their Spanish classes. Yet even though they usually choose English when given a choice, they are still invested in the cultural and familial aspects of the language. Marco states, "Spanish is an important language to our family," and Carolina says that she must speak Spanish to "understand my parents" (p. 25). I facilitate conversations with the family about each member's language preferences and the role of language in their lives and relationships with each other. We collaboratively determine my role throughout the session in navigating the multiple languages with them. This is a constant assessment as a family's preferences of my language participation may change and evolve in our work together.

My fluency and familiarity with Spanish, English, and Spanglish allow me to move between those languages. I am simultaneously bridging conversations within family members as therapist and interpreter, facilitating awareness of how language shapes their lives and identities (Santiago-Rivera et al., 2009). For example, a child may prefer to express themselves primarily in English yet turn to their parents and transition to Spanish in the middle of the session. I notice that children usually direct themselves toward me when sharing their feelings, thoughts, and experiences in English. Some bilingual therapists interviewed by Verdinelli and Biever. (2009) also observed how a person shifts from one language to another based on the topic or issue being addressed (p. 239). As multiple interactions are occurring and languages are spoken in the session, I am attentive and curious about how this may influence their relationships and familial experiences outside of therapy. In my experience, parents and children have expressed enthusiasm to engage in treatment when they can be present in the multiple languages that are part of their daily familial and cultural experiences. Crossing between languages in family therapy has brought insight into each family member's experience navigating an undocumented status.

Challenges and Solutions

When facilitating externalizing conversations by way of resources and referrals for undocumented families, a provider must be mindful not to externalize the undocumented status itself. Externalizing the undocumented status can minimize and perpetuate oppressive dominant discourses regarding undocumented immigrants (White & Epston, 1990, p. 49). A mental health provider cannot ignore the politics and systems of power that surround the experience of undocumented families in their communities and country when deciding how to move forward with externalizing. Also, externalizing is not limited to something that is an obstacle or challenge but can also include experiences such as a family's actions, hopes, and aspirations.

The following figure provides some guidance and ideas for the process of determining what to externalize concerning a family's undocumented status and experience.

- Moods, feelings, and emotions
- Ideas, thoughts, and feelings
- Memories and recollections
- Cultural practices and perspectives

- Skills and abilities
- Values and ethics
- Hopes, dreams, and aspirations,
- Expressions and ideas
- Personal behaviors or actions
- Experiences, struggles, or incidents

Conclusion

In many clinical practices situated within a community setting, providing referrals and resources is a common aspect of working with families. Undocumented families are systematically limited in the rights and benefits that they can access. They may view their providers as individuals who possess awareness and familiarity of available community resources. However, the process of sharing about resources and referrals and the conversations that evolve from that are not typically regarded as therapeutically significant. This chapter brings attention to the value of deepening conversations about the expressions of need and assistance undocumented families request for their lives. Narrative Therapy's externalizing practice offers an opportunity to meaningfully engage in discussions about a family's needs, hopes, and experiences. Undocumented families are already navigating a society, community, and dominant discourses that attempt to shame, dehumanize, and criminalize their existence. Beyond a practice, externalizing builds a foundation for every interaction with an undocumented family in the process of working together. Undocumented families are incredibly diverse, from the everyday experiences to the languages that each family member speaks. Through this introduction to externalizing and conversations about resources and referrals, I hope to inspire providers to attempt working from a stance that positions the children and families living with an undocumented status as agents and experts of their life. It takes practice to build on the skill of externalizing. Hopefully, learning how to begin this path will lead to new possibilities, understandings, and connections with and for families with undocumented status.

Resources

Externalizing Conversations: Statement of Position Map 1 by Mark Hayward
> *In this video, Mark Hayward presents a review of Michael White's statement of position map and its relationship to externalizing conversations. Hayward will demonstrate the process of charting an externalizing conversation and offers additional documents and a PowerPoint presentation for further reference. Here is the link to the video:* https://dulwichcentre.com.au/externalizing-conversations-statement-of-position-map-1-by-mark-hayward/

Externalizing Conversations Handout Developed by Kath Muller From Training Materials Created by Paul Montgomery
> *This information links Narrative Therapy's Statement of Position Map and the Scaffolding map. This is an easy step-by-step guide that provides ideas for further expanding on the different*

aspects of externalizing conversations. Here is a link to the handout: https://reauthoringteach-ing.com/pages-not-in-use/externalising-conversations-handout/

Journey of Metaphors and Metamorphosis by Aileen de Souza

In this video, Aileen de Souza presents her work with children and the creative use of meta-phors to speak about their problems and experiences. Souza presents several cases and discusses the effects on her work with her clients. Here is a link to the video: www.youtube.com/watch?v=qU4uQ-sxX_ 0&feature=emb_ title

Turns, B. A., & Kimmes, J. (2014). 'I'm not the problem!' Externalizing children's "prob-lems" using play therapy and developmental considerations Contemporary Family Therapy, 36(1), 135–147. https://doi.org/10.1007/s10591-013-9285-z

In this article, the authors present a playful approach to externalization with children and their families that considers their developmental level. This approach to externalization is organized in the psychosocial stage theory by Erik Erickson.

Informed Immigrant

Informed Immigrant is an English and Spanish online website that houses any infor-mation about policy, legal rights, mental health, and education for undocumented immigrants. The website is a collaborative project of diverse organizations and has tools to find national and local resources, information, organizations, and support.

Immigrants Rising

Immigrants Rising is an organization that focuses on uplifting the strengths, skills, abilities, and resilience of the undocumented immigrant community through its pro-jects, services, and spaces. Their website provides more information on their weekly mental health groups, entrepreneur guide, legal intake, financial assistance for college and more.

Bibliography

Babino, A., & Stewart, M. A. (2017). "I Like English Better": Latino Dual Language Students' Investment in Spanish, English, and Bilingualism, English. Journal of Latinos and Education, 16(1), 18–29. https://doi.org/10.1080/15348431.2016.1179186

Balderas, C. N., Delgado-Romero, E. A., & Singh, A. A. (2016). Sin Papeles: Latino parent–child conversations about undocumented legal status. Journal of Latina/o Psy-chology, 4(3), 158–172. https://doi.org/10.1037/lat0000060

Carey, M., & Russell, S. (2003). Re-authoring: Some answers to commonly asked ques-tions. International Journal of Narrative Therapy and Community Work, 3, 60–71. https://search.informit.org/doi/10.3316/informit.652291092639962

Cha, B. S., Enriquez, L. E., & Ro, A. (2019). Beyond access: Psychosocial barriers to undocumented students' use of mental health services. Social Science and Medi-cine, 233, 193–200. https://doi.org/10.1016/j.socscimed.2019.06.003

Cross, F. L., Agi, A., Montoro, J. P., Medina, M. A., Miller-Tejada, S., Pinetta, B. J., Tran-Dubongco, M., & Rivas-Drake, D., . . . Rivas-Drake. (2020). Illuminating ethnic-racial socialization among undocumented Latinx parents and its implications for adolescent psychosocial functioning. Developmental Psychology, 56(8), 1458–1474. https://doi.org/10.1037/dev0000826

Jill, M. S. W., & Combs, G. (1996). Narrative therapy: The social construction of pre-ferred realities. WW Norton & Company.

Madsen, W. C. (2014). Taking it to the streets: Family therapy and family-centered services. Family Process, 53(3), 380–400. https://doi.org/10.1111/famp.12089

Mathema, S. (2017, March 16). Keeping families together: Why all Americans should care about what happens to unauthorized immigrants. http://www.americanprogress. org/issues/immigration/reports/2017/03/16/428335/keeping-families-together/. Center for American Progress.

Raza, S. S., Saravia, L. A., & Katsiaficas, D. (2019). Coming out: Examining how undocumented students critically navigate status disclosure processes. Journal of Diversity in Higher Education, 12(3), 191–204. https://doi.org/10.1037/dhe0000085

Santiago-Rivera, A. L., Altarriba, J., Poll, N., Gonzalez-Miller, N., & Cragun, C. (2009). Therapists' views on working with bilingual Spanish–English speaking clients: A qualitative investigation. Professional Psychology: Research and Practice, 40(5), 436–443. https://doi.org/10.1037/a0015933

Soriano, M., & Gerrard, M. (2019). School-based family counseling: An overview. In B. A. Gerrard, M. J. Carter & D. Ribera (Eds.), School-based family counseling: An interdisciplinary practitioner's guide. Routledge.

Stanton-Salazar, R. D. (2011). A social capital framework for the study of institutional agents and their role in the empowerment of low-status students and youth. Youth and Society, 43(3), 1066–1109. https://doi.org/10.1177/0044118X10382877

United States Citizenship and Immigration Services. (2021, February 4). Consideration of deferred action for childhood arrivals. http://www.uscis.gov/humanitarian/ consideration-of-deferred-action-for-childhood-arrivals-daca

Verdinelli, S., & Biever, J. L. (2009). Spanish. Spanish-English bilingual psychotherapists: Personal and professional language development and use. Cultural Diversity and Ethnic Minority Psychology, 15(3), 230–242. https://doi.org/10.1037/a0015111

White, M. K. (2007). Maps of narrative practice. W.W. Norton & Company.

White, M. K., & Epston, D. (1990). Narrative means to therapeutic ends. W.W. Norton & Company.

Part 3
School Intervention

7 Counseling Undocumented Students

Stephaney S. Morrison

Due to the threat of deportation, many undocumented students and their families have remained invisible in the school system, being psychologically impacted by their challenges. This chapter describes the mental health challenges associated with undocumented immigrant students' status and describes the SBFC approach as an effective way to work with students and families. The SBFC practitioners stand poised as critical allies in implementing school-wide interventions to consider when advocating and counseling undocumented students. The chapter has several goals: (a) to provide background information on undocumented immigrant in schools and their mental health challenges; (b) to describe how SBFC practitioners can use a multitiered system of support with undocumented students and families; (c) to discuss multicultural considerations; (d) to describe the challenges and solutions to applying the SBFC model in a school setting; and (e) to provide additional resources.

Background

Referred to as the 1.5 generation, immigrant and undocumented youth arrived in the host country at a young age (Gonzalez, 2011). They are not citizens, but they grew up in the host country, went to school here, and identified with the culture. These students face incredible economic, legal, social and emotional, and educational barriers. It is imperative to consider the conditions of and interventions for undocumented children since limited evidence-based interventions exist. Undocumented children face many stressors that have negative consequences on students' socio-emotional well-being and educational achievement. The issues newly arrived immigrant students may face depend on the country of origin. For example, a student from Haiti may face discrimination for the first time, while a student from Central America deals with the aftermath of gang violence. Some students may be dealing with post-traumatic stress disorder from pre-migration experiences such as homelessness, war, separation from parents, or other close individuals. Other issues vary depending on the socioeconomic status of the families. Beyond the legal ramifications of their citizenship status, these

DOI: 10.4324/9781003097891-10

factors influence undocumented children's mental health in ways that negatively affect their academic performance and behavior. Yet many school mental health practitioners are unprepared or prefer to avoid the issue as too sensitive or complex for them to address. Too often, the lack of understanding of the legal, social, and psychological ramifications of undocumented students and families causes school staff and leaders to become silent on the issue. Therefore, SBFC practitioners must break the silence and work to bridge silos in the school systems to provide effective counseling care and provide a safe environment within the school system for undocumented students and their families. The following section will describe the various stressors that face undocumented students in the schools.

Stressors Faced by Undocumented Students

Many scholars have noted that stressors faced by undocumented immigrant students drain their coping capacities and leave them vulnerable to academic failure. Stressors include lack of documentation, mixed-status families, low socioeconomic status, family conflict, separation, and trauma (Martinez, 2014). Youths, in particular, may have experienced traumatic events pre- and post-migration. Many undocumented students deal with the psychological aftermath of strict Immigration and Customs Enforcement (ICE) in the United States. Typical adolescent versus parent discord is often intensified in immigrant families as the values and norms between home country clash with host country culture (Martinez, 2014). Parent-child conflict is a significant predictor of immigrant students' academic success (Perez, 2015). Family cohesion correlates with higher academic achievement. Research has shown that family conflict among Hispanic immigrant students leads to higher levels of depression and low self-esteem. Ultimately, undocumented immigrant students may feel depressed or alienated, leading them to look for the family unit elsewhere, such as in gangs (Spear, 2009). Therefore, SBFC practitioners need to understand the stressors in various phases of undocumented students' lives.

Acculturative stress and perceived discrimination (measured as experiences of prejudiced behaviors or observations of discrimination toward others in the school setting) are significant contributors to academic problems (Bryan et al., 2018). Anti-immigrant climate, xenophobia, and discrimination also exacerbate acculturative stress. In addition to these experiences, students' legal status also influences the post-migration acculturative experience for students and their families. The literature identified various ways in which undocumented children and their families are impacted by their undocumented status. The main areas are discussed in the next section.

Undocumented Status

The issue of legal status shapes the lives of immigrant children in many ways. For example, undocumented students are affected by immigration laws in the host country, integration and mobility, identity, sense of belonging, and health. For many undocumented students, these social and legal factors can affect access to education, health insurance, and public programs such as food stamps, family dynamics, and relationships with other social institutions. Even if children are citizens, their undocumented guardians may not entirely understand their child's eligibility and may also fear that seeking help puts them at risk for deportation (Martinez, 2014). Immigration laws and policies are commonly portrayed as necessary to restrict undocumented immigration. Yet research demonstrates this form of deterrence is mainly ineffectual, particularly given that individuals crossing the border are often refugees (Hiskey et al., 2016). Ultimately, immigration laws and policies often result in acute fear of deportation and a life of perpetual anxiety for undocumented immigrants (Suarez-Orozco, 2011).

Fear of Deportation

Another area of concern that SBFC practitioners need to attend to is the psychological impact of uncertainty, fear, and stress resulting from undocumented status. For example, fear of deportation increases the risk of depression, anxiety, and suicide ideation. Further, other writers suggest that the fear of deportation negatively shapes self-image and positively predicts stress (Arbona et al., 2010). This extended exposure to stress during the critical stages of childhood and adolescence creates long-standing consequences, and may involve decreased cognitive performance, decreased short-term and working memory, and poor impulse control.

Socioeconomic Status

Nearly 40% of undocumented children live below the federal poverty level (compared with 17% of native-born children) (Perez, 2015). Across many studies, poverty is associated with a range of adverse outcomes for children's physical health, language and cognitive development, academic achievement, educational attainment, and mental, emotional, and behavioral health (Yoshikawa et al., 2012). Furthermore, the effects of poverty are cumulative; consequences at one stage in a child's development can hinder development later (Gonzalez et al., 2017).

Children of immigrants are at higher risk of cognitive and language developmental issues and lower academic performance. They are at a disadvantage in school readiness compared to children of authorized individuals (Suarez-Orozco, 2011). Research demonstrates that undocumented status has a harmful influence on children's cognitive skills as early as 2 and 3. This influence is attributed to increased parental economic hardship and psychological distress combined with lower availability of social support and lower levels of information about public resources that could help children's cognitive development (Yoshikawa, 2011). The undocumented status of families can, directly and indirectly, hinder access to vital public programs, such as early childhood education, which can improve immigrant children's cognitive and behavioral development (Yoshikawa et al., 2012). In addition, to restricted access to resources, many parents work long hours or multiple jobs; thus, children are left unsupervised. Limited time with caregivers lessens exposure to language and nurturance, leading to less-developed cognitive and language skills and lower academic achievement (Morrison & Bryan, 2014). With these continued barriers, adolescents often face additional obstacles that may limit their daily lives, future career planning, and self-concept.

Pre-migration Experiences

Research clearly shows how pre-migration experiences can shape children's post-migration life. Further, scholars have noted how motivation for migration and events before the immigration experience constitute risk factors for immigrant youth. For example, Perreira and Ornales (2011) revealed that many immigrant school children (8–15 years old) are exposed to pre-immigration violence, which was prevalent and positively associated with post-traumatic stress disorder and depressive symptoms. Undocumented students may also experience psychological stress exacerbated by the entry experience. This process has become more dangerous due to increased border surveillance and the extreme crisis of separating families at the border. In addition, acculturative stress, which stems from challenges associated with adjusting to life in the host country, affects psychological well-being.

Post-migration Experiences

When undocumented students experience trauma or negative experiences before they arrive at their host country, these experiences can prompt further stress when they encounter new challenges. Studies find a positive association between acculturative stress and low self-esteem, depression, and more significant suicidal ideation (Perreira & Ornales, 2011). Additionally, undocumented children and families bear the additional burden of misinformation about themselves in the media that describes how society treats them. Regular experiences of perceived discrimination can cause psychological distress, major depression, and generalized anxiety (Yoshikawa et al., 2012). Informed SBFC practitioners can break the silence and lead school staff by suggesting and supporting effective interventions across the levels of a multi-tiered service delivery model.

Procedures

Multitiered Systems of Support Framework

The multitiered systems of support framework (MTSS) is a framework that helps educators provide academic and behavioral support for students with various needs. The significance of this framework is that instead of waiting for students to fail, educators take a proactive perspective and integrate support at three levels to help undocumented students succeed in the school system. The SBFC practitioners can use this system to lead school faculty and staff to integrate academic and socio-emotional support for students.

The SBFC practitioners need to hold as their value that all students, regardless of immigration status, must be given free public school education. Further, the SBFC practitioners must be culturally aware of their privilege and cultural differences as they work with families and children. Cultural awareness is the foundation to creating a culturally respective school environment in collaboration with the whole school system. Thus, encouraging cultural awareness in the school system becomes an issue of social justice in which taking action within a social justice framework reflects the need for all SBFC practitioners to engage in advocacy and equity work that both support the rights and opportunities of all and recognizes potential obstacles to this work, including system barriers that work against educational justice. Viewing undocumented students through this lens, SBFC practitioners can implement interventions directed at system-wide advocacy and individual equity and support.

Tier 1: Universal Systems of Support

At this first tier, the SBFC practitioners can include the entire school support system to provide supportive interventions to meet undocumented students. This structure involves creating support and positive interaction between staff and students. As noted earlier, undocumented immigrant students feel a lack of belonging and endure immense stress because of their status and especially because of the negative perceptions of their undocumented status. Therefore, it is essential to create a nurturing and supportive environment for all students, particularly undocumented students who need extra support and a positive and safe environment. Some ways schools can work together to support students include the following:

- Bridge Culture Between Home and School. To help students, SBFC practitioners need to collaborate with families. Undocumented status does not just impact students but the entire family unit. Most likely, parents are undocumented, or the students are documented, but their parents/guardians are undocumented. Students' psychological stress often is exacerbated by limited access to many social services at home, such as little parental supervision, low socioeconomic status, language barriers, and so on. Building relationships with families can give insight into the types of services practitioners can provide for families, such as food, housing, and other basic needs provided through community support, since undocumented immigrants cannot receive services through the state. Another way SBFC practitioners can be supportive is to help families feel welcome at the school. They can be encouraged to attend school activities and be included in academic decisions for their children. In addition, SBFC practitioners can seek language brokers through the community to assist with interpreting families' language and providing information to families. Sending letters home in the home language is also very important to provide information for families, as is holding workshops for families on immigrants' rights to public education.

- Provide Information for School Staff. The SBFC practitioners organize and promote school-wide workshops to highlight the strengths of undocumented families' cultures and the importance of teaching techniques to share their culture with their children, such as storytelling or talking about the significance of certain foods and traditions in their home country. Integrating family cultural values into school activities contributes to building trust. When trust is established, families can feel secure in accessing school resources such as counseling and other services that can reduce the sense of isolation created by the threat of deportation. Participating in school programs can increase acceptance and belonging that can help alleviate the feelings of persecution and isolation created by anti-immigrant rhetoric. When informed, undocumented families can access many school and community services, including orientation programs for new immigrants; free and reduced-price breakfast and lunch programs; after-school child care programs that provide homework support; family involvement programs that support the development of reading and mathematical reasoning; parenting workshops and parent support groups; language classes for parents; school interpreters; and community-based and culturally based social service agencies. Ideally, some school districts are providing workshops that share resources for legal assistance to undocumented immigrants and how to create emergency plans for the family in the case of deportation. SBFC practitioners should review the school's community interface to make sure parents can access information and resources. If school staff members are not bilingual, a bilingual community liaison needs to be identified and employed either as a volunteer or in a paid position.

In the United States, there has been consistent research that undocumented students are impacted psychologically by the actions of immigration enforcement. For example, according to a 2010 report by the Urban Institute, children who witnessed parents or family members apprehended in a home raid were more likely to experience symptoms of post-traumatic stress disorder and much higher degrees of fear and anxiety than children whose parents were arrested in other settings. SBFC practitioners can work with teachers to share general information about the topic of raids in a classroom setting instead of singling out individual students. Creating a culture of safety and trust in the classroom can encourage students to share critical information about their mental health needs with teachers. In addition, SBFC practitioners can work with teachers to encourage students to come to the SBFC practitioners for support.

- Provide Support for Teachers. It is recommended that SBFC practitioners work with teachers to incorporate equity, diversity, and inclusion in the classroom. Teachers may need help to practice reflective teaching and support for students. Teachers can provide resources such as books that include immigrant experiences. Another form of system-wide support entails incorporating culturally relevant books in language arts classes and in school library collections. Reading about characters who share experiences familiar to students whose families have immigrated is validating. It can help reduce feelings of isolation and alienation while adapting to a new way of life. Providing books with themes describing children's experiences of immigration can help students conceptualize their own experiences and provide references to further explore in class discussions and group counseling. The promotion of bilingual, dual language immersion and early learning dual-language learners' programs extends the idea of cultural and linguistic relevancy. By acknowledging a heritage language as an asset, immigrant students would benefit from the sense that they are well poised to become bilingual and help their monolingual peers achieve this valuable skill.

Tier 2: Secondary Level of Support

- Provide Small Group Counseling. On this level, students need extra support in meeting their academic and socio-emotional goals. Often this support is offered in a small group setting, such as friendship groups or reading groups. In addition, SBFC practitioners can promote group counseling for students with immigration issues in their families. Here, practitioners can collaborate with teachers to identify students who may have various socio-emotional challenges such as lack of belonging, appearing stressed out, anxious, or depressed.

- Additionally, SBFC practitioners can partner with English language (EL) program coordinators and teachers and help refer students who could benefit from group counseling explicitly designed to help undocumented students process their experiences as immigrants and minorities. Self-disclosure is more likely to happen if undocumented students are placed in groups with similar backgrounds and emotional struggles. The small group setting provides a space for undocumented students to normalize their situations. That is, they are not the only ones in that situation. Group counseling is ideal for easing some of the marginalization and creating a supportive setting.

To work effectively with immigrants, a staff member first needs to understand their cultural heritage, including its values and immigration history and must know what cultural values are embedded in their professional practices (Elizalde-Utnick, 2010). For example, (a) SBFC practitioners must be aware of their biases, assumptions, and discriminatory attitudes that may be conscious or unconscious. These biases can ultimately be barriers to providing adequate care to students and their families. (b) SBFC practitioners must be aware that undocumented families might not actively participate in school activities because of the fear of exposure and may not reach out for mental health help. (c) SBFC practitioners need to be aware of the help-seeking attitudes of immigrant families who may view mental health counseling in a negative light and feel that they will be stigmatized if they share their mental health concerns. With these points in mind, SBFC practitioners may need to explain the importance of group counseling to families and children. One way to introduce group counseling to families and students is to emphasize the psycho-educational benefits of understanding undocumented experiences and receiving information to help them develop strength-based strategies to cope with their situation.

- Accommodate Parents. Another way to build nurturing and trustworthy relationships is by going beyond the school walls and into the community. For example, if parents do not typically attend school functions due to scheduling or transportation issues, holding meetings in libraries, churches, or community rooms can better accommodate immigrant parents. Moreover, it is essential to communicate to parents that the practitioner is willing to do what is needed to develop a positive relationship with parents.

  Similarly, home visits are another way of showing intent to strengthen the home-school relationships. It is recommended that school support leaders (social workers or translators), who are familiar with the family situation, can be the first level of contact for parents and families. Supporting immigrant families includes home-school collaboration, linking families with school-based and community services, and providing specific instructional support to meet undocumented students' learning needs (Elizalde-Utnick, 2010).

Tier 3: Individual-Level Supports

- Undocumented students may need individual support, even with Tier I and Tier II supports. The SBFC practitioners can provide one-on-one counseling with undocumented students or students from mixed-status families. As mentioned previously, an internalization of behaviors, including a manifestation of depression and anxiety, can be seen in our immigrant students who live in a constant high-stress state. When students are impacted psychologically, this will affect their academic performance, interpersonal life (e.g., social withdrawal, conflict in relationships), and self-perceptions. In addition, disruptions in important social roles may be reflected in problems such as a high behavior referral rate, dropping out of school, and early pregnancy.

- Similarly, academic tasks may be interrupted by challenges to social bonds within the family (Lambert & Rudolph, 2007). The anxiety created by fear of detention and deportation can have acute or chronic mental health effects on children of immigrant families regardless of their legal status. These effects can result in post-traumatic stress syndrome (PTSD), anxiety disorders, or depression. An SBFC practitioner working with children dealing with these issues needs to know intensive individual or small group interventions that can help in these cases. Examples of Tier 3 interventions for practitioners include suicide prevention, threat assessment, or trauma-informed counseling for students.

Multicultural Considerations

The SBFC practitioner has an opportunity, and is in a pivotal position, to work with undocumented immigrants from a systems perspective. Understanding the various challenges associated with legal status is very important. This knowledge assists in how SBFC practitioners conduct clinical assessments, set goals, and develop culturally responsive treatment plans. SBFC practitioners ascribe to the ethical codes of their respective organizations, which have as their core value practitioners' attention to multicultural sensitivity when working with clients. SBFC practitioners must adhere to their ethical responsibilities as culturally aware providers and who will provide equitable access to students and their families.

Challenges and Solutions

To work with undocumented students, the SBFC practitioners need to be aware of the potential challenges that impact the systemic approach to implementing the multitiered levels discussed earlier. To overcome these barriers, the SBFC practitioners need (a) to be knowledgeable about existing laws and guidelines, (b) to gain support from other school staff, and (c) to reach out to undocumented immigrants.

Laws and Guidelines

SBFC practitioners need to be aware of the laws and policies that impact undocumented students and their families. In the United States, as a result of the denial of undocumented students from earning a public education, the supreme court in 1982 (Plyer v. Doe case) issued a critical decision that all undocumented students have constitutional rights to free public education. Further, schools cannot discriminate against undocumented students, request information regarding their immigration status, adopt policies or practices that discourage participation by undocumented students, and exclude students based on their parents' perceived citizenship or immigration status (American Immigration Council, 2006). The laws of the state usually paint an uncertain picture for undocumented students and their families. Therefore, SBFC practitioners must stay abreast of the latest educational opportunities available for undocumented immigrant students. Students and their families may not be aware of laws that can give them access to higher education. The SBFC practitioner can be a resource for these students, especially if there is no system for working with undocumented students.

Partnership With Other School Staff

As SBFC practitioners work with undocumented students, they may encounter barriers such as a lack of school support because of how undocumented students may be viewed. On the basis of these perceptions coming from school staff, the school might have concerns about providing help for these students due to perceived legal or political ramifications. Culturally aware SBFC practitioners can give voice to undocumented students by raising awareness among school staff. SBFC practitioners can do this by providing professional development days for school staff that draw attention to diverse student needs and by establishing partnerships in developing school policies that are inclusive of undocumented students. In addition, gathering pertinent information about each student's personal history, such as country of birth or residency status and that of the students' guardians, may help SBFC accurately determine the specific laws applicable for the students.

Supporting Undocumented Students

Many school staff have inaccurate perceptions about undocumented people, which can be a deterrent to how services can be offered in the school. Further, school staff can be oblivious to the struggles and needs of undocumented immigrant students. The SBFC practitioner who is culturally aware can give voice to undocumented students by engaging with other school staff members to raise awareness. The SBFC practitioner can call attention to the need for the school to provide services that meet the needs of diverse students in general and guide staff in building relationships with students from underserved and marginalized backgrounds. The aim is to create a trusting and safe place for students and encourage them to share any challenges they may be experiencing. The SBFC practitioner can encourage staff to refer students who need support based on their immigration status.

Reach Out to Students

As with any school-responsive service, it will be challenging to get students who need help to reach out, especially if students, such as undocumented students, are fearful of the ramifications of exposing their or their families' status. Lack of awareness of how the SBFC practitioner can support them could prevent students from participating in individual and group counseling programs. This applies especially to students who may come from a culture that stigmatizes help-seeking behaviors. The SBFC practitioner can best serve this population if they partner with school staff, such as teachers, parents, or others who play an essential role in students' lives. For example, in recruiting students for group counseling, the SBFC practitioner could request that teachers refer students who may benefit from the group. Further, the SBFC practitioner can advertise the group as an "education" group. It is noted that some immigrant families are more receptive to psychoeducation groups than individual counseling (Morrison & Bryan, 2014).

Conclusion

This chapter highlighted the various challenges faced by undocumented immigrants in the school system. In addition to the complex immigration status of these students and their families, they are confronted with many personal problems that impact their academic and socio-emotional development. A critical avenue for SBFC practitioners is to consider how they can use their role in a school system to partner with school faculty and staff in developing preventive and intervention programs such as the MTSS for students. At times much conversation is centered on only individual counseling or group counseling, without considering a whole-school approach. Everyone who works with undocumented immigrants is vital in this support system to provide a positive environment for all students.

Resources

www.sesameworkshop.org/what-we-do/refugee-response
www.sesameworkshop.org/what-we-do/social-impact-initiatives
   These two websites provide information about children and families in crisis and how Sesame Street resources can be used in this context.

www.onlinemswprograms.com/resources/social-issues/support-resources-immigrants-refugees/
   This website describes 60 resources that can be useful when working with undocumented immigrants.

Bibliography

Arbona, C., Olvera, N., Rodriguez, N., Hagan, J., Linares, A., & Wiesner, M. (2010). Acculturative stress among documented and undocumented Latino immigrants in the United States. Hispanic Journal of Behavioral Sciences, 32(3), 362–384. https://doi.org/10.1177/0739986310373210

American Immigration Council. (2006). Public education for immigrant students. Understanding Plyler v. Doe. http://www.americanimmigrationcouncil.org/research/plyler-v-doepublic-education-immigrant-students

Bryan, J., Williams, J., Jungnam, K., Morrison, S., Caldwell, C. H., & Jackson, J. S. (2018). School bonding and family support as predictors of academic achievement among African American and Caribbean Black adolescents. Urban Education, 10.117/0042085918806959. DOI

Elizalde-Utnick, G. (2010). Immigrant families: Strategies for school support (pp. 12–16). National Association of Secondary School Principals.

Gonzalez, R. G. (2011). Learning to be illegal: Undocumented youth and shifting legal contexts in the transition to adulthood. American Sociological Review, 76(4), 602–619. https://doi.org/10.1177/0003122411411901

Gonzalez, R. G., & Chavez, L. R. (2012). "Awakening to a Nightmare": Abjectivity and Illegality in the Lives of Undocumented 1.5-Generation Latino Immigrants in the United States. Current Anthropology, 53(3), 255–281. https://doi.org/10.1086/665414

González, J. J., Kula, S. M., González, V. V., & Paik, S. J. (2017). Context of Latino students' family separation during and after immigration: Perspectives, challenges, and opportunities for collaborative efforts. School Community Journal, 27(2), 211–228. http://arktos.nyit.edu/login?url=https://search.   http://-proquest-com.arktos.nyit.edu/docview/2052790994?accountid=12917

Hiskey, J. T., Cordova, A., Orces, D., & Malone, M. F. (2016). Understanding the Central American refugee crisis: Why they are fleeing and how U.S. policies are failing to deter them. American Immigration Council.

Lambert, S. F., & Rudolph, K. D. (2007). Child and adolescent depression. In E. J. Mash & R. A. Barkley (Eds.), Assessment of childhood disorders (4th ed., pp. 213–242). Guilford Press.

Martinez, L. M. (2014). Dreams deferred: The impact of legal reforms on undocumented Latino youth. American Behavioral Scientist, 58(14), 1873–1890. https://doi.org/10.1177/0002764214550289

Morrison, S., & Bryan, J. (2014). Addressing the challenges and needs of English-speaking Caribbean immigrant students: Guidelines for school counselors. International Journal for the Advancement of Counselling, 36(4), 440–449. https://doi.org/10.1007/s10447-014-9218-z

Perez, W. (2015). Americans by heart: Undocumented Latino students and the promise of higher education. Teacher's College Press.

Perreira, K. M., & Ornelas, I. J. (2011). The physical and psychological well-being of immigrant children. Future of Children, 21(1), 195–218. https://doi.org/10.1353/foc.2011.0002

Suárez-Orozco, M. M., Darbes, T., Dias, S. I., & Sutin, M. (2011). Migrations and Schooling. Annual Review of Anthropology, 40(1), 311–328. https://doi.org/10.1146/annurev-anthro-111009-115928

Spear, L. P. (2009). Heightened stress responsivity and emotional reactivity during pubertal maturation: Implications for psychopathology. Development and Psychopathology, 21(1), 87–97. https://doi.org/10.1017/S0954579409000066

Yoshikawa, H. (2011). Immigrants raising citizens: Undocumented parents and their children. Russell Publishing Sage Foundation.

Yoshikawa, H., Aber, J. L., & Beardslee, W. R. (2012). The effects of poverty on the mental, emotional, and behavioral health of children and youth: Implications for prevention. American Psychologist. American Psychological Association, 67(4), 272–284. https://doi.org/10.1037/a0028015

8 Using Solution-Focused Brief Counseling

Carol E. Buchholz Holland

The main focus of this chapter is to describe how to use solution-focused brief counseling (SFBC) with refugee and immigrant students in school settings. It will provide (a) a brief overview of this counseling approach, (b) a description of the basic tenets and assumptions of SFBC, (c) a case example, which illustrates the application of this approach, (d) a description of SFBC multicultural consideration, and (e) information about challenges and solutions for using this approach with refugee and immigrant students. Additional resources are included at the end of this chapter.

Background

Working with children and adolescents in school settings can present unique challenges for school-based family counseling (SBFC) practitioners, and working with students who are refugees or immigrants can add another layer of complexity. It is important for an SBFC practitioner to find an effective counseling approach, which is developmentally appropriate and a good fit within a school setting. In addition, the chosen approach ideally would meet the following criteria: (a) it is culturally sensitive; (b) it is evidence based; (c) it helps connect with and engage students in the counseling process; (d) it does not increase the likelihood of retraumatizing students who have experienced past traumas; (e) it helps students identify their personal strengths and coping strategies; and (f) it helps build students' hope and resiliency. Although this is a fairly long list of criteria, there is one counseling approach, which meets all of them and stands out from the crowd. That approach is the solution-focused brief counseling (SFBC).

How SFBC Fits Within the SBFC Meta-Model

SFBC is a good fit for work with students who are refugees or immigrants. In addition, SFBC fits within the SBFC meta-model for several reasons because both

- are strength-based;
- are collaborative;

DOI: 10.4324/9781003097891-11

- engage individuals in counseling process;
- are culturally sensitive;
- help students and families identify their own resources;
- emphasize respect, caring, and humility;
- promote student success and wellness; and
- are action-oriented (Gerrard et al., 2020).

Although this chapter only focuses on using the solution-focused approach in the "School Intervention" quadrant of the SBFC meta-model, it is important to note that this approach can also be adapted and used in the other three quadrants (School Prevention, Family Prevention, and Family Intervention). Unlike most other counseling approaches and theoretical approaches, the solution-focused approach can be easily adapted for a variety of applications within school setting. It can also provide a common strength-based language that can be used both in and outside of counseling sessions.

Brief Overview of SFBC

Many traditional counseling approaches focus efforts on discovering the explanations for why problems occur in order to resolve problems (Birdsall & Miller, 2002). Furthermore, these approaches tend to use a deductive problem-solving method when searching for the causes of problems. In contrast, SFBC (commonly called *solution-focused brief therapy*) emerged in the early 1980s when Steve de Shazer, Insoo Kim Berg, and their colleagues at the Brief Family Therapy Center in Milwaukee, Wisconsin, experimented pragmatically and used an inductive manner to identify effective therapeutic techniques and determine what worked in therapy sessions (Berg & Steiner, 2003). They concluded that it was more effective for mental health practitioners to help their clients identify and co-construct solutions instead of concentrating on how to resolve their clients' problems. During solution-focused counseling sessions, clients' preferred futures became the focus of the sessions instead of clients' past or current problems. In other words, the solution-focused approach redirects attention and energy to efforts designed to identify what possible solutions may already exist in the clients' lives instead of concentrating on the clients' problems. Clients' existing strengths and past successes are also highlighted in counseling sessions, and they help create "a foundation for formulating solutions" (George, 2008, p. 147).

Using SFBC With Children and Adolescents

SFBC is a future-oriented, goal-directed, and evidence-based approach, which works well with children and adolescents. For example, the inductive process infused within the solution-focused approach is similar to the trial-and-error method that children use to learn. In contrast, insight-oriented approaches may not be the best fit to use with children and adolescents. On the basis of her experiences working with children, Insoo Kim Berg concluded that children did not need or want to know what caused their problems (Berg & Steiner, 2003). Instead, children would rather experiment to see what works and what does not work for them. Not surprising, this approach has been found to be effective when used with children because it is congruent with "how children think and view the world" (Berg & Steiner, 2003, p. xv). Because SFBC is an action-oriented, strengths-based approach, it is very appropriate for use with this population, and it works well when SBFC practitioners collaborate with their clients to identify individualized tools and strategies. Examples of evidence-based support for SFBC are shown in Box 8.1.

Box 8.1   Solution-Focused Brief Counseling Evidence-Based Studies

Beauchemin, J. D. (2018). Solution-focused wellness: A randomized controlled trial of college students. Health & Social Work, 43(2), 94–100. doi:10.1093/hsw/hly007

Franklin, C., Moore, K., & Hopson, L. (2008). Effectiveness of solution-focused brief therapy in a school setting. Children & Schools, 30, 15–26.

Franklin, C., Streeter, C. L., Kim, J. S., & Tripodi, S. J. (2007). The effectiveness of a solution focused, public alternative school for dropout prevention and retrieval. Children & Schools, 29, 133–144. doi:10.1093/cs/29.3.133

Froeschle, J. G., Smith, R. L., & Ricard, R. (2007). The efficacy of a systematic substance abuse program for adolescent females. Professional School Counseling, 10(5), 498–505.

Gong, H., & Hsu, W. (2017). The effectiveness of solution-focused group therapy in ethnic Chinese school settings: A meta-analysis. International Journal of Group Psychotherapy, 67(3), 383–409. https://doi.org/10.1080/00207284.2016.1240588

Wallace, L. B., Hai, A. H., & Franklin, C. (2020). An evaluation of Working on What Works (WOWW): A solution-focused intervention for schools. Journal of Marital and Family Therapy, 46(4), 687–700. https://doi.org/10.1111/jmft.12424

Whitehead, L., Allan, M. C., Allen, K., Duchak, V., King, E., Mason, C., . . . Tully, S. (2018). "Give us a break!": Using a solution focused programme to help young people cope with loss and negative change. Bereavement Care, 37(1), 17–27.

Its time-limited nature is especially useful for SBFC practitioners who might have large caseloads but do not have large amounts of time to work with students (Littrell et al., 1995). In addition, students are more likely to become engaged in a counseling session that focuses on their positive traits instead of their deficiencies (Sklare, 2005). Because SFBC is a strength-based and conversation-based approach, it helps create a relaxed and positive atmosphere, which helps build rapport between the student and the practitioner during the counseling session. Children and adolescents may also be more likely to feel heard and valued when practitioners use conversation-based approaches such as SFBC. Furthermore, the collaborative nature of this approach helps build therapeutic relationships between young clients and practitioners. Engaging students in the counseling process is especially important when working with students who are in crisis.

SFBC Tenets and Assumptions

SFBC is based on several tenets and assumptions, which have created a foundation for this approach. In addition, they help inform SBFC practitioners on how to work with clients of all ages. Here are some examples that help practitioners develop a deeper understanding of SFBC:

1. *Every client is resourceful and has the capacity for change.* Solution-focused practitioners believe that all clients are capable of changing and have inherent strengths and resources to help themselves—regardless of their level of functioning (Berg & Miller, 1992; Murphy, 2008). One role of the solution-focused practitioner is to help clients identify these strengths and resources that they may have forgotten they possess them, may be underutilizing them, or may not be using them at all.
2. *Every client is unique and is the expert of his/her life.* Because solution-focused practitioners believe that clients are the experts of their lives, they encourage clients to identify their own goals for counseling. Client's goals—not the practitioner's—provide the direction for counseling sessions (Murphy, 2008). In addition, solutions are generated in a collaborative process and are individually tailored to fit each client. SFBC is respectful of the client's experiences and strives to empower them in the solution-building process.
3. *If it isn't broke, don't fix it. If it works, do more of it. If it doesn't work, do something different* (de Shazer et al., 2007, pp. 1–2). In other words, there really is not a need to spend much time or effort in a session talking about things that are not "broke." Instead, solution-focused practitioners devote more time helping clients identify things that the clients have done in the past that works for them. In addition, practitioners encourage clients to do more of things that personally worked for them. On the flip side, there is a popular quote that says the definition of *insanity* is doing the same thing over and over but expecting different results.

That definition fits with this solution-focused tenet. Asking a simple question such as "How's that working for you?" can prompt clients to self-evaluate and determine if their actions are helping them achieve their goals. It is more effective when a client is the one who decides that something is not working for them instead of the practitioner making this judgment especially when working with children and adolescent. Instead of continuing to do same things that have not worked for clients in the past, the clients are encouraged to try something different.

4. *You don't need the details or the cause of a client's problem in order to help them find a solution.* One striking difference between SFBC and traditional counseling approaches is that SFBC does not believe it is necessary to gather a detailed description of a client's past. In addition, obtaining details about a client's past problems may be more about satisfying a mental health practitioner's curiosity rather than benefiting the client. Since a client's past cannot be changed, the client's *preferred future* (what they want to see happen in their future) becomes the focus of solution-focused counseling sessions. In a recorded interview with Arnoud Huibers, Insoo Kim Berg gave a brief description of her work with a client who was ashamed to share a problem in the counseling session (see Resources at the end of this chapter for this video link). Berg stated that she did not need the client to share the problem with her. Instead, Berg only needed to know what the client's goals and preferred future were so that they could work collaboratively to identify a solution. Berg also noted that needing a solution implies that there is a problem even if the client never reveals the problem. Since clients are not required or expected to share possible painful details about their pasts, they are likely to experience SFBC as a much less intrusive form of counseling. Refugee and immigrant students may also find this approach less threatening and may be more likely to engage in the counseling process.

5. *No problem is constant* (Murphy, 2008). The solution-focused approach believes that there are times when a problem is not present, or at the very least the problem fluctuates in intensity and/or in its duration. These times when the problem wasn't present or less intense are called *exceptions.* The solution-focused approach believes that a person can find an exception to any problem. For example, a student explains to a practitioner that the student has difficulty focusing in class. The practitioner then works with the student to identify times when the student was able to focus in class (or even just a little bit more). Within each exception lies a potential solution.

6. *Small change can lead to bigger changes.* In a situation where a client feels stuck or overwhelmed, it is helpful to encourage the client to identify small changes that he/she believes to be more realistic or manageable to achieve. Being successful at taking small steps toward a desired goal can help energize the client, generate hope, and lead to bigger changes. This slow and steady process for accomplishing goals is also a good fit

for refugee and immigrant students who may have limited resources or have limited power to change their situations on a big scale. It is important to remember that small changes accumulate over time, and they help create a positive forward momentum in counseling.

7. *People are more invested in goals and solutions they generate.* Co-constructing goals and solutions with clients is an effective way to engage clients (Murphy, 2008). In addition, there is a greater chance that clients will actually implement solutions they helped generate especially if they have been successful using these solutions in the past.

Procedure

Solution-focused practitioners realize the importance of language, and they use carefully crafted questions as tools to facilitate the identifications of clients' strengths and solutions (Berg & Steiner, 2003). Solution-focused questions and Socratic questioning are the main tools/techniques of this approach. The following fictional case example is provided to illustrate the use of the solution-focused approach with a student who is a refugee. This case example provides an example of commons steps a solution-focused practitioner would take during a first session with a student.

Case Example: Amal

Amal is a 16-year-old student who is originally from Iraq. Amal and her family arrived in the United States when she was 10, and they were resettled in a small North Dakota community. Until recently, Amal had maintained an "A" average in school. However, Amal has been experiencing several somatic symptoms such as headaches, stomach aches, and dizziness over the past couple of months. In addition, it has been difficult for Amal to focus in class and complete her homework on time. A week ago, Amal met with her family physician and had a complete physical. Fortunately, no underlying health conditions were found. Amal's family physician recommended that Amal meet with a mental health practitioner in her school.

Here is a description of steps taken during Amal's first session with the solution-focused SBFC practitioner:

1. Develop Rapport With the Student by Using Problem-Free Talk

When first working with a student, it is important to develop rapport and join with them (Berg, 1994). Encouraging "problem-free talk" such as asking about the student's interests and/or preferred activities is one way of connecting with a student. The first few minutes of a session are a critical period in the development of a counseling relationship (Henden, 2008). Without rapport, it becomes more difficult to develop trust between the student and the mental health practitioner. Here are two basic *problem-free questions* that can also be utilized to gather some useful information about the student:

Practitioner: Amal, what is your favorite thing to do in your free time when you are not in school?

or

Practitioner: What is one small thing you recently did that you enjoyed (even a little bit)?

In addition, it is helpful to note that problem-free talk is not just small talk. It is a valuable therapeutic tool, which can be used to increase client engagement. In this case, the practitioner may also begin learning about Amal's coping strategies, strengths, skills, and/or resources, which can be applied later in the conversation during solution-building phase.

2. Begin the Goal-Setting Process With the Student

After briefly engaging in problem-free talk with Amal, the solution-focused practitioner asks her a *goal-setting question* such as the following:

Practitioner: Amal, what are you hoping we can accomplish today by working together?

or

Practitioner: Amal, what are your best hopes for our meeting today?

Instead of asking Amal to describe the problem that brought her to counseling, the practitioner words the question so that it prompts Amal to begin formulating what she hopes to get out of counseling. In other words, Amal is encouraged to articulate her own goal that will provide direction for the counseling session. Even though the practitioner initially only asks Amal what she hopes to achieve by meeting with the practitioner and does not ask about Amal's problem, Amal still has the opportunity to share the details of her problem with the practitioner if she chooses. When asking Amal a goal-setting ("best hopes") question, the solution-focused practitioner also takes a "not knowing" stance, which may help counter any preconceptions that the practitioner may have about Amal's situation or what Amal might need (De Jong & Berg, 2008). In addition, the "not knowing" stance allows the practitioner to be open to Amal's own goals for counseling and to decrease the likelihood of making assumptions about Amal's problems or the causes of her problems.

   The goal-setting process is an important part of a counseling session and should not be overlooked. After all, clearly defined goals can help improve the likelihood for positive counseling outcome. Surprisingly, many traditional counseling approaches do not emphasis this step as much as the solution-focused approach does. An important role of a solution-focused practitioner is to assist clients in formulating concrete and measurable goals. Henden (2008) suggested that practitioners help clients create SMART+ goals (small [and specific], measurable, achievable, realistic, and time limited). The word "small" was added to the common SMART goal acronym because it emphasizes the recommendation of forming small goals, which can be achieved more easily, which in turn can help build the client's levels of confidence and hope.

It is common for individuals unfamiliar with the solution-focused approach to initially develop what is termed as "avoid goals" (aka negative goals) (Bannink, 2012). Avoid goals focus on what the client does not want such as "I don't want to procrastinate" or "I don't want to feel anxious." However, Bannink (2012) recommends that mental health practitioners help clients turn avoid goals into "approach goals" (aka positive goals). Approach goals focus on what the client wants instead or in place of the problem. For example, an approach goal is formed when the client describes his/her preferred future and what he/she wants to be doing or feeling such as "I want to turn in all of my assignments on time" or "I want to feel more relaxed." One quick way to convert an avoid goal into an approach goal is to ask the client this question: "What would you like to be doing (feeling) instead of your problem?" "Instead" is a very useful and powerful word, and it is frequently used in solution-focused conversations.

3. Ask the Miracle Question to Help Identify and Describe Student's Preferred Future

If Amal was to struggle with identifying or providing details about her goal for the counseling session, it would be helpful to ask her the *miracle question*, which is a hallmark of the solution-focused approach. The miracle question was designed to help a client visualize what his/her life would be like when his/her problem no longer existed. Here is an example of how the solution-focused practitioner can use the miracle question to help Amal clarify her goal(s) and make them observable.

Practitioner: Now, I want to ask you a strange question. Suppose that while you are sleeping tonight and the entire house is quiet, a miracle happens. The miracle is that the problem that brought you here is solved. However because you were sleeping, you don't know that the miracle has happened. So, when you wake up tomorrow morning, what will be different that will tell you that a miracle has happened and the problem that brought you here is solved? (de Shazer, 1988, p. 5).

After asking the miracle question, the practitioner encourages Amal to provide as many details about her "miracle" as possible. The richness of these details can provide valuable information, which can be used to assist Amal in developing her SMART+ goals and help her identify potential coping strategies and solutions. In addition, the practitioner asks questions intended to uncover what Amal would be doing after the miracle and what others would see her doing. The reason the practitioner focuses on asking about what Amal would be doing after her miracle occurred is because her actions/activities help make things more concrete and specific. In addition, these actions can provide insight into possible solutions that Amal might be willing to try. For example, the practitioner could ask Amal:

Practitioner: Amal, what is the first thing you would notice you are doing after this miracle happened? What else? What else?

Asking "What else?" prompts is a very effective and subtle method for encouraging the student to dig deeper and provide more details without being too pushy/intrusive. The focus is on identifying the student's observable positive behaviors and actions.

It is also helpful to ask a relationship question such as the following:

Practitioner: What would other people notice you are doing after this miracle happened?

Relationship questions encourage students to view things from a different perspective. Using a third-person perspective can often help bring attention solutions that are present in the student's life but were not on the student's radar. Taking a third-person perspective can also help tap into more creative ideas because it puts some distance between the student and his/her problem.

4. Assist Student With Identifying Exceptions and Past Successes

A basic assumption of the solution-focused approach is that no problem is constant, and its intensity fluctuates over time (Murphy, 1997). Solution-focused practitioners are interested in helping clients identify the times when the problem is not occurring, is less frequent, or is less severe (aka *exceptions*). Henden (2008) noted that it is helpful to look for *exceptions* after the client describes his/her *miracle*. For example:

Practitioner: Tell me about a time when a little bit of your miracle (being relaxed and focused) has already occurred. What did you do to make this happen?

Follow-up questions may include the following:

Practitioner: How did you make that happen? What else? What else?
How did you decide to do that?
What did you discover by doing that?
What would happen if you tried that again?

The practitioner can also ask questions such as these:

Practitioner: What time of the day are you most productive?
Where are you most productive?
What did (teacher, family, friends, and so on) do or say that
was most helpful for you?

The follow-up questions serve the purpose of amplifying the exceptions. Murphy (1994) described the 5-E method of utilizing exceptions that was designed to recognize and use exceptions that exist in students' lives. Solution-focused practitioners using the 5-E method can assist students to (a) elicit times when the problem is absent, less intense, or less frequent, (b) elaborate on the conditions and features of these times, (c) expand these identified exceptions to other contexts, (d) evaluate these exceptions using pre-established goals, and (e) empower the client to maintain positive change over time (Murphy, 1994). Since exceptions are often overlooked, solution-focused practitioners need to be very intentional in identifying and amplifying these "micro-solutions" (Sharry et al., 2002, p. 392).

Solution-focused practitioners are also interested in drawing attention to the student's past successes. A past success question specifically asks what the student has done in the past that has led the student to success. It focuses on what was in the student's control to achieve this success (and hopefully still in the student's control to do again). For example, the practitioner may ask:

Practitioner: What have you done in the past that has helped you (even a
little bit) with this problem?
                                          or
Practitioner: Think of a time in the past when you initially felt very anxious
but then found a way to calm yourself. What did you do that
helped you to be successful in calming yourself down?

In addition to past success questions, the practitioner can encourage a "coping dialogue" in which the practitioner helps the student identify past coping strategies that the student has found to be helpful in the past. Remember, "if it works, do more of it." Sometimes people don't readily recall things they have done in the past that were helpful. They need someone else to prompt them to explore and remember/identify previous coping strategies. This can be done by asking a simple coping question such as this:

Practitioner: When you are feeling anxious, what is your favorite thing to
do and which helps you relax a little bit?

This type of question encourages the student to identify things he/she has done in the past that have helped him/her. These identified exceptions and coping strategies help create an individualized map for the student, which can lead to more solutions and successes in the future.

5. Ask Scaling Questions

The *scaling question* is one of the most frequently utilized solution-focused techniques because it is easy to use, and it can be adapted to serve multiple purposes. For example, scaling questions can assess (a) how a student is feeling; (b) a student's commitment/investment in change; (c) a student's confidence about finding a solution; or (d) a student's progress toward implementing a solution. In addition, it can be used to assess different perceptions of the problem (or solution) as viewed by others such as teachers, parents, friends, and so on. Furthermore, a scaling question can help a student set goals by identifying what the student would be doing differently when things were going a little better in his/her life and the student moved up one number on the scale (McConkey, 2002).

Sometimes it is challenging for younger clients to provide verbal descriptions for how they are feeling especially during times of heightened emotions. On the other hand, the use of scaling questions is a non-threatening and easy way for the student to share things about him-/herself such as how he/she is currently feeling or has felt in the past. Surprisingly, a number on a scale can provide a great deal of information to the practitioner. For example, the solution-focused practitioner may ask Amal:

Practitioner: On a scale of "0" and "10", with "10" being extremely focused and "0" being the complete opposite, how would you rate your level of being focused today?

If Amal responds by saying "4," the practitioner then asks:

Practitioner: Can you think of a time when you felt a little more focused and you were a '5' instead of a '4' on this scale?

If Amal says yes, she will be asked additional follow-up questions such as this:

Practitioner: What is different between your "4" day and your "5" day?, What were you doing differently on your "5" day?, What else?, and so on.

If Amal struggles to identify differences between her "4" day and "5" day, Amal will be encouraged to look for even very small differences. The practitioner can also use prompts such as "What," "How," "Where," or "When" to gather as many details about the difference as possible. Using these questions, the practitioner helps Amal make these differences more observable and transferrable to other situations.

6. Identify Potential Challenges (aka "Flag the Minefield")

After Amal has identified exceptions and possible solutions to her problem, she is encouraged to "flag the minefield" (Sklare, 2014, p. 64). *Flagging the minefield* is a basic solution-focused technique designed to help prepare students for challenges they might encounter in the future when implementing their solutions. In addition, it is easier to think of effective strategies when the things are relatively calm instead of trying to come up with a solution in the heat of the moment. In this case, the solution-focused practitioner creates a scenario or two and asks Amal how she might respond to it and what coping strategies she might use. For example, the practitioner may ask:

Practitioner: Although you have identified some things that help you calm down, what will you do the next time you have multiple assignments due in the same week?

Amal and the solution-focused practitioner then work collaboratively to identify effective ways to overcome these challenges.

7. Provide Student With Direct and Indirect Compliments

Providing compliments to students is an effective method for highlighting and reinforcing students' strengths and resources. The solution-focused practitioners often use direct compliments and indirect compliments (Fiske, 2008). A *direct compliment* is a positive reaction or evaluation by the solution-focused practitioner in response to what the student has shared in a session. For example:

Practitioner: Wow Amal! From how you describe to me, you have been really busy with school, your part-time job, and watching your younger siblings, and yet you have also been able to complete several assignments on time.

An indirect compliment is presented in the form of a question. It invites the student to describe what he/she did that has led to a successful outcome. For example:

Practitioner: Wow Amal, how did you manage to focus and complete all of your assignments on time?

or

Practitioner: What did your teachers (parents) appreciate about how you approached completing all of your assignments?

Both types of compliments encourage Amal to reflect on her own competence. In addition, these compliments may encourage Amal to give herself a self-compliment when she explains how and what she did to make things happen. Compliments that are given near the end of a session can also serve the purpose of getting a student's attention and encouraging the student to become more receptive to carrying out therapeutic tasks after the session (Henden, 2008). For example:

Practitioner: Amal, a couple of things that really stands out to me from our conversation today is how determined you are to find things that help you focus more and help you complete your work on time. I am impressed by insightfulness because I know how important getting good grades are to you.

8. Provide Bridging Statements and Identify Tasks

As the solution-focused practitioner begins the process of wrapping up the session and has given Amal compliments, he/she will use *bridging statements*, which are linked to therapeutic tasks. Henden (2008) noted that a *bridging statement* often pertains to something that was discussed in the session and is then used to encourage the student to complete a small task (aka "homework") before the student's next session. The purpose of these identified tasks is to encourage the student to begin implementing small parts of his/ her solution. For example:

Practitioner: During our discussion today, you mentioned that you were able to focus a little more on your homework after you took your dog for a walk in our neighborhood. Is that something that you would be willing to do again this week?

The practitioner can also ask a Formula First Session Task such as this:

Practitioner: Between now and the next time we meet, I want you to look at what is happening at home, in class, and in your life that you would like to see continue happening (de Shazer & Molnar, 1984).

or

Practitioner: Pay attention to the times when you are feeling a little more relaxed and focused. Ask yourself what is different about those times? What are you doing during those times? Where are you? Who are you with?

9. Summarize and Wrap-Up Session

The session wrap-up/summary is an important part of the counseling process that should not be overlooked. Part of the session summary includes highlighting Amal's current coping skills and her past successes in dealing with challenging times. The practitioner also confirms with Amal therapeutic tasks that she plans to complete. Amal is also encouraged to co-summarize the session with the practitioner. Finally, this initial solution-focused counseling session is designed to build hope, to empower Amal, and to encourage further solution-building activities.

Multicultural Considerations

SFBC is inherently a culturally sensitive approach. Furthermore, SFBC assumptions and strategies help build strong therapeutic relationships with refugee and immigrant students and promote a respectful and empowering solution-building process. Here are brief explanations as to why several SFBC assumptions and strategies mentioned earlier in this chapter are culturally responsive.

1. *The solution-focused practitioner takes a non-expert and "not knowing" stance.* In SFBC, the practitioner is described as taking a *non-expert stance* and *leading from one step behind* (Pichot & Dolan, 2003). Furthermore, it is the client who is the expert of his/her life and is the one who identifies the goals for counseling. By taking a "not knowing" stance and not making assumptions, the practitioner invites the client to share how the client experiences and views the problem.

2. *SFBC is a collaborative strengths-based counseling approach, which seeks to empower clients through competence-seeking activities.* Instead of focusing on a client's problems, a solution-focused practitioner spends a significant amount of the session working collaboratively with the client to identify the client's past successes, strengths, resources, and coping strategies. In addition, competence-seeking activities help to minimize the shame a client may initially feel when he/she begins counseling and help the client gain a sense of empowerment (De Jong & Berg, 2008).

3. *SFBC is designed to be a short-term solution-building approach, which emphasizes the importance of the goal-setting process.* Since SFBC focuses on goal-setting and solution-building instead of concentrating on the client's problems, it may be the ideal fit for clients who may be anxious about seeking support outside of their families (Ali et al., 2004). In addition, some individuals may not even view SFBC as "therapy." Instead, they may associate SFBC as a fast and easy method for solving their problems (or finding solutions) with the assistance of a trained practitioner.

4. *Minimal self-disclosure about the client's past is needed, and the practitioner introduces the concept of pride in the counseling session.* As discussed earlier in this chapter, SFBC does not require a client to provide a detailed history of the client's problems and/or past trauma in a counseling session (De Jong & Berg, 2008). Instead of spending a significant amount of time in the session talking about "what happened to the student" (i.e.,

trauma), the majority of time in a SFBC session is focused on discussing "what the student did" to help him-/herself deal with the problem and/or trauma. By asking past success, exception-seeking, and coping questions, the solution-focused practitioner helps introduce the concept of *pride* into the conversation and encourages the client to identify things he/she feels proud for doing. Pride is a powerful protective and resiliency-building asset.

5. *Relationship questions help bring family and friends "into" the counseling session.* In some cultures, there is a strong interconnectedness and closeness within a client's family and/or community. By asking the *relationship question*, the practitioner helps include people who are important to the client in the counseling session even though they are not physically present in the room. For example, the practitioner may ask: "What would be the first thing your mother would notice you doing when you are feeling more focused?" or "What would your grandfather say is your greatest strength?"

Challenges and Solutions

Making the Solution-Focused Approach Developmentally Appropriate for Use With Children and Adolescents

When working with younger clients, it is important to use interventions that are developmentally appropriate. Even though SFBC is a good fit for use with children and adolescents, its techniques and questions sometimes need to be adapted for this population. Since children and some adolescents are concrete thinkers, they may struggle with "abstractions, such as exception-finding" and "applying exceptions to problem behavior" (Corcoran, 2002, p. 301). Here are a few examples of how to enhance solution-focused activities for younger clients who have not yet reached the formal operations developmental stage.

• Berg and Steiner (2003) recommend using creative solution-focused activities with children because they can help unleash children's resources. In addition, children naturally communicate through play so why not incorporate it into counseling sessions?

• King (2017 recommends adding an experiential component to scaling questions. She suggests using toys or other objects to "represent points along the scale" (p. 313). There are a wide variety of items that can be used such as buttons, nesting dolls, animal figurines, toy cars, trucks, planes, and so on. Children also love to use props such as a Hoberman sphere when asked to answer a scaling question. A Hoberman sphere is an isokinetic, expandable, geodesic dome structure, which has been turned into a colorful plastic children's toy. It comes in several sizes.

However, one of the popular sizes starts at 9.5 inches, expands to 30 inches, and then contracts back to 9.5 inches (refer to Wikipedia's "Hoberman Sphere"). Because it can also expand and contract over and over, the Hoberman sphere is also a good tool to use for "belly breathing" activities.

- De Jong and Berg (2008) recommend drawing activities because drawing can slow down the conversation and provide the child or adolescent an opportunity to think. In addition, drawing helps make thoughts and ideas more concrete and easier to share with the practitioner.
- Using whiteboards during a counseling session is a helpful tool, which encourages the client and the practitioner to co-create visual representations of the client's goals and solutions.
- Games such as Jenga, Pick-Up Stick, or Sorry can be turned into solution-focused activities with the simple addition of solution-focused questions (refer to Bannink's 1001 Solution-Focused Questions book).

Several books included in this chapter's Resources and References sections provide numerous examples of creative methods for adapting the solution-focused approach for use with children and adolescents.

Focusing on a Student's Strengths May Not Be Congruent With the Student's Culture

For some students, focusing on strengths may be contrary to their cultures' values such as humility. Instead of focusing on identifying the student's strengths, the culturally sensitive conversation can be shifted to identifying available resources within the student's life such as strong personal relationships, spiritual beliefs, or school activities. In addition, it may be difficult for the student to hear *direct compliments* from the solution-focused practitioner. One alternative would be to use *indirect compliments*, which encourage the student to identify actions he/she took that were helpful. For example, a practitioner could utilize an indirect compliment by asking, "Wow! How did you complete all of your assignments on time?"

Making the Miracle Question Culturally Sensitive

In certain situations, it may not be appropriate to ask the *miracle question* as it was originally worded. Using the word "miracle" may feel too religious for some students. However, there is an easy fix for this. Instead of encouraging a discussion about the student's miracle, the practitioner can ask the student about what they would be doing after they wake up and start having a "really awesome day." Even though the question's wording is a little different, similar information can be gathered from both versions of the miracle question.

Conclusion

Even though using SFBC with children and adolescents in school settings may present a few challenges, it can readily be adapted for this population. Through the use of carefully crafted questions, solution-focused practitioners help students identify their past successes, exceptions, coping skills, and resiliency. The true value of these questions is highlighted in the following adapted quote from French anthropologist, Claude Levi-Strauss:

The wise person is not the person who provides the right answers, but the one who asks the right questions.

Fortunately, the solution-focused approach provides the right questions for SBFC practitioners to ask.

Resources

Bannink, F. (2010). 1001 Solution-focused questions. W.W. Norton & Company.
    This book provides examples of 1001 solution-focused questions, which are categorized based on the purpose of the question.
Bannink, F. (2015). Solution-focused questions for help with trauma, 101. W.W. Norton & Company.
    This book provides useful examples of solution-focused questions that can be used when working with clients who have experienced trauma.
Berg, I. K., & Steiner, T. (2003). Children's solution work. W.W. Norton & Company.
    The authors provide numerous examples of creative solution-focused activities that are developmentally appropriate to use with children.
De Shazer, S. (1985). Keys to solutions in brief therapy. W.W. Norton & Company.
    This book provides an excellent overview about the solution-focused approach and how to use it effectively with clients.
Kim, J. S. (2014). Solution-focused brief therapy: A multicultural approach. Sage Publications.
    Contributors to this book provide practical applications of the solution-focused approach with a wide variety of clients from different cultural groups.
Kim, J. S., Kelly, M. S., & Franklin, C. (2017). Solution-focused brief therapy in schools: A 360-degree view of research and practice (2nd ed). Oxford University Press.
    This book provides examples of how to apply the solution-focused approach in several areas within a school setting.
Metcalf, L. (1995). Counseling toward solutions: A practical solution-focused program for working with students, teachers, and parents. Jossey-Bass.
    The author provides practical examples of how to use the solution-focused approach with students, teachers, and parents in school settings.
Murphy, J. J. (1997). Solution-focused counseling in middle and high schools. American Counseling Association.
    The author provides practical examples of how to use the solution-focused approach with middle and high school students.

Selekman, M. (1997). Solution-focused therapy with children: Harnessing family strengths for systemic change. Guilford Press.
This book provides creative and developmentally appropriate methods for adapting the solution-focused approach to use with children.

Sklare, G. B. (2005). Brief counseling that works: A solution-focused approach for school counselors and administrators (2nd ed.). Corwin Press.
The author provides numerous examples of how school counselors and administrators can apply the solution-focused approach to their work in schools.

YouTube Video

Arnoud Huibers' interview with Insoo Kim. http://www.youtube.com/watch?v=kWifZOBuxIU. Berg Publishers.
In this YouTube video, Arnoud Huibers interviews Insoo Kim Berg who helped develop the solution-focused approach.

Websites

Dr. Linda Metcalf's website: https://solutionfocusedschool.com/
Dr. Metcalf provides excellent free solution-focused resources and training webinars on her website.
Dr. Russell Sabella's website: https://schoolcounselor.com/
Dr. Sabella's website provides numerous free solution-focused resources for practitioners.

References

Ali, S. R., Liu, W. M., & Humedian, M. (2004). Islam 101: Understanding the religion and therapy implications. Professional Psychology: Research and Practice, 35(6), 635–642. https://doi.org/10.1037/0735-7028.35.6.635

Bannink, F. (2010). 1001 Solution-focused questions. W.W. Norton & Company.

Bannink, F. (2012). Practicing positive CBT: From reducing distress to building success. Wiley-Blackwell.

Berg, I. K. (1994). Family-based services: A solution-focused approach. W.W. Norton & Company.

Berg, I. K., & Miller, S. D. (1992). Working with the problem drinker: A solution-focused approach. W.W. Norton & Company.

Berg, I. K., & Steiner, T. (2003). Children's solution work. W.W. Norton & Company.

Birdsall, B. A., & Miller, L. D. (2002). Brief counseling in schools: A solution-focused approach for school counselors. Counseling and Human Development, 35(2), 1–10.

Corcoran, J. (2002). Developmental adaptations of Solution-Focused Family Therapy. Brief Treatment and Crisis Intervention, 2(4), 301–314. https://doi.org/10.1093/brief-treatment/2.4.301

De Jong, P., & Berg, I. K. (2008). Interviewing for solutions (3rd ed). Brooks/Cole.

de Shazer, S. (1988). Clues: Investigating solutions in brief therapy. W.W. Norton & Company.

de Shazer, S., Dolan, Y., Korman, H., Trepper, T., McCollum, E., & Berg, I. K. (2007). More than miracles: The state of the art solution-focused brief therapy. Hawthorne, FL.

de Shazer, S., & Molnar, A. (1984). Four useful interventions in brief family therapy. Journal of Marital and Family Therapy, 10(3), 297–304. https://doi.org/10.1111/j.1752-0606.1984.tb00020.x

Fiske, H. (2008). Hope in action: Solution-focused conversations about suicide. Routledge.

George, C. M. (2008). Solution-focused therapy: Strength-based counseling for children with social phobia. Journal of Humanistic Counseling, Education and Development, 47(2), 144–156. https://doi.org/10.1002/j.2161-1939.2008.tb00054.x

Gerrard, B. A., Carter, M. J., & Ribera, D. (2020). School-based family counseling: An interdisciplinary practitioner's guide. Routledge.

Henden, J. (2008). Preventing suicide: The solution-focused approach. John Wiley & Sons.

King, P. K. (2017). Tools for effective therapy with children and families: A solution-focused approach. Routledge.

Littrell, J. M., Malia, J. A., & Vander Wood, M. (1995). Single-session brief counseling in a high school. Journal of Counseling and Development, 73(4), 451–458. https://doi.org/10.1002/j.1556-6676.1995.tb01779.x

McConkey, N. (2002). Solving school problems: Solution-focused strategies for principals, teachers, and counselors. Solution Talk Press.

Murphy, J. J. (1994). Working with what works: A solution-focused approach to school behavior problems. School Counselor, 42, 59–68.

Murphy, J. J. (1997). Solution-focused counseling in middle and high schools. American Counseling Association.

Murphy, J. J. (2008, March). Solution-focused counseling in schools. Based on a program presented at the ACA Annual Conference and Exhibition. Retrieved June 27, 2008. http://counselingoutfitters.com/vistas/vistas08/Murphy.htm. Honolulu, HI.

Pichot, T., & Dolan, Y. M. (2003). Solution-focused brief therapy. Routledge. (leading from one step behind).

Sharry, J., Darmody, M., & Madden, B. (2002). A solution-focused approach to working with clients who are suicidal. British Journal of Guidance and Counselling, 30(4), 383–399. https://doi.org/10.1080/0306988021000025690

Sklare, G. B. (2005). Brief counseling that works: A solution-focused approach for school counselors and administrators (2nd ed). Corwin Press.

Sklare, G. B. (2014). Brief counseling that works: A solution-focused therapy approach for school counselors and other mental health professionals (3rd ed). Corwin Press.

9 A Trauma-Informed Approach to Help Immigrant and Refugee Children in Schools

Stephaney S. Morrison

Traumatic experiences can alter immigrant and refugee children's development and affect their academic, behavioral, and socio-emotional development. However, to help these children, school-based family counseling (SBFC) practitioners who work with immigrant and refugee children need to know how to recognize the impact of trauma and use a systemic approach by working with other professionals in the school and community to promote resilience in academics and socio-emotional development. The SBFC practitioner can lead other school staff to change the school culture and provide trauma-informed services to immigrant and refugee children, youth, and families. The principal purposes of this chapter are (a) to give a background of immigrant and refugee children who suffer from trauma, (b) to describe how SBFC practitioners can use a trauma-informed approach in the school system in partnership with all school staff from a whole school system perspective, (c) to discuss multicultural considerations, (d) to describe the challenges and solutions to applying the approaches in a school setting, and (e) to provide additional resources.

Background

Over the past decades, there have been increasing migration rates for children and families across international borders. In 2017 approximately 30 million children and youths under the age of 18 were forcibly displaced. Of this amount, 17 million have experienced violence or conflict in their home country, and approximately 13 million were eligible for refugee status (Sidhu, 2017). Many of these children experienced significant trauma before migration, through civil war or unrest, destructive effects of climate change, gang or drug-related violence, or poverty (Sidhu, 2017). Children also face vulnerability during the migration journey and may be the victims of physical or sexual abuse, unsafe travel conditions, separation from family members, and human trafficking (MacLean et al., 2019). Furthermore, upon arrival in new countries, immigrant youth and families may experience xenophobia and discrimination (Sidhu, 2017). While these children possess remarkable resilience and strength, the experiences of repeated and

DOI: 10.4324/9781003097891-12

prolonged exposure to trauma place them at risk for adverse academic and psychosocial outcomes. Trauma and toxic stress are associated with higher rates of depression, anxiety, and post-traumatic stress syndrome (PTSD), among other health-related issues. For this chapter, trauma is defined as a deeply distressing or disturbing experience that robs a person of a sense of power and control over his or her life. Mental health practitioners are aware that the guiding principle to recovery from trauma is to restore the power and control survivors have lost through their experiences.

When children experience trauma, their experiences can impact behavior inside and outside the classroom. Immigrant and refugee children often experience stressful or traumatic events that significantly impact their ability to function in school. Some students may be dealing with post-traumatic stress disorder from pre-migration experiences, such as homelessness, war, separation from parents or other close individuals, or dealing with the effects of being refugees. Other issues vary depending on the families' financial and/or social status (González et al., 2017). Immigrant and refugee children experience high rates of traumatic events before, during, and after migration, leading to inimitable mental health challenges for families, schools, and communities (González et al., 2017). However, some of these mental health issues can be mitigated if traumatized students are provided mental health and educational support in schools to improve psychosocial, behavioral, and academic functioning.

Trauma-Informed Interventions

There are many school mental health service providers for students in the school system. Among these are school social workers, school psychologists, drug and alcohol counselors, and outside mental health consultants. However, many of these practitioners are not part of the day-to-day operations of the school. Given the extent and nature of trauma exposure, it is critical that the primary individual supporting trauma-informed practices is physically present in the school daily, integrated within school routines, and has ongoing relationships with students, teachers, and staff. The SBFC practitioner is involved in individual and group counseling interventions, as well as other responses that take into consideration partnership with teachers, families, communities, and other school staff.

Importantly, given these criteria, the SBFC practitioner is well positioned to enact the American Institutes of Research's (2016) guiding principles for school-wide implementation of trauma-informed programs in five key domains: (a) supporting staff development; (b) creating a safe and supportive environment; (c) assessing needs and planning services; (d) involving consumers; and (e) adapting practices.

Finally, SBFC practitioners facilitate change in the school system by changing school culture, assessing policies, training staff, working with community partnerships, and assisting families. These tools help the SBFC practitioner accountable for the programs and services provided for students in the class-rooms and the entire school community. The trauma-informed approach allows SBFC practitioners to connect across the school to ensure a safe, inclusive environment with consistent policies and practices. SBFC practitioners emphasize using consultation and collaborative models to include staff members at every grade level to coordinate responsive services across all levels.

The Role of the SBFC Practitioner

The care required to support the development and success of immigrant and refugee children can overwhelm parents, who themselves are experiencing challenges based on their refugee and immigrant status. It requires knowledge of connected systems that include, but are not limited to, school, family, and community systems. Gerrard (2008) highlights the need for school-based family counseling (SBFC) due to the inadequacy of traditional school counseling and family counseling in supporting students who experienced difficulty in school. He further wrote (2008, p. 2):

> SBFC is an integrated approach to mental health intervention that focuses on both school and family in order to help children overcome personal problems and succeed at school. SBFC is practiced by a wide variety of mental health professionals, including: psychologists, social workers, school counselors, psychiatrists, and marriage and family therapists, as well as special education teachers. What they all share in common is the belief that children who are struggling in school can be best helped by interventions that link family and school.

Gerrard and Soriano (2013) have identified SBFC as a culturally responsive modality, effective with diverse populations. The SBFC practitioners work together from their specific expertise to provide effective solutions for students and their families in a school setting. Soriano (2017, pp. 4–5) made a compelling case about the convenience of utilizing the SBFC model in a school system.

> First, when services are brought to the school, they can be easily coordinated and monitored. This avoids duplication of services when different providers are working with the same child or family. It also helps to provide for a more streamlined and effective services plan. Second, when services are wrapped around the child and family's needs, gaps in service can be readily identified and addressed. Third, when multiple services are provided at the school site, children and families do not have to go from agency to agency for help. This convenience makes it more likely for them to follow through with referrals.

With the understanding that SBFC practitioners are critical allies in the school system, it is recommended that using a trauma-informed approach can be effective in working with immigrant and refugee children and their families. The following sections will discuss elements of the trauma-informed approach and how an SBFC practitioner can involve a whole school approach to work with immigrant and refugee children and families. The procedure section outlines how the SBFC practitioners can work across levels that integrate trauma-informed responsive services to students and families, such as classroom interventions, individual counseling, group counseling, community, and family engagements.

Procedure

Strength-Based Classroom Intervention

SBFC practitioners need to help traumatized children feel a sense of safety and teach them how to reconstruct a life that is not controlled by the traumatic experiences they have had in their homeland, en-route to the new host country, or while they are in the host country. The SBFC practitioner is encouraged to emphasize children's ability to bounce back and to be resilient in the face of their challenges. That is, children can deal with the experiences of the trauma they had encountered. In helping children through their traumatic experiences, the SBFC practitioner attends to the stories that children have based on their experiences. However, the SBFC practitioner will not dwell for very long on the details of the stories. The primary purpose of allowing children to tell their stories is to help children see the immense strengths they have despite conditions they have encountered and see the strengths that have kept them alive. Strength-based counseling is an approach that allows clients to identify what makes them able to cope with life challenges. Strengths are lenses we use to process information, experience others, view time and structure, accommodate to make change in our lives, and communicate with others (Jones-Smith, 2019).

Further, SBFC practitioners are aware that the guiding principle to recovery from trauma is to restore the power and control survivors have lost through their experiences. SBFC practitioners need to help traumatized children feel a sense of safety and teach them how to reconstruct a life that is not controlled by the traumatic experiences they have encountered. The SBFC practitioner, in his/her work with educators, is encouraged to emphasize children's ability to bounce back and to be resilient in the face of their challenges. Any interventions used are geared toward directing children to overcome the effects of psychological pain and experience safety. This is with the knowledge that trauma is manifested in various ways, such as excessive anger, unusual startle reaction, loss of appetite, physical/verbal aggression, defiance, alienation from peers, or troublemaking (González et al., 2017).

The following fictional case example is provided to illustrate the use of the trauma-informed strength-based approach with an immigrant student who has behavioral problems resulting from his experiences with instability at home and the violence he had encountered. The traditional mode of working with students in the school system is to employ a behavioral response as consequences. Trauma-informed interventions use a more positive response, taking into consideration that trauma influences how children behave. It is important to note that students who encounter trauma can respond negatively to punishment from a behavioral perspective. This case example in the next section provides an example of the trauma-informed cultural strength-based approach to working with a student. As a result of the whole school approach, the SBFC practitioner will also include responses in individual and group counseling, family engagement, community engagement, and resources that can meet the needs of students who have encountered trauma.

Case of Nayib

Nayib (a refugee student) is standing in the classroom when his class-mate Sam bumped into him. The students' eighth grade English teacher, Ms. Damon, heard Nayib and Sam yelling at one another and intervened just as Nayib punches Sam in the face. Ms. Damon and another teacher, Ms. Carter, stepped in to break up the fight. This has been the fifth time Nayib has been in a fight this school year. The strength-based approach helps educators and SBFC practitioners work with the students in a more culturally responsive way because of the knowledge of the impact of trauma on students' mental health and academics. (See Box 9.1).

Box 9.1   A Comparison of the Traditional Approach and the SBFC Trauma-Informed Strength-Based Approach

	Traditional approach	*SBFC trauma-informed strength-based approach*
Response	Ms. Damon and the other teacher verbally reprimanded Nayib and Sam and called the school resource officer. The boys are sent to the principal's office, and Ms. Damon returns to her classroom.	Ms. Damon and Ms. Carter separated the boys and brought them each to an empty classroom to calm them down. In the meantime Ms. Damon developed a relationship with Nayib, and once he was calmed down, she asked, "What's going on with you?" After a few minutes Nayib eventually opens up to her that he is feeling "on edge" due to instability in his home and violence he had experienced in his home country. While Ms. Damon met with Nayib, Ms. Carter calms Sam and began a conversation about his behavior.

	Traditional approach	SBFC trauma-informed strength-based approach
Action	Both students met with the principal who gathered the facts and determined that the level of severity of the alteration warranted a 3-day out-of-school suspension for Sam (as this was his first offense) and a 10-day out-of-school suspension for Nayib. Since Nayib is a repeat offender he was told that he will be expelled for his next offense. The parents were called in and told that the boys have a discipline problem.	After the individual conversations with the boys, Ms. Damon, Ms. Carter, Nayib and Sam met with the school principal. The boys were encouraged to apologize to each other. Additionally, in accordance with school policy each boy received an in-school suspension (ISS). ISS is a disciplinary technique, which is designed to penalize problem students for their behavior while still ensuring that they participate in the academic community in some way. Each boy will report to school in a special suspension classroom led by a teacher. The students serve the entirety of their suspension in that classroom, while completing assignments, homework, and so on. Sam received 3 days as this is his first offense, and Nayib received 6 days for his fifth offense.
Implications	Sam missed 3 days of class and Nayib missed 10 days. As a result, both boys fell behind in their classwork, and their grades suffer. Sam and Nayib felt that the school has negatively labeled them, and their parents began to feel that they are working in opposition to the school staff, as opposed to cooperating to better meet the children's needs.	During their time in ISS, Nayib and Sam are able to complete their classwork while receiving extra supports. Ms. Damon and the SBFC practitioner met with Nayib together during the ISS to discuss the instability at home and violence he experienced in his home country. They learned that Nayib was recently placed with his grandmother due to his parents' alcohol use problems. The SBFC practitioner reached out to the grandmother to involve her in developing a behavioral plan for Nayib at school, and Nayib was referred* to mental health services at a community non-profit. The SBFC practitioner also recommended an after-school program in the community that also provided mentoring for young immigrant boys focusing on social skills development and academic support.

*Most SBFC practitioners would provide the student with the mental health counseling at the school site as referred to later and only refer out if they (a) lacked skills or (b) wanted to refer the entire family for counseling.

Strength-Based Individual Counseling Intervention

Immigrant and refugee children have strengths that can be used to promote positive counseling outcomes. In the case of Nayib, in addition to the interventions utilized with the teachers, in partnership with the SBFC practitioner, the SBFC practitioner also conducts counseling sessions to explore trauma experiences, intending to identify strengths that Nayib can use at school and also to provide a safe space for him to explore his feelings about violence or abuse he encountered. The following box describes trauma-informed strength-based questions that can aid in attending to Nayib's story that can delineate his experience with trauma (see Box 9.2).

SBFC practitioners need to be aware that while they are counseling someone like Nayib, there is a possibility that he could be re-traumatized if he is forced to share information about traumatic events prematurely. Therefore, it is recommended to work within the "window of tolerance": that is, the practice of sharing emotions within a tolerable range (Miller et al., 2019). Exceeding the window of tolerance too quickly can result in unacceptable levels of emotional pain and is unlikely to be therapeutic. Utmost sensitivity is important to his healing. With guided questions that place ownership on the client (Nayib), it gives him control of his narrative and empowers him to only share information that he feels comfortable sharing or avoid sharing

---

Box 9.2 An Example of Trauma-Informed Strength-Based Individual Counseling With Nayib

Strength-based approach goal	Examples of strength-based questions to promote discussion
To gather information about family and self	• Tell me a little bit about yourself. • What are some things that you're really proud of? • What is something you're good at? • What do you like best about your family?
To gather information about systems support	• If something difficult were to happen, who would be available to help you? • If something really good were to happen, who would be cheering for you?
To acknowledge accomplishments	• I'm so glad to hear that you are fighting less— that's wonderful! That's a really challenging task. • I can tell that you are really trying to form friendships and are motivated to fit in with your peers. You should be really proud of your hard work.
To acknowledge specific strengths	• That's pretty great that you play football. It's a huge advantage when looking for extra curricula activity—make sure you try out at the upcoming trials.

details that cause stress. It is recommended that the SBFC practitioner share with Nayib why they are asking for information, followed by request to ask additional questions. For example,

> I want to make sure that we're giving you the best care possible. To make sure I understand your history, I would like to ask a few additional questions about your family experiences before, after, and currently in your journey. Is that okay with you?
>
> (Miller et al., 2019)

As the SBFC practitioner works with Nayib the SBFC practitioner should validate him for his experiences and emotions.

3. Trauma-Informed Interventions for Younger Children

A number of creative activities can be adapted when working with young immigrant and refugee children who have suffered trauma. These activities include art, dramatization, pantomiming, puppetry, role-playing, and written responses. It is important to consider how to work with all children, including those children who cannot read. For children who can read, the SBFC practitioner can include books in their language. Books that meet language needs can be used to allow students to read aloud, construct collages, and compose letters to a book character as valuable activities to engage students on a more personal level with the story. For those children who cannot read, resources such as videos in the language of choice can allow them to learn language responses that represent how they are feeling. In addition to creative activities, the SBFC practitioner can use questioning to help children identify with the characters, recognize their coping strategies, and relate the story to their own experiences. Nicholas and Pearson (2003) provide some guidelines as to how SBFC practitioners can ask questions when working with students:

- What are some of the things that you like most about this book?
- Who would like to draw a picture of a favorite character?
- Who can say something or make a noise like a character?
- If you could be like one of the characters, who would it be?
- What do you think you'll remember about this story?

4. Strength-Based Group Counseling Intervention

The SBFC practitioner can also conduct weekly group sessions with Nayib and other students who have suffered trauma by utilizing trauma-informed counseling questions to identify the students' (clients') strengths. Group counseling allows students to normalize their situation within the safety of a group context with other group members who have experienced trauma. In this group, students share their stories, gain support, and engage with each other through trauma-informed conversations and activities (see Box 9.3).

**Box 9.3   An Example of Trauma-Informed
Group Counseling With Nayib**

Example of trauma-informed strength-based questions in a group
counseling session

- Share experiences you have had with negative experiences in
  your home country and at home.
- Can you share some of those experiences or memories?
- What memories are most difficult for you to remember?
- Did you leave any family members behind?
- Tell us a little bit about those you have left behind? How do you
  feel about leaving them behind?
- What did you do when you experienced negative experiences in
  your country? Who did you talk to when you wanted to feel better?
- What did you do when you experienced negative experiences?
- How would you like to feel better from these experiences?
- What support can I give to you?

---

5. Strength-Based Trauma-Informed School Culture and Infrastructure

A trauma-informed school uses a whole systems approach that includes teachers, administrators, and the SBFC practitioner who work from a strengths perspective that promotes healing and dispels deficit views of children and youth. Creating a trauma-sensitive, safe, and supportive school requires a paradigm shift by practitioners in the school, such as teachers, administrators, and school staff. It also involves changing the whole school system by transforming the school culture, building supporting infrastructure, and altering curriculum content and interventions. For example, SBFC practitioners can follow the following guidelines suggested by Cole et al. (2009) to promote trauma-informed approaches school-wide:

- Prepare strategic planning
- Provide staff with training that addresses trauma issues and strengthen relationships between staff, traumatized students, and families
- Confidentially review and plan for individual cases
- Review policies (e.g., school discipline policies) to ensure they reflect an understanding of the role of trauma in students' behaviors
- Partner with appropriate community providers to identify and access supports
- Evaluate these efforts on an ongoing basis
- SBFC practitioners can guide teachers to attend to instruction for students, such as building on academic competencies, providing safe structure, language-based teaching, and providing support for students' speech and psychological needs.

6. Community Resources for Trauma-Sensitive Intervention

Partnerships with other individuals and agencies in your area outside of the school can be an invaluable resource for refugee and immigrant youths who are traumatized. Immigrant and refugee youth and their families may have past experiences of trauma that impact their trust or engagement with various services and may be unfamiliar with how to access services in an unfamiliar environment. The SBFC practitioners may be the first professionals to interact with immigrants and refugee youth and families and, as such, can play a vital role in bridging interrelated systems and services. SBFC practitioners can advocate for students and partner with other practitioners to create a community-based support system for students and their families. For example:

- Connecting with experts in immigration law, counselors, and psychologists practicing trauma-informed mental health care in the youth or caregivers' first language, community centers for community building and physical activity, and resources for nutritious food and safe housing.
- Legal assistance, in particular, can be helpful if immigrants are undocumented. Children and adolescents who live with undocumented family members have been shown to have high anxiety levels about the fear of deportation. Lack of documentation can result in additional barriers resulting in poorer psychosocial outcomes.
- Thus, it is crucial to refer to low-cost or free legal services to promote health for the entire family.

7. Trauma-Informed Family Engagement Intervention

SBFC practitioners have potential opportunities to engage parents and children with services that would benefit them. When children and youth complete the transnational journey with most of the close family, remember that each family member has experienced the same traumatic events (war, extreme poverty, persecution, and so on). Parents are one of the most protective factors for children in surviving stress and trauma. Supportive and consistent relationships with a caring adult can protect children from the negative impacts of trauma (Toppelberg & Collins, 2010). Given the role parents and caretakers play in managing childhood trauma, SBFC practitioners should extend their service to caregivers by supporting parents in navigating a new and unfamiliar education system. Doing so will ensure that they can access the same services by connecting them to community providers, such as social workers or community mental health practitioners. When parents and caregivers are empowered and find a community of support, they are invaluable for the trauma-sensitive healing of their children and adolescents.

Multicultural Considerations

Culturally responsive SBFC practitioners are familiar with, and respect, their students' culture, language, and trauma experiences. This level of awareness creates pathways for understanding strengths through awareness of (a) knowledge of the life experiences of migrant/refugee children who are traumatized and the long-term effects of trauma on the children, families, communities, and professionals who work with them and (b) gaining cultural skills or competence with traumatized children (The Center for Victims of Torture, 2005). All of these principles are incorporated into a trauma-informed approach when working with refugees and immigrants. By adopting a trauma-informed approach, educators and SBFC practitioners undertake a paradigm shift at the school level to recognize, understand, and address children's learning and behavioral needs impacted by trauma. This also includes a commitment to shaping the school culture related to discipline practices and policies sensitive to the needs of the traumatized students. The essential competencies for culturally responsive counseling and teaching can be grouped into three categories: (a) awareness, (b) attitudes, and (c) skills. Culturally responsive SBFC practitioners (a) are aware of their values and biases, (b) develop knowledge of students' cultural backgrounds, and (c) gain skills to work with students.

Challenges and Solutions

Although the trauma-informed model has been widely accepted and has shown promise in working with immigrants and refugee students, some challenges may impede the trauma-informed work in the school system. Several ideas on how SBFC practitioners can work with other practitioners is to understand the challenges and anticipate culturally specific solutions:

- Systemic Inequality: Most refugees experienced extreme conflict and persecution in their home country, yet they may not understand the inequality in the host country. Schools can mitigate the ramification of inequality and discrimination by teaching students about the history of racism and oppression in the host country. Schools cannot deny that discrimination and inequality will impact students in their daily lives. Teachers can engage students in engaging activities so that their awareness can be heightened about these challenges and how to confront them. One way to do this is to include in their reading list books on persons from different cultures and the challenges they face.
- Connections to Diverse Peers: Social connection is critical in all students' development. This developmental phase is especially helpful to immigrants and refugees who are still developing socially and need to be integrated into schools with students who are similar to them, as well as with peers who are long-time residents or native-born, who may be of different socioeconomic or racial backgrounds. These connections can build the kind of social capital that is vital to students' post-school opportunities.

- Culturally Aware Teachers: Most teachers in the school system are White, relatively affluent women with limited experience teaching immigrants and refugees and may not know how to prepare refugees and immigrant children to deal with and navigate poverty, racism, and xenophobia. Schools with refugee students must actively recruit more teachers with backgrounds and experiences similar to their refugee students. They can also seek opportunities through after-school programs, internships, and visiting speakers to connect students with adults who can help them navigate barriers they will face post high school.

Other challenges that are equally important to consider when SBFC practitioners are working with immigrant and refugee students are the following:

- Differences in School. The host country's education system may not be easy to understand for immigrants or refugee families, particularly those for whom English is a second language. Many families may have waited years in refugee camps with limited access, if any, to education. Even for those with formal education before resettlement, the host country's education system often differs widely from what they knew. From the requirements made of students, parents, and teachers, the curricula and school structures, to lockers, textbooks, computers, and desks; from school bells and fire alarms to classroom changes and cafeterias, all may be new. Adjusting to such changes in their environment is a daunting task.
- Linguistic Challenges. A simple instruction from the teacher can be quite complex for refugee students. It takes time to translate what the teacher said, figure out the English names of the animals, and write the names of the animals in an unfamiliar alphabet. Refugee students have to take these extra steps constantly to keep pace with their peers all during the school day.

From the first day refugee students arrive in the host country, they are constantly learning English. Most refugee students have separate English for Speakers of Other Languages (ESL) classes built into their school day, which helps advance their skills. Still, other subjects, such as math and social studies, are typically taught in English. The first year is extremely challenging as they struggle to understand what people around them are saying and how to communicate their thoughts and ideas.

- Bullying. Developing positive peer relationships is crucial, yet refugee students may have difficulties making friends in schools. They might be teased and bullied for differences in how they speak, dress, or look or for behaviors unfamiliar to the host country. Often, such situations can escalate into physical fights or leave refugee students in constant fear. Persistent bullying and teasing are difficult to endure daily and can lead some refugee youth to drop out of school. Schools can emphasize anti-bullying programs in the school system and model good behaviors in the classrooms.

- Family Pressures and Dropout. The entire family copes with many changes while refugees adjust to their new environment. Refugee students are acutely aware of their parents' challenges in seeking employment, learning English, or understanding medical, transportation, and school systems, all the while keeping the family together. Since children tend to pick up new languages quicker than their parents, they may take on the role of interpreters for their parents. This adds to the pressure refugee students experience. They may miss class to help their parents or be privy to information not usually discussed with children, such as medical and financial situations. As a result, refugee children often assume a more adult role than they would if interpretation services were provided or circumstances were different. Older refugee youth appear to be particularly vulnerable to family pressures, especially those of working age. Although refugee parents often place great importance on education, some refugee high school students may drop out because they feel obliged to help with family expenses and taking care of younger siblings. Schools can collaborate with community partners who may offer sliding scale or free child care services to low-income or immigrant families. Additionally, there may be government programs and assistance that families can access but are not aware that they are available to them. It is vital to bridge the gap between school and families to know what challenges they face and how the school can help them negotiate for children's academic and socio-emotional development.

Conclusion

In this chapter, the trauma-informed approach was introduced as an effective mode of practice for SBFC practitioners in the school system who work with immigrants and refugees impacted by trauma. The chapter explained the role of the SBFC practitioners, discussed how students and families are impacted by trauma, and provided procedure on how this approach can be implemented via classroom, individual, and group counseling. The chapter also discussed possible challenges and solutions and provided resources that practitioners can use to help them better understand how to work with this vulnerable population in the school system.

Resources

American School Counselor Association. (2016). The school counselor and trauma informed practice. http://www.schoolcounselor.org/asca/media/asca/Position-Statements/PS_ TraumaInformed.pdf
  The American School Counselor Association website indicates the position statement about the importance of trauma-informed work in the school.
American Institutes of Research. (2016). Trauma-informed care in service systems. https://www.air.org/resource/trauma-informed-care-service-systems

National Institute of Mental Health. (2017). Coping with traumatic events. http://www. nimh.nih.gov/health/topics/coping-with-traumatic-events/index.shtml
This website gives practitioners information and resources about trauma and coping.

Bibliography

American institute for research. (2016). Trauma informed care curriculum. http://www. air.org/resource/traumainformed-care-curriculum

Center for Victims of Torture. (2005). Working with torture survivors: Core competencies. In Healing the heart: A guide for developing services for torture survivors. http://www.cvt.org/main.php/healingthehurt (pp. 20–49).

Cole, S. F., O'Brien, J. G., Gadd, M. G., Ristuccia, J., Wallace, D. L., & Gregory, M. (2009). Helping traumatized children learn: Supportive school environments for children traumatized by family violence. Massachusette Advocates for Children.

Gerrard, B. (2008). School-based family counseling overview, trends, and recommendations for future research. International Journal for School-Based Family Counseling, 1(1), 1–30. http://dx.doi.org.arktos.nyit.edu/10.1108/AEDS-01-2015-0002

Gerrard, B., & Soriano, M. (2013). School-based family counseling: An overview. In B. Gerrard & M. Soriano (Eds.). http://dx.doi.org.arktos.nyit.edu/10.1108/AEDS-01-2015-0002, School-based family counseling: Transforming family-school relationships (pp. 2–15). Institute for School-Based Family Counseling.

González, J. J., Kula, S. M., González, V. V., & Paik, S. J. (2017). Context of Latino students' family separation during and after immigration: Perspectives, challenges, and opportunities for collaborative efforts. School Community Journal, 27(2), 211–228.

Howell, P. B., Thomas, S., Sweeney, D., & Vanderhaar, J. (2019). Moving beyond schedules, testing and other duties as deemed necessary by the principal: The school counselor's role in trauma informed practices. Middle School Journal, 50(4), 26–34. https://doi.org/10.1080/00940771.2019.1650548

Jones-Smith, E. (2019). Culturally diverse counseling: Theory and practice. SAGE.

MacLean, S. A., Agyeman, P. O., Walther, J., Singer, E. K., Baranowski, K. A., & Katz, C. L. (2019). Mental health of children held at a United States immigration detention center. Social Science and Medicine, 230, 303–308. https://doi.org/10.1016/j.socscimed.2019.04.013

Miller, K. K., Brown, C. R., Shramko, M., & Svetaz, M. V. (2019). Applying trauma-informed practices to the care of refugee and immigrant youth: 10 Clinical pearls. Children, 6(8), 3–11. https://doi.org/10.3390/children6080094

Nicholas, J., & Pearson, Q. (2003). Helping children cope fears: Using children's literature in classroom guidance. Professional School Counseling, 7(1), 15–19.

Sidhu, S. S. (2017). Impact of recent executive actions on minority youth and families. Journal of the American Academy of Child and Adolescent Psychiatry, 56(10), 805–807. https://doi.org/10.1016/j.jaac.2017.07.779

Smith, E. J. (2006). The Strength-Based Counseling Model. Counseling Psychologist, 34(1), 134–144. https://doi.org/10.1177/0011000005282364

Soriano, M. (2017). When leadership and vision fail: The dismantling of a school-based family counseling leadership program. http://www.instituteschoolbasedfamilycounseling.com/journal.html (pp. 4–5). International Journal of School-based Family Counseling

Toppelberg, C. O., & Collins, B. A. (2010). Language, culture, and adaptation in immigrant children. Child and Adolescent Psychiatric Clinics of North America, 19(4), 697–717. https://doi.org/10.1016/j.chc.2010.07.003

10 A Holistic, Strengths–Based Approach to Mental Health Intervention Development and Implementation for Immigrant and Refugee Students

Maisha M. Syeda, Natasha Robinson-Link, Claire V. Crooks, and Sharon Hoover

The chapter focuses on the co–development of a program and a system–wide implementation model of a resilience-enhancing, school-based mental health intervention (falling in the "school intervention" quadrant of school-based family counseling [SBFC] meta-model; see Figure 1.2) for immigrant and refugee students, Supporting Transition Resilience of Newcomer Groups (STRONG; [Hoover, 2019]). STRONG has been implemented in Ontario (Canada), New York, Illinois, and Massachusetts. The chapter describes the rationale and processes for the co–development of STRONG, details the training and procedure for STRONG, and highlights the culturally responsive initiatives and strategies incorporated to create a holistic and strengthening experience for immigrant and refugee students participating in STRONG. The chapter concludes with a list of resources associated with STRONG.

Background

Supporting the mental health of immigrant and refugee students and families is now being recognized as a public health priority in high–income countries. In Canada, for example, between January 2015 and March 2018, nearly 100,000 refugees resettled, and among them, 42.7% were under the age of 18 (Miller & Rasmussen, 2017). Immigrant and refugee students have many strengths and exhibit resilience. Yet refugee students are at higher risk of developing mental health issues due to the many stressors and traumas they are exposed to throughout their migration journey (Durà-Vilà et al., 2013; Fazel et al., 2009;Miller & Rasmussen, 2017). Immigrant and refugee students may face many post-migration stressors, like acculturation, language differences, separation from families, uncertainty about status, and racism. These stressors and traumas may impair immigrant and refugee students' mental health functioning, underscoring the need for culturally responsive

DOI: 10.4324/9781003097891-13

and accessible interventions to address their psychosocial needs and bolster coping skills to ease their transition to schools and related settings.

Existing School-Based Interventions With Immigrant and Refugee Students

The UN Convention on the Rights of the Child emphasizes the urgent need to develop interventions to support trauma, healing, and resilience promotion among immigrant and refugee youth populations (Hettich, 2020). However, there is limited published literature on school-based mental health interventions specifically designed to support immigrant and refugee youth who have experienced multiple traumas (Fazel, 2015). Of those mental health interventions reported in the literature, many were evaluated with refugee youth. They primarily employed cognitive behavioral or narrative strategies to promote resilience, adaptive coping, and overall well-being Sullivan & Simonson, 2016; Tyrer & Fazel, 2014).

There are effective school-based interventions for students with a history of trauma and adversity (e.g., Cognitive Behavioural Intervention for Trauma in Schools [CBITS]; Jaycox et al., 2012). These interventions primarily aim to decrease trauma and psychopathological symptoms in participants. However, there are problems with exclusively using the Westernized trauma model to design and deliver interventions with immigrant and refugee youth (Bracken, 2002; Summerfield, 1999). Cultural factors could influence youth's reaction and experiences with trauma. Scholars and clinical experts of immigrant and refugee mental health have promoted a shift away from using trauma processing as the central mechanism of action for resettlement interventions and toward therapeutic processes that foster strength, capacity, and resilience. Specifically, resettlement intervention models are called to acknowledge immigrant and refugee students' inner capacity and strengths to cope with their suffering and the external supports and relationships they had that contributed to their psychosocial recovery and growth during and post traumas (Gozdziak, 2004).

Development of a New Intervention

In response to the increasing number of students arriving in Canadian schools displaced from Syria, there was a provincial effort in Ontario, Canada, during 2015–2016 to monitor, assess, and respond to the mental health needs of these student populations (Crooks, Smith et al., 2020). Specifically, the Ontario Ministry of Education asked the School Mental Health Ontario (SMHO), an intermediary organization that supports mental health programming in 72 publicly funded school boards, to provide universal, school-wide, Tier 1 resources and strategies to create welcoming and safe environments for refugee students. Over time, mental health professionals in Ontario schools recognized that many refugee students were exhibiting signs of distress in schools for whom these universal resources and strategies were not sufficient: more specific mental health services individualized to the transitional needs of these students were needed. In alignment with the SBFC meta-model emphasizing integrating multitiered school-based mental health services (i.e., school-based preventions versus interventions), it was urgent to have a Tier 2 group intervention in Ontario schools for the refugee student populations (Crooks, Smith et al., 2020). Tier 2 interventions teach preventative strategies to promote healthy coping and problem-solving skills among students at risk of possibly developing psychosocial disorders (Fazel et al., 2014).

To address the need for unique Tier 2 intervention for immigrant and refugee students, SMHO collaborated with the co-director (one of the co-authors of the chapter) of the National Centre for School Mental Health (NCSMH) at the University of Maryland to explore possible options for structured programming. The exploration phase involved consulting the existing literature on evidence-based strategies developed for immigrant and refugee students and school-based mental health programs addressing trauma, psychosocial distress, and resilience. As inferred from the earlier sections, the cross-agency literature review conducted by SMHO and the NCSMH team did not locate any interventions conceptually developed to address pre-and-post-migration resilience for immigrant and refugee youth. Due to the gaps in the literature and obvious needs in schools, a collaborative team was established to co-develop a manualized, group intervention, STRONG (Hoover, 2019). The development team engaged a multidisciplinary team that consisted of researchers, immigrant and refugee community members, and school- and community-based mental health professionals servicing immigrant and refugee youth to co-develop STRONG.

STRONG Description

The STRONG intervention is a Tier 2, group, ten-session manualized intervention that aims to strengthen immigrant and refugee youth's resilience and reduce distress following their transition to the resettlement country. The principles of SFBC center on a child advocacy approach in which professionals collaborate with different social systems (e.g., schools, families) to create structures, resources, and equitable opportunities and aim for the child to be empowered (Gerrard & Soriano, 2019). Similarly, the development of the STRONG program centered on an advocacy principle to highlight the strengths and resilience of immigrant and refugee students instead of having the predominant focus on "fixing" their challenges that might have resulted from pre- and post-migrations stressors and adversities. Like the SBFC advocacy approach, the STRONG program asserts that enhancing children's strengths and resilience is essential to their positive development and empowerment.

STRONG takes a holistic, strength-based approach in supporting immigrant and refugee youth to identify their inner strengths to cope with their distress and recognize the external supports and relationships they have that would help their psychosocial healing and growth (Crooks, Kubishyn et al., 2020). Table 10.1 details the overview, objectives, and structure of the STRONG program. STRONG has two manuals: one for elementary students (5–12 ages) and another for secondary students (13–18; Hoover, 2019). Both manuals feature the same topics and core concepts, but the activities and language have been adapted to meet each age group's developmental needs, interests, and capacities. The developers recommend that STRONG be implemented by licensed mental health professionals such as school psychologists, mental health counselors, and social workers. See Table 10.1 and Table 10.2.

Following the launch, STRONG was piloted in two Ontario school boards in 2018 and 2019. The pilot evaluations collectively suggest that participants in STRONG learned important coping skills (e.g., relaxation skills), enhanced their resilience, developed a sense of belonging in schools, and accessed an accepting and interactive space to make friends (Crooks, Kubishyn et al., 2020). Furthermore, school mental health professionals implementing STRONG saw clear benefits for students and reported professional and personal benefits (Crooks, Hoover et al., 2020). School mental health professionals implementing STRONG indicated learning new therapeutic strategies to support students with stress and trauma and perceived increases in their confidence to support students in developing and processing personal narratives to build resilience. They indicated enjoyment and appreciation in having the opportunity to connect with immigrant and

Table 10.1 STRONG: Overview, Objectives, and Structure

Overview	• A school-based group intervention that aims to promote resilience and reduce psychological distress among refugee and immigrant children and youth
Objectives	• Understanding and normalizing distress
	• Building resilience and coping skills (e.g., relaxation skills, switching to helpful thoughts)
	• Teaching goal-setting and problem-solving skills
	• Increasing positive sense of identity and buffering from impact of racism and xenophobia
	• Identifying inner strengths and outside supports that helped to cope before, during, and after migration journeys
	• Creating a safe and welcoming space with students who might share similar lived experiences
	• Supporting teachers and parents in understanding the transition experience of immigrant and refugee children and youth
Structure	• Ten, 1-hour group sessions, facilitated by licensed school mental health professionals (e.g., social workers, school psychologists)
	• One additional, individual session with each STRONG participant to help them take a strength-based approach to process their journey narrative
	• One teacher/interpreter and one parent/caregiver group informational session

refugee students, hear about their migration journeys, and learn about their cultures and lived experiences. Currently, SMHO offers STRONG training to all Ontario school boards, and its delivery and evaluation have been extended to New York, Illinois, and Massachusetts.

Procedures

The STRONG program has the flexibility to be delivered in different settings, including schools, hospitals, and community organizations. The development team reviewed existing school-based mental health interventions that have been effectively scaled up in numerous school boards (e.g., CBITS) in the United States to structure STRONG's length and session duration in efforts for easier integration in schools. STRONG has also been implemented in a community-based resource center for immigrant youth and families and delivered virtually since the onset of Covid-19.

Training and Implementation in Ontario

SMHO provides training and implementation consultations to support school boards across Ontario to implement STRONG. Initially, mental health leaders and clinical supervisors of mental health professionals in Ontario school boards were invited to assess their needs for immigrant and refugee support services and their existing capacity to deliver STRONG. This initial assessment aimed to determine whether their mental health professionals should participate in one of the annual STRONG trainings. Mental health leaders are senior mental health professionals in an Ontario school board responsible for coordinating the board's mental health strategy (Short, 2016). To implement the STRONG program in a new school district, we recommend that school administrators and mental health service managers engage in an initial need and capacity assessment to determine whether they will train their licensed school mental health professionals in STRONG.

The SMHO collaborates with the STRONG developers to train licensed mental health professionals working in Ontario schools. SMHO also partners with cultural brokers to enhance trainees' awareness of and preparation to engage in culturally responsive ways to implement STRONG (see details in the section on Cultural Considerations). The training modules include providing information about migration and settlement patterns and pathways to Canada, trauma experienced during pre-, during, and post-migration, and an orientation to the STRONG manual (Crooks, Hoover et al., 2020). Then trainees are divided into elementary and secondary groups to walk through each STRONG session and participate in relevant role-plays and small-group interactive discussions.

A specific component of STRONG training involves supporting mental health leaders and clinical supervisors of the participating Ontario school boards to support their school mental health professionals and schools in implementing STRONG. Specifically, SMHO and the STRONG training team provide consultation on building partnerships with school administrators (e.g., principals), teachers, and school-based settlement workers. These consultations aim to establish referral pathways for STRONG and promote the program's overall acceptability in schools for smoother implementation processes. The final component of STRONG training offers a planning session for school boards to (a) create tentative timelines for program delivery, (b) identify potential schools where STRONG could be implemented based on needs and interests, and (c) consider barriers or challenges to be addressed before or during STRONG delivery.

SMHO offers consultation support and resources to school boards and STRONG facilitators (i.e., licensed school mental health professionals implementing the program) to improve implementation successes and the program's impact on immigrant and refugee students. Three community of practice calls are arranged during the implementation of STRONG to consult with experts (e.g., developers, evaluators, previous implementers). Mental health leaders and clinical supervisors also have the opportunity to have regular consultations with SMHO to seek clinical support, share programming experiences, and problem-solve implementation challenges. In summary, Box 10.1 also describes the procedural steps and considerations for school boards before STRONG delivery to support schools in optimizing both student impacts and implementation successes of the program.

Box 10.1 STRONG: Pre-implementation Planning and Considerations for School Boards

1. Assess the school board's need

   • Prevalence and mental health supports needed for immigrant and refugee students.
2. Evaluate the school board's capacity
   • Availability, professional experience and preparedness, and workload of licensed school mental health professionals
   • Funding and resources (e.g., private space in schools).
3. Train licensed school mental health professionals on STRONG.
4. Identify schools, establish corresponding timelines for STRONG delivery, and determine referral procedures to identify STRONG students.
5. Engage with school administrators, teachers, school settlement workers, and counselors to familiarize them about STRONG and identify their roles and scopes to optimize STRONG success on students and school well-being.

Create board-level consultation opportunities and community of practice calls for licensed school mental health professionals implementing STRONG.

Implementing STRONG

Group Sessions. Table 10.2 lists the materials and logistics to run the STRONG program in schools. Each group session for STRONG has the following components: (a) conduct check-in and icebreaker activity, (b) practice the relaxation activity from the previous session, (c) teach core concepts and facilitate relating activities and discussions, (d) introduce and practice a new relaxation activity. In addition to these cognitive-behavioral interventions, STRONG sessions are grounded in resilience and socio-therapy frameworks. These frameworks help students identify their internal strengths and external resources to problem-solve, learn, practice, and integrate new coping strategies in their daily lives while simultaneously providing peer support in the STRONG space to help each other learn (Crooks, Kubishyn et al., 2020). Box 10.2 lists the STRONG group session topics.

Table 10.2 STRONG: Implementation Materials and Logistics

Materials	Logistics
• STRONG manuals • STRONG certificate for students • Print-outs of programming materials (e.g., relaxation scripts, visuals) • Participant worksheets • Parent and teacher letters	• Creating a referral procedure (e.g., a referral form) to identify potential students who may benefit from STRONG • Interpreters, if needed • Private space in the school for the sessions • Peer consultation for STRONG facilitators (if possible)

Box 10.2   Topics of STRONG Group Sessions

Session 1: My Inside Strengths and Supports
Session 2: Understanding Stress
Session 3: Common Stress Reactions and Identifying Thoughts
Session 4: Measuring and Managing Feelings
Session 5: Using Helpful Thoughts
Session 6: Steps to Success
Session 7: Problem-Solving
Session 8: My Journey Part I
Session 9: My Journey Part II
Session 10: Graduation

Group Sessions

Individual Session

The purpose of the individual journey narrative session is to engage immigrant and refugee students in a strength-based approach to cohesively reflect and re-construct their personal narratives of their migration journey and pre- and post-migration experience. The SBFC practitioner (i.e., the STRONG facilitator) guides students in an interactive conversation with structured questions to help students identify inner strengths and outside supports that helped them navigate difficult situations and reflect on how they have grown and built resilience from those experiences (Hoover, 2019). The SBFC practitioner then supports the student in choosing a part of the narrative they would like to share with the group. The SBFC practitioner also screens students for post-traumatic stress disorder (PTSD) and makes referrals for more intensive community- or school-based services if necessary. We provide a sample script from a segment of the journey narrative conversation between a facilitator and a student here.

The SBFC practitioner begins the session by familiarizing the student with the rationale and intended objectives of sharing stories of the student's migration journey.

SBFC practitioner:	I would first really like to hear a little bit about your time in Syria and some of the things you enjoyed or liked about Syria.
Student:	Yeah, I miss Syria so much. I used to live in the same building with my cousins and we really enjoyed our time. We went to school together and then sometimes we did our homework together.
SBFC practitioner:	You lived in apartments with your cousins and I know you probably played with them. What are some of the things that you played and did with them?
Student:	Yeah, we were in the same building. We would go to the park together and, you know, to have those family gatherings. And we had, like, a big family of cousins and friends.
SBFC practitioner:	So you had a lot of good times and family support and a lot of things that you miss about Syria.
Student:	Absolutely. Because we were together and we were going through the same kind of difficult times. I'm glad we were all together. Nobody died.
SBFC practitioner:	Yeah. Tell me a little bit about some of the difficult times that you went through that kind of led up to you leaving Syria.

Student:	Bombings went on and on for so long. But then there was like this very intense month when it became so intense. It [bombings] was close to where we lived. So, everybody had to go to the basement and stay there. We had to stay there for like over 30 days. Everybody would come down. Some buildings didn't have basements, so they would come to us.
SBFC practitioner:	They [people from other buildings] would come to stay with you?
Student:	Yeah. And all the children were crying. And it was very, very hard. And we never know if we're going to go out, if we still have our home or not. So, it was very, very scary.
SBFC practitioner:	I'm sure it was scary. You must have been really brave to go through that.
Student:	That's what I'm learning in this [STRONG] group that I'm brave, but I, I don't know. I think many people [who were with us] brave. And I didn't think about it that way. I just felt like, OK, how can I help the younger kids who were crying? I like kids so I try to teach them some things. I try to play with them or sing. Sometimes I just have the time pass.
SBFC practitioner:	So, you really took care of the people around you in addition to kind of making sure you got through it, OK?
Student:	I tried. I mean, I mean, you just forget about yourself in such a situation.
SBFC practitioner:	Well, it sounds like you did in the sense that you were able to take care of other people. So, you kind of have a helper nature.
Student:	Yeah.
SBFC practitioner:	I have seen that in the group. When other people are feeling unsettled in the group, you try to help.
Student:	I just feel like I can do that, and I'm happy to do that. And a lot of people help me as well.
SBFC practitioner:	Who are some of the people that you remember being helpful to you?
Student:	My mom, she was very strong, and she always made sure that, you know, that I'm OK. She's would check up on me. Yeah, you know, she's like my rock, like, she would just keep praying. I feel when you don't know what's going to happen, you just keep praying for safety. And whatever happens, she would say we were together. It doesn't matter. We'll stay together.

As this sample illustrates, the SBFC practitioner repeatedly emphasizes the student's strengths to help them re-construct a cohesive personal narrative while recognizing their resilience.

Virtual Adaptation

In response to the interruptions of school-based services due to the Covid-19 pandemic, there was an urgent need to explore how STRONG could be adapted virtually in Ontario and the United States. The Covid-19 pandemic might be particularly distressing to immigrant and refugee families due to their increased risks of experiencing financial challenges and social isolation. Furthermore, the physical distancing and lockdown measures might remind them of their migration journeys with long periods of isolation and uncertainty, emphasizing the continuous need for culturally responsive mental health services to support immigrant and refugee families. A Tier 2 intervention like STRONG that focuses on skill and resilience development rather than trauma exposure and processing reduces risks for harm to emotional safety in virtual settings. With appropriate supports (e.g., digitalizing worksheets) and safeguards (e.g., doing pre-screeners to identify immigrant and refugee students who are not experiencing significant levels of self-harm, mood, or trauma symptoms) in place, STRONG appears to be a promising fit for virtual implementation.

Multicultural Considerations

Focusing on Resilience and Community Connections

Scholars and mental health professionals supporting immigrant and refugee communities have called for more strength- and resilience-building approaches in services to support immigrant and refugee students. Helping immigrant and refugee students recognizes and celebrates their strengths, external supports, and relationships promote their sense of identity, self-efficacy, successful acculturation, and coping with transitional challenges. From the beginning, the principles of strength-based and holistic approaches were at the forefront of STRONG's development. Specifically, STRONG developers collaborated with immigrant and refugee community members and refugee mental health, trauma, and resilience experts in efforts to ensure that the program's core concepts and activities (e.g., individual journey narrative) are culturally responsive and commensurate with immigrant and refugee students' lived experiences.

Culturally Responsive Icebreakers

STRONG group sessions begin with an icebreaker (a "warm-up" activity as indicated in the STRONG manuals) to promote connectedness among students, social inclusion, and cultural identity. The warm-up exercises invite students to learn and reflect on commonalities and have a safe and accepting space to share and hear about others' cultural rituals and traditions. For example, the warm-up activity five invites students to share and show an object (e.g., photograph) that symbolizes a pre-migration region (e.g., birthplace). SBFC practitioners implementing STRONG are asked to have a globe or world map at the session so that students could use it to elaborate on their pre-migration social locations with their peers. However, SBFC practitioners have to be aware that due to wars, political unrest, and events risking families' safety, it is not uncommon for some refugee families to be abruptly displaced from their homes. Hence, some STRONG students may not have photographs or personal objects from pre-migration. Still, SBFC practitioners could use other inclusive strategies to engage students in celebrating and sharing their identity and journey.

Collaboration With Cultural Brokers

During our STRONG training in Ontario, we invited cultural brokers to share their personal narratives (e.g., if they were an immigrant or refugee themselves) or experiences supporting immigrant and refugee communities (e.g., if they were a community-based clinician and also of similar cultural backgrounds). In the third year, we expanded this section of Ontario's training to highlight specific information about different immigration pathways to Canada to familiarize STRONG trainees with potential students' migration experiences. We recognized that such storytelling would be important in supporting our STRONG trainees to critically reflect on their social locations and privileges and take a curious stance about others' unique experiences, adversities, and resilience. These are essential components to developing cultural humility to work with immigrant and refugee students and families (Captari et al., 2019). STRONG trainees described these culturally responsive sections of the training to be highly beneficial.

Creating a System of Care

Immigrant and refugee students and families face many challenges accessing mental health services (Bean et al., 2006). While having Tiers 1 and 2 interventions is one initial culturally responsive step in promoting the mental well-being of immigrant and refugee students, we also need to recognize the possibility that some students may be experiencing more significant distress for which more individualized and intensive Tier 3 services are needed (e.g., psychotherapy). STRONG facilitators screen for PTSD symptoms during the individual journey narrative session to determine whether more follow-up services are required for certain students. Providing parents with only resources and contacts for tertiary mental health services may be ineffective. Parents are likely to continue to experience similar accessibility issues for tertiary care (e.g., cost, language differences, stigma, culturally responsive mental health professionals or care, not knowing how to navigate wait-lists best). Therefore, STRONG implementation teams are encouraged to explore how to integrate Tier 3 services in their local settings (e.g., schools) or build partnerships with tertiary care providers (e.g., community mental health clinics).

Challenges and Solutions

Creating Clear and Consistent Referral Pathways

During the first 2 years of the STRONG pilot, our schools in Ontario did not have a formalized procedure to identify potential students who might benefit from the program. School mental health professionals were offered an eligibility form that included several categories of possible distress (e.g., sadness, anger) and problems with functioning (e.g., academic, social). But we left inclusion criteria quite broad to allow for local tailoring of referral pathways and decision-making about group composition. Referrals for the STRONG program largely depended on school administrators' and teachers' discretion. For example, one teacher referred her entire English as a Second Language class to participate in STRONG. In another school, a school principal selected a group of adolescent boys for the STRONG program, whom he deemed to be having behavioral problems. As a Tier 2 intervention, STRONG is intended for immigrant and refugee students experiencing some degree of mental health, interpersonal, or transition challenges. Immigrant and refugee students have diverse migration experiences, strengths, and resilience skills. Hence, instead of using an ambiguous referral procedure for STRONG, we need to take a holistic, data-driven, non-biased approach to identify students who might benefit from a structured intervention.

Using a Program-Specific Referral Form

In the third year of STRONG programming in Ontario, we developed a program-specific referral form to guide school mental health professionals and schools to select potential students for the STRONG program. Along with asking for students' demographic and mental health information, the STRONG referral form inquires about their functional needs and circumstantial stressors to take a more holistic approach to assess whether they are experiencing distress and would benefit from participating in STRONG. We also encourage school boards to consider how STRONG can be integrated into their existing referral pathways to identify students for Tier 2 mental health programming. From an evaluation viewpoint, using a referral form could also help determine for whom the STRONG intervention is more effective as we continue to research the program to understand its scopes and impacts better.

Using Interpreters

Immigrant and refugee students participating in STRONG might not have attained fluency to converse in the first language (e.g., English) of the resettlement country. Thus, the SBFC practitioner may choose to have interpreters in the sessions. However, the decision to use interpreters could have variable impacts on access, delivery time, and student engagement. There are some advantages to using interpreters, including enabling students of different language skills to participate in STRONG and not excluding students that are not yet proficient in the program delivery language. However, requiring interpreters could slow down the group (i.e., longer sessions) and contribute to student disengagement and barriers to building a quality therapeutic alliance between SBFC practitioners and students. In our Ontario evaluation, we learned that some STRONG students wished to have more access to interpreters. Others indicated that they enjoyed the safe and accepting space of the STRONG program to practice their English skills (Crooks, Kubishyn et al., 2020). The availability of school boards' resources and participating students' preferences and language skills could help decide whether to utilize interpreters. If using interpreters, it may be beneficial to have students from one language group (i.e., having one interpreter) for each STRONG group. Having multiple interpreters could hinder the flow, dynamic, and process of STRONG sessions. Ideally, SBFC practitioners will have access to one regular interpreter and will have the opportunity to orient them to the STRONG program and materials before the group.

Engaging Teachers and Parents

School-level buy-in is critical to the acceptability and successful delivery and scale-up of school-based mental health interventions. School administrators and teachers need to be informed of the importance of targeted mental health interventions. During the first 2 years of STRONG programming, some teachers were concerned with their students missing instructional time to participate in the program. Anxiety about missing instructional time (or disappointing teachers) could hinder students' acceptability and engagement in the school's mental health program. In the third year, we created program materials for school staff, including administrators and teachers, to communicate the importance of school-based mental health care for immigrant and refugee students and how they could support their students' learning from the STRONG program. Notably, we linked how improved well-being contributes to academic success to reduce the perception that STRONG competes with academic achievement.

Parental involvement contributes to youth's mental well-being and enhanced school functioning (Cureton, 2020). We recognize that parents engaging and supporting their youth's learning in the STRONG program could also lead to more enhanced outcomes. At the same time, we are aware of the barriers that might limit parental involvement among immigrant and refugee families, including language differences, work schedules, child care demands, transportation, and potential anxiety about interacting with school personnel due to seeing them as an authority (Cureton, 2020). School teams must create open communication spaces to encourage ongoing parental involvement. We encourage SBFC practitioners implementing STRONG to arrange individual and group sessions with parents, and there are guidelines for these sessions in the STRONG manuals. During these parent sessions, SBFC practitioners familiarize parents with an overview of the STRONG program. Session content includes the program's rationale, processes, and intended outcome of the individual journey narrative session and discusses how parents could participate in the program. SBFC practitioners also send home letters after each STRONG session to describe the activities and skills taught. For these parent interactions, we encourage schools and SBFC practitioners to arrange for language support whenever needed and translate the weekly letter or related program information fliers in parents' first language.

Conclusion

Access and availability of strength-based, holistic, culturally responsive interventions should be an essential component of resettlement and positive adjustment efforts for immigrant and refugee students experiencing psychosocial distress. The STRONG program provides a socio-therapeutic space for immigrant and refugee students to develop cohesive and resilient personal narratives and learn critical coping skills to enhance their adjustment and mental well-being. As STRONG expands in Ontario, New York, Illinois, Massachusetts, and elsewhere, we continue to build on our initial research with more rigorous school- and community-engaged evaluations to enhance our understanding of long-term student impacts, effective ways to involve parents and families, and the expansion of existing culturally responsive strategies.

Resources

STRONG website. http://www.strongforschools.com/
   This website allows eligible SBFC practitioners (i.e., licensed mental health professionals) to register (for free) and download the STRONG manuals and other program materials.
STRONG impact videos. http://www.strongforschools.com/impact
   These videos show STRONG facilitators describing their experience with STRONG. They include examples of what benefits they observed among students, some of the lessons they learned, and what they enjoyed about the program.
STRONG Canadian evaluation site. http://www.csmh.uwo.ca/research/strong.html
   This site provides access to several plain language evaluation reports and our published articles.

Holmes, M. M. (2000). A terrible thing happened (Pillo, C. Illustrator). American Psychological Association.

This book uses a gentle narration to illustrate the emotional and physical effects of witnessing any violent or traumatic event in childhood. We recommend STRONG facilitators use this book as an accompanying tool with elementary-level students participating in the program to introduce and explain the effects of trauma on thoughts, feelings, and actions.

Bibliography

Bean, T., Eurelings-Bontekoe, E., Mooijaart, A., & Spinhoven, P. (2006). Factors associated with mental health service need and utilization among unaccompanied refugee adolescents. Administration and Policy in Mental Health, 33(3), 342–355. http://doi.org/10.1007/s10488-006-0046-2

Bracken, P. J. (2002). Trauma: Culture, meaning and philosophy. Whurr Publishers.

Captari, L. E., Shannonhouse, L., Hook, J. N., Aten, J. D., Davis, E. B., Davis, D. E., Van Tongeren, D., & Ranter Hook, J. . . . Ranter Hook. (2019). Prejudicial and welcoming attitudes toward Syrian refugees: The roles of cultural humility and moral foundations. Journal of Psychology and Theology, 47(2), 123–139. https://doi.org/10.1177/0091647119837013

Crooks, C. V., Hoover, S., & Smith, A. C. G. (2020). Feasibility trial of the school-based STRONG intervention to promote resilience among newcomer youth. Psychology in the Schools, 57(12), 1815–1829. https://doi.org/10.1002/pits.22366

Crooks, C. V., Kubishyn, N., Syeda, M. M., & Dare, L. (2020). The STRONG resiliency program for newcomer youth: A mixed-methods exploration of youth experiences and impacts. International Journal of School Social Work, 5(2). https://doi.org/10.4148/2161-4148.1059

Crooks, C. V., Smith, A. C. G., Robinson-Link, N., Orenstein, S., & Hoover, S. (2020). Psychosocial interventions in schools with newcomers: A structured conceptualization of system, design, and individual needs. Children and Youth Services Review, 112. https://doi.org/10.1016/j.childyouth.2020.104894, PubMed: 104894

Cureton, A. E. (2020). Strangers in the school: Facilitators and barriers regarding refugee parental involvement. Urban Review, 52(5), 924–949. https://doi.org/10.1007/s11256-020-00580-0

Durà-Vilà, G., Klasen, H., Makatini, Z., Rahimi, Z., & Hodes, M. (2013). Mental health problems of young refugees: Duration of settlement, risk factors and community-based interventions. Clinical Child Psychology and Psychiatry, 18(4), 604–623. https://doi.org/10.1177/1359104512462549

Fazel, M., Doll, H., & Stein, A. (2009). A school-based mental health intervention for refugee children: An exploratory study. Clinical Child Psychology and Psychiatry, 14(2), 297–309. https://doi.org/10.1177/1359104508100128

Fazel, M. (2015). A moment of change: Facilitating refugee children's mental health in UK schools. International Journal of Educational Development, 41, 255–261. https://doi.org/10.1016/j.ijedudev.2014.12.006

Fazel, M., Hoagwood, K., Stephan, S., & Ford, T. (2014). Mental health interventions in schools 1: Mental health interventions in schools in high-income countries. Lancet Psychiatry, 1(5), 377–387. https://doi.org/10.1016/S2215-0366(14)70312-8

Gerrard, B. A., & Soriano, M. (2019). School-based family counseling: The revolutionary paradigm. In B. A. Gerrard, M. J. Carter & D. Ribera (Eds.), School-based family counseling: An interdisciplinary practitioner guide (pp. 1–15). Routledge.

Gozdziak, E. M. (2004). Training Refugee Mental Health Providers: Ethnography as a Bridge to Multicultural Practice. Human Organization, 63(2), 203–210. https://doi.org/10.17730/humo.63.2.mh8fl2hl8d1f2qnf

Hettich, N., Seidel, F. A., & Stuhrmann, L. Y. (2020). Psychosocial interventions for newly arrived adolescent refugees: A systematic review. Adolescent Research Review, 5(2), 99–114. http://doi.org/10.1007/s40894-020-00134-1

Hoover, S. (2019). Policy and practice for trauma-informed schools: Comprehensive mental health support makes students safer and better able to learn. https://nasbe.nyc. http://3.digitaloceanspaces.com/2019/01/Hoover_ January-2019-Standard.pdf

Jaycox, L. H., Kataoka, S. H., Stein, B. D., Langley, A. K., & Wong, M. (2012). Cognitive behavioral intervention for trauma in schools. Journal of Applied School Psychology, 28(3), 239–255. https://doi.org/10.1080/15377903.2012.695766

Jaycox, L. H., Langley, A. K., & Hoover, S. A. (2018). Cognitive behavioral intervention for trauma in schools (CBITS). https://www.rand.org/content/dam/rand/pubs/tools/TL200/TL272/RAND_ TL272.pdf. Rand Corporation.

Lustig, S. L., Kia-Keating, M., Knight, W. G., Geltman, P., Ellis, H., Kinzie, J. D., Keane, T., & Saxe, G. N., & . . . Saxe. (2004). Review of child and adolescent refugee mental health. Journal of the American Academy of Child and Adolescent Psychiatry, 43(1), 24–36. https://doi.org/10.1097/00004583-200401000-00012

Miller, K. E., & Rasmussen, A. (2017). The mental health of civilians displaced by armed conflict: An ecological model of refugee distress. Epidemiology and Psychiatric Sciences, 26(2), 129–138. https://doi.org/10.1017/S2045796016000172

Short, K. H. (2016). Intentional, explicit, systematic: Implementation and scale-up of effective practices for supporting student mental well-being in Ontario schools. International Journal of Mental Health Promotion, 18(1), 33–48. https://doi. https://doi.org/10.1080/14623730.2015.1088681

Statistics Canada. (2017). Immigration and ethnocultural diversity: Key results from the 2016 census. https://www150.statcan.gc.ca/n1/daily-quotidien/171025/dq171025b-eng.htm

Sullivan, A. L., & Simonson, G. R. (2016). A Systematic Review of School-Based Social-Emotional Interventions for Refugee and War-Traumatized Youth. Review of Educational Research, 86(2), 503–530. https://doi.org/10.3102/0034654315609419

Summerfield, D. A. (1999). A critique of seven assumptions behind psychological trauma programmes in war-affected areas. Social Science and Medicine, 48(10), 1449–1462. https://doi.org/10.1016/s0277-9536(98)00450-x

Tyrer, R. A., & Fazel, M. (2014). School and community-based interventions for refugee and asylum seeking children: A systematic review. PLOS ONE, 9(2), e89359. https://doi.org/10.1371/journal.pone.0089359

Part 4
Family Prevention

11 Developing Collaborative Relationships Between Teachers, Parents, and Families

Sudia Paloma McCaleb

The goal of this chapter is to introduce school mental health professionals, administrators and teachers to an educational partnership approach that integrates families into the education of their children. This approach explores ways that parents can share their lives, cultures, values, and struggles not only with their own children but with the people in the school who are working with the children. You will discover specific activities and processes that can be followed as ways to build strong and supportive learning communities.

Background

My life as an educator began as a child growing up in our apartment above the preschool that my parents operated throughout my young life. I can still remember the swings, slide, and climbing bars in our front yard. My career took many twists and turns, but I eventually ran an innovative preschool in my own home, completed a Master's degree in Education at Bank St. College in NYC, was the educational director at four childcare centers on the UC Berkeley campus, and became a professor of education after earning my EDD at the University of San Francisco. I created and directed a Teacher Education Credential program in San Francisco, California, accredited by the Commission on Teacher Credentialing for the state. My learning is always evolving in collaboration with my students and their families and with the international educators I have worked with and have come to know. Through participatory action research I came to respect and love the groups of parents and educators with whom I have done my most important and personally fulfilling work. I began to see participatory research as a "philosophical and ideological commitment which holds that every human being has the capacity of knowing, of analyzing and reflecting about reality so that she or he becomes a true agent of action in her or his own life" (Ada).

For many years I have worked with families in California public schools, engaging in dialogues with young people and their parents. Many students in our classrooms have been uprooted from their home countries and as a result don't feel wholly connected to their new country's culture. Most of their families have neither the resources nor the traditional family support

DOI: 10.4324/9781003097891-15

systems formerly available to them in their own countries or native communities. For the past 25 years I have coordinated projects with educators and indigenous communities in Guatemala, Cuba, El Salvador, Romania, Hungary and Oaxaca, Mexico. When immigrants arrive and settle in the United States they often feel helpless and lacking in personal or group validation. When I work with parents I invite them to tap into their internalized traditional sources of knowledge and wisdom, and by sharing and being heard, they begin to feel whole again while contributing to their children's educational well-being and self-confidence.

In an early research project, my initial question was:

> How can educators create partnership with parents and young students that will nurture literacy and facilitate participation in the schools while celebrating and validating home culture and family concerns and aspirations?

Many cultural and linguistic minority parents have not experienced the school as a welcoming environment. Both individual and group dialogues provide an opportunity to hear from parents. I have developed a series of approaches or activities that school counselors may use and also guide classroom teachers to implement. I believe and have found that these activities can help develop a sense of belonging and pride as parents and student voices and experiences are incorporated into the classroom community and learning environment. These are some of the questions that guide my work.

- What have been the educational experiences of linguistic and ethnic minority parents in formal schooling and out-of-school learning?
- How do parents view their own children's educational experiences in the context of family, community, and school?
- How can educational bridges be built between the home and the school that validate the home culture and community?

Procedure

In this section you will find six activities that will support SBFC practitioners and teachers in building relationships with students, in an effort to connect with parents, adults and the home community or environment of students. The instructions for students are phrased in terms of how a teacher might use them; however, an SBFC practitioner could the same instructions.

Activity #1: Proverbs (Dichos)

Overview: This activity seeks to explore with parents and young people phrases they have heard throughout their lives from a parent, grandparent, or other family member. What do these words mean? How do they communicate values, a philosophy of life, or advice about some proper way to live or how to be a good person?

1. A common proverb is: An apple a day keeps the doctor away (now children don't forget to eat your fruits and veggies if you want to stay healthy).
2. The squeaky wheel gets the grease (make sure to stand up for what you need or for what is right).
3. Don't wear your heart on your sleeve (be cautious about how you share your emotions and your love so you don't get hurt or abused).

Ask parents to share a proverb (share one from your own family as an example (when you are willing to share, others will be more open to sharing of themselves), or you may ask children if there is anything they always hear their parent or grandparent say. Children may also be asked to go home and ask their parents to share a proverb with them and bring it back to the classroom. Each child has a turn to share what they heard, what they think it means, and then to illustrate it. Sometimes children (and adults) may reveal something in a simple drawing that they cannot easily articulate. There can be a lively and often humorous discussion both among adults and young people as they discuss the meaning of proverbs and whether or not they believe these are good lessons or not. Every culture has its own popular proverbs, and we can learn a lot about the way people think and act by listening to these seemingly simple aphorisms.

For many years I have worked with communities in an agricultural region in Oaxaca, Mexico, where everyone was a farmer and a common dicho was: "Cada quien cosecha lo que siembra." That is, each one harvests what he sows. In El Salvador, after many years of civil war, the former combatants would say, "Mas vale morir de pie que morir de rodilla" (It is better to die standing up on your feet than on your knees) and "El que no oye consejos no llega a viejo" (He who does not listen to advice will not reach old age).

This activity can help to build a strong classroom community of sharing in which parents also feel more valued. It can also be fun and bring on deep conversations and often positive laughter. One memorable example was a dicho that said, "If you keep your mouth closed, the flies will not enter" (Con boca cerrada no entran moscas). There was loud disagreement here. Some thinking it had to be about not gossiping while some more vocal participants said, "No, we have kept our mouths closed for too long and now is the time to speak out." There is no right or wrong here. In this case the discussion motivated new thinking about an old proverb and whether or not it was something we wanted to preserve or change in our ways of behaving. A skilled teacher or school psychologist could facilitate the conversation.

Teacher may begin like this: (to students) Are there any words of wisdom you have heard many times from one of the adults in your life; like mom or dad or grandparent or auntie or uncle? . . . some words that may tell the kind of person they want you to be or a certain way they want you to act. I will give you an example. "Do onto others like you would have others do onto you." In your own words, what do you think that means? Does anyone in your family say something like this? Hands . . . no one can think of anything? OK, another idea; Tonight, I want you to ask a grown-up what kind of special or important words someone said to them many times in their life growing up. By asking about significant sayings in the lives of your adult family members, we will better understand the kinds of ideas/messages that were communicated to them in their earlier lives. Let's all bring one saying to school tomorrow and then I will take out some art materials and you can each illustrate what we call a proverb . . . and then we can turn each of your illustrated pages of a proverb into a class book and share it with others, including our parents and other family members. Wow! I think we will learn so much about how people think and what is important to parents and grandparents and more.

When teachers follow up with students about this activity they should positively reinforce students work and emphasize the importance of the ideas that are important to their parents, grandparents, or guardians.

Activity #2: Childhood Friendships

Overview: This activity seeks to understand what friendship means to both young people and adults and how they relate to friends. Participants begin by brainstorming what is important to them in friendship. Children hear about the childhood friendships of their parents and grow quite interested. Adults talked about friends they walked to school with along country roads. Some parents expressed concerns about the kinds of friendships their children might develop that would lead them down the "wrong path." The children focused on friendship qualities as "they are nice, you can play with them, they can come to your house, they share and they hug."

Teacher may begin like this:
We all have friends and I would like you to think about some of the things that are important to you in having a friend. Let's make a list on this chart paper of some of the qualities of a person you would wish to be your friend. Now let's make another list of things you like to do together with a friend. Close your eyes and think about that for a minute and then each of you will take piece of paper and some art material from that table and draw a picture of you doing something special with your friend and write a few sentences about what you are doing together. We can put it all together as a book of Friendships in Our Class and then put it on the bookshelf and everyone can have a chance to read it.

Tonight, I want you to try the same thing at home with a grown-up in your house. Make a list as they tell you what is important about being a friend. Then ask them to think back about a childhood friend they had and what they liked to do together. Ask them to make a drawing of them doing something with their friend or if they prefer, you can do the drawing for them. On Friday we will share their words and drawings, which gives you a few days to complete the activity at home.

When the words and pictures are returned from home, have the children compare and contrast what is important to them in friendship and what is important to the adults. Ask them what they think of the activity drawing pages that the grown-ups did.

Activity #3 Families Building Together

Overview: This is an activity that uses blocks and building accessories to create a living space or community. Children can do this in the classroom and also do this at home with adults. Parents spoke about wanting to do things with their children that are fun: like watch TV or play Nintendo games. I developed an activity where a family would receive a small suitcase or shoebox filled with small blocks, little cars, trains, trucks, tracks, farm and forest animals, and a multiracial group of persons. They were asked to build a structure or scene and create a story with members of the family where they could be the main characters. The building was the stimulus for the story, and then they were asked to take a picture of the building with the builders. Everyone said they did have a camera. Each family photo and story were to be put in a group book.

Teacher may begin like this: I have put together a small box/suitcase of objects/things you might see in a small town, city, or community. I am going to lay the things out on the table. We have three groups in our classroom, and each group will have a chance to arrange the contents of the suitcase in their own way and then to write a story about the scene that they have created. Each group will get a big piece of chart paper, and you can take turns being the scribe or the writer. Then we will share each group's story. We will observe how we can use the same object to create different stories. Isn't it amazing how everyone's mind and creative thinking works in different ways? I will take a picture of each group's arrangement and put it together with the story. Then, surprise, we will have a sign-out list, and each one of you will have an opportunity to take the suitcase home for a night and do the activity with your family. There is a little camera in the suitcase to take ONE picture of your completed building and the story you write accompanied by the people who participated. I will have the pictures printed. I think it will be amazing to see how many different versions of the story emerge. It will also be interesting to see if and how the grown-up's stories differ from ours. We can put all of the photos and stories together in a big book and even share with other classes. What do you think of this idea?

Activity #4 Families as Problem Solvers Through Struggle and Change

Overview: What does it mean to solve problems or to struggle? Are the challenges that adults have different than those of young people and how may these differ with migrant families or families that have different cultural roots? In a group conversation we spoke about the word "struggle" and what it means to each. Many parents of children in urban schools have had only limited formal schooling, but this does not mean, as educators sometimes believe, that they have not experienced many challenges and struggles in their lives. All parents are by nature problem solvers and while coming up with solutions weave many pieces of information together and reflect on them before making a decision. Children can come to learn about their parents as problem solvers and need to hear about their struggles. During my dialogues with parent participants, all of them described how they have struggled in their lives and continue to struggle in the present. The children made drawings of what they heard from their parents.

Teacher may begin like this:

> What does it mean to struggle or face challenges? What does the word "struggle" (or challenge) mean to you? Do you know the word for struggle in the language you speak at home or that your parents and grandparents speak at home? Let's make a list on this chart paper on the wall about what it means to struggle. Some examples? Have you ever struggled in your life? What did that look and feel like? Brief discussion. Do you think your parents or other adults you know have struggles? What do you think they might be or look like? Discussion. Tonight I would like you to go home and ask a grown-up what struggle means to them. You can write down what they say so tomorrow we can share their thoughts. Then ask the grown-up to share with you a struggle that they may have at the present time or one they have had in the past. Parents who are immigrants may relate stories of struggle in their country of origin, which may connect to reasons they have come to this country.

The following day: Let's talk about what we heard or learned from speaking with grown-ups last night. Can someone share some thoughts about the word "struggle"? Can someone share some examples of present grown-up struggles? Can someone share an example of a struggle in a grown-up's native country? Were there any surprises? What kinds of emotions did grown-up struggles generate? In what ways were lives changed because of struggle?

Activity # 5 The Most Frightening Time in My Life

Overview: When people speak about fears in a safe and supportive environment they are able to overcome some of their fears and also to see that they are not alone with their fears. Fear is a common feeling in most children and young people's lives. Adults may consider a child's fear unimportant or irrational, but for the child, it seems very real and may cause great anxiety. This can take the form of fear of strangers, the unknown, new situations, or bad dreams. Some children's fears prevent them from learning. During Halloween season when scary images appear everywhere, children cling more to their parents to be assured that some things are just pretend. When parents are asked to share times in their lives when they were frightened, children become more aware of fear as a common human emotion. When both children and adults share experiences of fear in a supportive community sometimes they can eliminate the fears that immobilize them. A teacher may make a list of the fears that students share and talk about ways for dealing with or overcoming them. Ask students to ask parents to share with their children fears they have experienced in their lives and what have been some of the scariest moments they can recall from their childhood and then of course how they have overcome them. An illustrated book of fears can be put together by children and parents and becomes a very popular classroom reading text based on information gathered through dialogue.

Teacher may begin like this: Boys and girls, it is almost Halloween and we can feel it all around. Have you noticed? What have you seen around the neighborhood or on TV that makes you a little scared? Let's talk about fear and what we may be afraid of; about not only Halloween but other things too. Who would like to share something that they feel afraid of? Raise your hand if you are also afraid of that. Let's break into groups of three and have a small conversation. Each person in your triad can tell of something they are afraid of or something they used to be afraid of but are not any more. What did they do to overcome that fear? Bring the groups back together to a circle and ask: Who heard something about a fear they would like to share? Who has a fear of their own they would like to share? Does anyone have a good idea about how to get rid of or overcome something they are frightened about? Discussion

Tonight I would like you to go home and ask a grown-up to remember something they were afraid of when they were a child. Are they still afraid of this thing or what did they do to stop being afraid? Did someone help them or comfort them? Did they just get older and not be afraid anymore?

Next day: Can anyone share something they heard from a grown-up about a fear? Discussion. Today we are going to make a drawing of fears. You may choose to make a drawing of your own fear or something you heard from someone else in the class or that you heard from a grown-up. On the bottom of your drawing you will write a sentence or two about the fear and how it was perhaps overcome or ended. Finally we can put our drawings together in a class book. Do you think a book like this will help us to be less fearful or maybe make us feel more scared? Let's see!

During class discussion the teacher can point out that in different families there may be different ways of coping with fears and that while there are many different things that cause fear, there are also hopeful and effective ways of dealing with them.

Activity # 6 Words of Advice From Our Parents

Overview: The transmission of values has been at the core of every civilization and culture. Students need to know what their elders think is important and what expectations they have for their children. What words of wisdom do parents feel obligated to pass on? What words does each new generation receive from its family or cultural group through advice, ritual, and tradition? In our work, a letter was sent home to parents asking them to pretend that they were going on a long journey and weren't sure when they were returning and wanted to give their children some important advice before leaving. For some parents this was very matter of fact while for others it brought tears or caused them to do some deep thinking. When the responses were brought back children shared with others in the class the similarities and differences and talked about whether they knew these things before and if they felt they could meet their parents expectations. Turning the responses into a class book reminded the students each day of who they are and how much they are loved.

Teacher may begin like this: Let's pretend that your parents had to go away for a few months. Maybe to visit a relative that is sick and lives far away and they need to help take care of them. They don't really want to leave you but they have to. You will be staying with a friend of the family for a few weeks or months. Your parent wants to give you some good advice while they are away about ways they want you to act or behave while they are away. Let's think for a minute. What do you think they would tell you? Some ideas . . . let's talk about those words of advice. Do you think that you can follow your parents' expectations while they are gone? Discussion . . .

Tonight I would like you to go home and ask a parent, if they had to go away for a few months, what words of advice or expectations would they give to you? Write down what they say and we will talk about those things tomorrow.

Next day: How did you feel about the things they said? Were there any surprises? Did they differ from what you thought they would say? Do you think you can meet your parent's expectations?

An extension of this activity could include something about teachings from childhood or memories from childhood. This project can give adults the opportunity to think and talk about memories of the place they spent their childhood. Memories may be vivid, nebulous, or even painful. Thinking about these memories gives the children the opportunity to know more about their parents but also to think about their own communities with guiding questions like these: Is the community multiethnic or multilingual? Where do people get their food? Where do people go when they want to have fun? What may be dangers in the community and how do young people learn to protect themselves?

Another extension might look at the concept of "wisdom." Through this research children will recognize and come to know a person who possesses "wisdom," and parents will also take time to think about someone they have known who possessed a nontraditional form of knowledge. It can be a way of honoring and validating alternative knowledge gained through living and reflection. Begin by brainstorming the meaning of the word "wisdom." You may look up the meaning in several dictionaries. Read some folk tales where an important character is a wise person in a village and think about where do her/his powers lie? Children can ask their parents about wise people they have known and children in class can share and compare qualities and abilities that the parents shared with them at home. Invite a person to the classroom that is considered "wise" in the community and generate questions in advance to ask them. Most of the activities spoken about in this chapter have been created to include work with immigrant families. The activities highlight ways to find out about experiences and values that exist in the home countries and communities.

Multicultural Considerations

This chapter recognizes and acknowledges the multiple cultures and languages that we find in many schools. The activities are designed to hear voices from all cultural and linguistic perspectives and to support parents in feeling included in the school of their new community. All parents, whether refugees or immigrants, are encouraged to share memories and experiences from their childhood and their country of origin.

Challenges and Solutions

Building trust may be the biggest challenge. Parents do not automatically trust the school or the teachers. This may be a result of their own experiences in schooling in their home country or feelings of isolation or perceived or actual marginalization in this country or in the community in which they are living. One way to begin to build trust is by inviting parents to small events where they can share coffee/tea and snacks together. It is important that the counselor and teacher share something of themselves, their lives, their families, and ask parent participants to do the same. They can even share photographs. Parents can be asked to share what they miss most from their home country. Also they can be asked to share ways in which they think their children are special. Potluck dinner get-togethers where parents are asked to cook a dish from their country are also popular and create a feeling of acceptance, sharing, and inclusion.

Resources

The following resources may not directly connect with the activities mentioned earlier, but they have inspired our thinking and the ways we approach learning along the way.

Books

Ayers, B. (2016). Demand the impossible: A radical manifesto. Haymarket Books.
This ambitious and exuberant book perfectly matches its historical moment. Ayers fearlessly confronts the interesting crises of our age—endless war, surging inequality, unchecked White supremacy, and perilous planetary warming—while mapping emancipatory new possibilities.

Igoa, C. (1995). The inner world of the immigrant child. St Martin's Press, Inc.
This book cuts through much current thinking in this field by going right to the central point, namely that the human relationships established between teachers and students are central to academic achievement and student engagement.

McCaleb, S. P. (1994). Building communities of learners: A collaboration among teachers, students, families and community. Lawrence Earlbaum Associates. Inc.
This book is an analysis of the dangers inherent to traditional schooling processes and examines some compelling alternative possibilities. Although it is most likely unintentional, teachers often make parents feel that they are not worthy enough to be active participants in their children's education because of their cultural differences. This book offers various ways of identifying, respecting, and welcoming parents of children as a way to break down barriers between a child's world at home and at school.

Orr, D. (1994). Earth in mind: On education, environment, and the human prospect. Island Press.
As a rule, economists understand economics, ecologists the environment, and educators teaching. Orr is one of the rare authors who understand all three, and in these finely etched essays, he delivers the revolutionary credo necessary for the long-term survival of our species.

Shor, I. (1987). Freire for the classroom: A sourcebook for liberatory teaching. Heinemann.
This book is an anthology of chapters by teachers using Paolo Freire's methods in their classrooms. These are some examples of experimental teaching done to adapt Freire's liberating pedagogy to North American classrooms. Many teachers share here their creative enthusiasm gained from Freire's ideas as well as the political awareness gained by this approach.

Skutnabb, K., & Cummins, J. (1988). Minority education: From shame to struggle. Multilingual Matters Ltd.
In both Europe and North America during the past many years, controversy has surrounded the education of children from linguistic minority backgrounds. An increasing number of minority children are experiencing difficulties at school, and many leave school without graduating. There are fears that an entire generation of alienated youth with no future prospects is being produced by Western educational systems. This book analyses policy issues regarding the education of minority students in Western industrialized societies and presents a number of case studies of programs that have been successful in reversing the patterns of academic failure.

Films

The Apple Pushers (2001). The inspiring story of five immigrant push-cart vendors who are rolling fresh fruits and vegetables into New York City neighborhoods where finding a ripe apple is a serious challenge. They are sometimes called "food deserts" (Laurie Tisch Illumination Fund).

Schools That Change Communities (2013). The film re-imagines what education can be by engaging students.in learning by solving real-world problems in a variety of communities. Administrators, teachers, students, and local residents discuss their projects and the value they find in place—and community based education—an interdisciplinary approach that emphasizes hands-on, curiosity-based investigation using surrounding neighborhoods as "living" classrooms (Bob Gliner).

No Grades, No Homework, Better Learning (2009). Research consistently finds that giving students letter or number grades leads them to think less deeply, to avoid challenging tasks, and to become less enthusiastic about what they are learning. Home work only proves frustrating for kids (and their families) but also turns learning into a chore. Alfie Kohn makes a compelling case that grades and homework are counterproductive (Alfie Kohn).

Race to Nowhere: The Dark Side of America's Achievement Culture (2009). Concerned mother-turned-film maker turns her camera to the high stakes, high-pressure that has invaded our schools and our children's lives, featuring the heartbreaking stories of young people across the country that have been pushed to the brink, educators who are burned out and worried that students aren't developing the skills they need, and parents who are trying to do what's best for their children (Vicki Abeles).

12 Supporting Immigrant and Refugee Family Cohesion

Using the Kako'o Family Mentorship Model

Erwin D. Selimos

Immigrant and refugee family resettlement[1] can have adverse effects on family cohesion. Given that strong family life is a critical factor in children's development, a practical question arises as to what the SBFC practitioner can do to promote family cohesion and stability within the context of resettlement. This chapter, which addresses the family prevention sector of the SBFC meta-model, focuses on this question. The chapter begins by addressing two critical questions: (a) what produces family cohesion? (b) How might the resettlement process undermine it? After addressing these two questions, the chapter then discusses how the SBFC practitioner can adapt Fryxell's (2013) Kako'o family mentoring program as a prevention measure to support immigrant and refugee families in the context of their resettlement.

Background

Family Cohesion: Shared Values, Division of Labor, and Social Support

Social cohesion has been a fundamental topic of inquiry in sociology since the beginning of the discipline. One of sociology's most significant early thinkers—Emile Durkheim—spent much of his academic career exploring the question of what produces group cohesion.

While Durkheim was not theorizing family cohesion in particular, as a heuristic device, the factors and dynamics that he suggested contribute to social cohesion are helpful when thinking about issues of family cohesion.

Durkheim (1960) proposed that a social group will demonstrate higher levels of cohesion if its members share common values and an organized division of labor. Shared values and an organized division of labor contribute to the predictability of social life, promote group membership, and enhance the capacity for different individuals to coordinate their actions.

In addition to shared values and an organized division of labor, I would like to add one more factor contributing to family cohesion: social support.

DOI: 10.4324/9781003097891-16

Personal networks and connections provide family members with emotional and instrumental support during times of stress. Our social supports also provide social control: they remind us of norms and values that can reinforce the commitment to our family, exerting pressure that helps maintain family cohesion.

Resettlement and Family Cohesion

Unfortunately, migration and resettlement can undermine these factors. The disorganizing effects of resettlement on the family are recurrent observations in sociological research, dating back to Thomas and Znaniecki's (1918) foundational examination of Polish immigrants' migration and acculturation processes in Chicago.

Resettlement and Value Gaps

The tendency for children to adopt new host society norms faster than their parents can produce value gaps within immigrant families (Degni et al., 2006). By listening closely to their clients, the observant clinician will detect tensions due to value gaps within the family. Immigrant and refugee parents may express fear of losing connection with their children. They may speak about a diminishment in their sense of parental authority and a deeply felt fear of being unable to communicate with their children. Children will talk about a sense of estrangement produced by the tension of having to "live in two worlds." They will express an ambivalence produced by, on the one hand, a sense of duty to their parents, but, on the other hand, a feeling that their parents do not understand their struggles and are unable to assist them in solving these struggles. These feelings, experiences, and tensions are symbolic of the uneven and differently directed resocialization experiences of immigrant family members within the context of resettlement.

In Chapter 2 of this volume, Gerrard presents a case study of Amira and her family that illustrates possible tensions emerging from gaps in values within immigrant and refugee families. One sees, for instance, a tension between Amira and her mother's desire to form new traditions and the father's desire to maintain established practices. If not discussed and negotiated, such value gaps could produce tensions within the family, leading to more substantial family functioning issues. What traditions does Amira's father want to uphold? What types of new traditions does Amira wish to establish? Why do these family members differ concerning these values? How can they mediate these orientations of continuity and change within the family?

However, while resettlement may produce generational value gaps within immigrant and refugee families, other research shows that family migration can also create intergenerational integration (McGovern &

Devine, 2016; Selimos, 2017; Taylor & Krahn, 2013; Tyyska, 2008). Collectively experienced struggles, trials, and tribulations, if handled well, can be a great source of group integration. One needs only to think about the group affinity expressed by a "band of brothers" or a well-run social support group to realize that the school-based family counseling (SBFC) practitioner can harness collective struggles to promote group cohesion.

Resettlement and the Division of Labor

By its very definition, resettlement also produces changes in immigrant and refugee families' division of labor, as families re-organize their role relationships in their attempt to adapt to life in a new society (Degni et al., 2006). In this conceptualization, resettlement constitutes resocialization (Fein, 1989). Renegotiating roles is inherently stressful because at its root is the renegotiation of identity. A father used to being the family breadwinner, competent and in control, may confront unemployment. Wrapped up in this status inconsistency, he may feel angry at his inability to perform his role. These feelings may lead to lashing out toward his family members, depression, and even alcohol or substance abuse. In his difficulty in managing his role transformations, the father may lose his authority in the eyes of his children (Degni et al., 2006).

Sociologists remind us of the conservative nature of roles: people often respond to change by doubling back on familiar roles and behaviors (Fein, 1989). This is true among immigrant and refugee families. For example, within immigrant and refugee families, the tendency toward role maintenance may be observed in parents' difficulties with changing their disciplinary practices to meet the legal expectations of the new host society, even though their parenting strategies are ineffective.

In addition to problematic role maintenance, families may develop new role relationships to address immediate needs, but these relationships may be harmful to certain family members in the long run. Think of cases where a child takes on extra caretaking responsibilities at the expense of their schoolwork, personal enjoyment, or personal development. While immigrant and refugee youth see assisting parents in caretaking, in the family business, or as interpreters as an honor and duty (Selimos, 2017), such obligations can pull them away from investing in their development in the new host society.

Resettlement and Social Isolation

The SBFC practitioner should also keep in mind that resettlement can lead to social isolation. In such a case, families face their problems and pressures with no one to turn to for guidance, emotional release, or instrumental support. It does not take much effort to imagine how stressful and painful such loneliness would be, especially for a family new to a country. Some immigrant families, of course, will already have pre-existing connections they can draw on for social support. But this might not be the case for all families or family members. Rebuilding this support network is a key feature of the resettlement process.

Implications for SBFC Practice

The SBFC model defines prevention as interventions that "help parents, guardians, and families to develop skills that prevent future problems" (Gerrard & Soriano, 2013, p. 13). The preceding discussion of how migration and resettlement may negatively impact family cohesion highlights several important implications for SBFC prevention practice.

Firstly, the possible effects of resettlement on value gaps within the family raise the question of how to assist families in utilizing the migration and resettlement experience to strengthen their commitment to each other and reaffirm common values. Thus, prevention measures may require offering programs to assist families in examining and negotiating aspects of their value systems in the context of their new situation and future dreams. Some families may need more assistance in doing this than others. For instance, families emigrating from societies with significantly different cultural norms than the new host society will probably express more struggles with intergenerational value gaps than those migrating from a milieu culturally similar to the new host society.

Secondly, because resettlement produces and necessitates a change in the familial division of labor, struggles with the renegotiation of roles may be at the root of many clients' troubles. From the standpoint of prevention, the practical question is how to encourage the renegotiation of familial roles to be more functional to the new host society, and that draws an appropriate balance between continuity and change for the family members. Related to the question of role negotiations include issues of employment and access to education. Again, one could predict that families emigrating from cultures and societies with significantly different norms than the new host society will demonstrate more difficulty with role change than those migrating from a culturally and socially similar milieu. The clinician, therefore, must keep in mind the diversity of migratory, cultural, and social experiences of immigrant and refugee families.

Thirdly, the resettlement process can lead to the social isolation of the family. Therefore, the prevention question arises as to how to build the family's social support networks. Assisting immigrant families in building social support within the new community of residence and their families can be viewed as an essential measure to buffer resettlement stress and promote family cohesion.

Table 12.1 offers a summary of the preceding section.

Table 12.1 Summary of Preceding Section

Factors producing family cohesion	How resettlement can undermine family cohesion	Implications for prevention
Common values and orientations **Adequate division of labor** **Social support**	Resettlement may lead to value gaps between members of the family, especially parents and children. Resettlement may disrupt the division of labor, and families may have difficulty renegotiating roles. Resettlement may lead to social isolation.	Opportunities to reaffirm and promote core family values. Assistance in the renegotiation of the division of labor or resolving conflict related to issues in the division of labor. Cultivating social supports.

Procedures: A Proposal for an Adaptation of the Kako'o Family Mentoring Program

Given the preceding discussion of family cohesion and resettlement stressors, I believe that an adaptation of the Kako'o (meaning "to support") Family Mentoring Program described by Fryxell (2013) in *School-Based Family Counseling: Transforming Family-School Relationships* provides a fruitful prevention program for supporting immigrant and refugee family cohesion. The Kako'o Family Mentoring Program provides a model to support families in the resettlement program that could simultaneously address problems related to value gaps, role negotiations, and social support. Still, it does so through a non-therapy, social support model more palatable to the sensibilities of immigrant and refugee families.

Short Description of the Kako'o Family Mentoring Program

The Kako'o Family Mentoring program was a 3-year initiative developed at an elementary school in Hawaii to serve a multicultural, relatively high-poverty population. According to Fryxell (2013), after a series of community-based discussions related to the needs of the community, students, parents, and school staff expressed a desire for the school to assist in strengthening families in the community: "This decision was based on the premise that strong families will in turn nurture, healthy, confident, and successful children" (p. 571). The project's coordinating body decided to employ a mentoring model to assist in strengthening families. The most significant innovation of the mentoring model was that it used a family-to-family mentoring approach. That is, instead of matching individuals with mentors, the Kako'o Family Mentoring program matched families with other families, where "entire families were trained to be mentor families who were then paired with mentee families" (p. 573).

Organizers implemented the project over 3 years. The first year involved the selection, recruitment, and training of mentor families. Mentor families (twelve families were selected in the original project) received training over a year that focused on strengthening their own family and equipping each member with the skills necessary for mentoring other families. Fryxell describes the core components of the project's first year:

1. developing communication skills
2. problem-solving
3. conflict resolution
4. conducting family meetings
5. building trust and respect
6. promoting responsibility
7. successful child-rearing strategies
8. supporting children to be active learners
9. relieving stress

In addition to these topics, mentor families also participated in training sessions related to concerns, such as preventing drug and alcohol use and friendship skills.

The second year of the program involved pairing trained mentor families with mentee families, who either were referred to the program by school staff or volunteered to join. During the second year, mentor and mentee families participate in workshops to learn new skills, develop relationships, and strengthen their families. Mentor and mentee families also met outside these monthly meetings during pre-planned events such as a weekend family retreat and a community service project. In addition to the workshops and pre-planned events, program coordinators encouraged mentors and mentees to meet on their own for informal activities. The final year of the project saw its expansion from the elementary school to the entire school district.

While Fryxell admits that measuring the project's impact was difficult, evaluation of the workshops and qualitative data suggests that families enjoyed the program and found it helpful in improving their family lives. He also identifies ten core features to achieve positive mentoring outcomes. I reproduce these ten key points in Box 12.1 because they undergird the essential features an SBFC practitioner should consider if they decide to retool this model to assist immigrant and refugee families.

Box 12.1   Core Elements to Achieve Positive Mentoring Outcomes (Fryxell [2013])

1. Mentoring is particularly effective when intervening with children and their families as early as possible and before major problems arise.
2. Maintaining a consistent level of contact between mentor families and mentee families, typically involving meetings 3–4 times per month for one or more hours per meeting.
3. The mentoring program has a well-thought-out structure, which includes a project management plan, policies, and procedures.
4. Standards and procedures are established for screening mentor families, orientation and training of mentor families, matching of the mentor and mentee families, and the required frequency of meetings between mentor and mentees families.
5. Mentor families are trained in behavioral skills, behavioral management skills, interpersonal skills, and evaluation skills enabling them to identify needs of the mentee families.
6. Mentor families are matched with mentee families taking into account the preferences of both families. Consideration regarding appropriate matches is based on factors such as the racial, cultural, and religious backgrounds of the families.
7. In addition to providing friendship and social support, mentor families are encouraged to assist their mentee families in developing specific competencies (i.e., problem-solving skills, conflict resolution skills), which will increase positive relationships and interactions in families.
8. Efforts are made to ensure that caring relationships are developed between the mentor and mentee families that promote improvement in all areas of the family's life.
9. Ongoing supervision and support of each mentoring match is provided by project personnel who maintain frequent contact with all the families.
10. When assistance is requested or when difficulties arise, extra support and referral services are provided.

The Kako'o Model and Immigrant and Refugee Families

When I read about this model, I was immediately struck by its applicability to immigrant and refugee families. One of the most essential elements of the model is developing social support and connections among families. The resocialization involved in resettlement is taxing and difficult. Immigrant and refugee families would benefit significantly from working through these issues with other families that have successfully settled. An adaptation of the Kako'o model would assist in building these connections and providing opportunities for essential social support, both instrumental and emotional. Immigrant and refugee families often need guidance in negotiating resettlement. Who better to assist than those families who have experienced it!

Another attractive and significant feature of the Kako'o model is its flexibility regarding training for both mentor and mentee families. The model has training sessions dedicated to essential family strengthening but has the flexibility to include additional workshops explicitly related to immigrant and refugee family issues. For example, in the second year of the program, I could easily see targeted workshops that encourage families to collaboratively work through resettlement-specific challenges (such as value gaps, division of labor issues, and so on). In other words, the model provides a base of cultivating skills and dispositions that constitute universal features of strong families and the ability to target interventions to the specific needs of immigrant and refugee families.

While the formal training and planned sessions are in their own right important, the informal information exchanged between mentor and mentee families represents a critical component of the Kako'o model. Newly settled immigrants and refugees draw extensively on informal ethnocultural connections to access resources. A re-tooling of the Kako'o also provides immigrant and refugee families the opportunity to expand their ties to the larger community. As I argue in Chapter 19, an SBFC practitioner can assist immigrant and refugee children and their families by finding routes to expand their clients' social participation in community life. Newly arrived families need to learn about the exciting opportunities in their community and establish a sense of place and belonging to their new locality. The Kako'o model, which involves both formally and informally planned trips to local areas, provides the opportunity for new families to be introduced to their new place of residence by other families.

Multicultural Considerations

Perhaps the biggest strength of the Kako'o family mentorship program is its sensitivity to cultural diversity through its emphasis on a non-medicalized model of prevention. As Fryxell rightly discusses, non-Western families, the bulk of immigrants and refugees to North America, often perceive a stigma attached to receiving professional help, especially from psychologists or therapists. The Kako'o model avoids this trap, as it emphasizes community self-help, mutuality, and guidance. Most of the issues and struggles that immigrant and refugee families are related to the interpersonal struggles produced by migration and resettlement and are resolutely not medical problems. These families need assistance in problem-solving, and in the

Kako'o model, they can receive this assistance from new friends with similar backgrounds and experiences. Such an approach reduces the potential for cultural misunderstanding and is consistent with the multiculturally sensitive approach of SBFC, which treats parents as partners.

Challenges and Solutions

The Kako'o family mentorship model provides a unique approach to supporting immigrant and refugee families. However, the model does present the SBFC practitioner with important logistical and programmatic questions that will need to be resolved.

1. **Coordinating the Complexity of the Project.** An individual-to-individual mentorship program requires a lot of management in its own right, and the complexity intensifies with family-to-family mentorship. The first step in implementing the program would be to organize a steering committee or advisory board to design and promote the project. The SBFC practitioner needs to spend some time deciding who should sit on this body. A diverse representation of school staff, local social service agencies, and community members would be ideal. Most likely, securing funding for the program would require collaboration among the school and other local agencies, so members of these organizations will presumably make up most of the composition of the advisory board.

   If the program involves a partnership among schools and community agencies, a discussion will have to be made about where the program is housed. Funding arrangements will most likely determine this decision. The Kako'o model was implemented through a school, but the model could be implemented by a community agency as well.

   The successful implementation of the program requires at least a full-time program coordinator who has strong understanding of immigrant and refugee issues and mentoring scholarship, excellent organizational skills, and the ability to design and implement evaluation tools. Hiring the right person is a critical and essential task of the advisory board, as the project coordinator will be responsible for the daily operations and implementation of the program.

   The advisory board and program coordinator will need to do a lot of pre-planning before the recruitment for the project begins. I would recommend spending an entire year drafting a project management plan. Such a plan would outline, among other points, the project's scope, the roles of the partners involved in the project, the screening procedures for identifying mentors and mentees, recruitment, workshop curriculum, additional events, and program evaluation methods. In designing the program, the advisory board and the program coordinator will have to spend significant time discussing the screening and matching procedures for mentees and mentors. For example, what criteria should be used to select mentor families? Should mentees be placed with mentors from the same ethnocultural community? There are or can be significant social and class divisions within and between immigrant and refugee groups. Organizers will need to consider these differences in the matching process.

2. **Commitment.** Fryxell identified changes to the school's leadership and maintaining funding as two of the biggest challenges to the mentorship program. I would anticipate that leadership instability and funding to be two main challenges that the SBFC practitioner would encounter in re-tooling the mentorship model for immigrant and refugee populations. Of course, these are often complex problems to solve. One way to ensure that leadership instability does not impact the delivery of the program is to have a clear project management plan to ensure that any changes to the project coordinator or the advisory board would not change the general direction of the program. Maintaining funding is perhaps the most difficult challenge. Grant-funded programs are typically time-limited and easily cut or not renewed. Ideally, if a school was interested in implementing such a program, funding for it could be written into the school budget. Those, too, are subject to change.

3. **Measuring Impact.** An essential element to stable funding is constantly championing the necessity of the program. School and community leaders must see the value in offering this mentorship program. This necessitates a thorough evaluation plan and an effective method of communicating the project's impact. As Fryxell demonstrates, documenting the impact of a mentorship program is quite difficult and requires multiple methods: surveys, interviews, observations, and photo and video—elicitation techniques. The SBFC practitioner could draw on the growing body of evaluation research techniques to document the program's impact (see, for instance, the website betterevaluation. org). It is a great idea to invest in developing an excellent evaluation plan, as future funding may require demonstrating the program's effectiveness, as marketing the value of the program to the school and community will require documenting its successes. If expertise is an issue regarding how to implement an effective evaluation plan, one thing the SBFC practitioner could do is contacting a local university's School of Social Work, School of Education, Psychology department, Sociology department, or Anthropology department. There may be faculty members and graduate students who specialize in evaluation research or who could design a research project around the evaluation of the mentorship program. I imagine that they would jump at the opportunity to be involved in such a project.

Conclusion

After documenting some of the settlement processes that undermine immigrant and refugee family cohesion, I argued that re-tooling the Kako'o Family Mentorship Model to address the needs of immigrant and refugee families represents one fruitful avenue for providing this resettlement support. While such a project requires sorting out significant logistical challenges, the benefits are well worth it. I hope that reading about this project has inspired you to develop a mentorship program in your community for immigrant and refugee families. The strength of these families is a fundamental factor in promoting the well-being and success of immigrant and refugee children.

Note

1 Immigrant and refugee families are varied, multifaceted, and dynamic, encompass modalities beyond the nuclear model, and include a wide range of blood and fictive kin. Furthermore, they often span national borders (Menjivar et al., 2016, p. 1). This chapter examines immigrant and refugee families resettling in a new "host" country together with their parents, grandparents, children, and other kin. This delimitation leaves out important considerations, including unaccompanied child migrants, who often leave or are sent away, either within their countries of origin or across borders, to earn money for their family.

Resources

Fryxell, D. R. (2013). Promoting school success through mentor families. In B. Gerrard & M. Soriano (Eds.), School-based family counseling: Transforming family-school relationships (pp. 571–578). San Francisco: Institute for School-Based Family Counseling.
Fryxell provides an overview of the Kako'o Family Mentorship model, which is thoroughly referenced in this chapter and is a must-read for those interested in family-to-family mentorship programs.

Degni, F., Pöntinen, S., & Mulki, M. (2006). Somali parents' experiences of bringing up children in Finland: Exploring social-cultural change within migrant households. Forum Qualitative Sozialforschung. Forum: Qualitative Social Research, 7(3), Art. 8. http://www.qualitative-research.net/index.php/fqs/article/view/139
This article provides interesting insights into how migration impacts family relationships.

National Mentoring Resource Center

The National Mentoring Resource Center website provides a variety of resources on mentoring and establishing mentoring programs, including evidence reviews, training materials, and evaluation resources. In fact, the National Mentoring Resource Center even provides technical assistance for program evaluation. The website includes specific information on mentoring programs for immigrant and refugee youth. The website can be accessed here: https://nationalmentoringresourcecenter.org/index.php

Bibliography

Degni, F., Pontinen, S., & Molsa, M. (2006). Somali parents' experiences of bringing up children in Finland: Exploring socio-cultural change within migrant households. Forum Qualitative Sozialforschung. Forum: Qualitative Social Research, 7(3), Art. 8. http://www.qualitative-research.net/index.php/fqs/article/view/139

Durkheim, E. (1960). The division of labor in society. Glencoe, IL: The free press of Glencoe, Illinois.

Fein, M. (1989). Role change: A resocialization perspective. Praeger.

Fryxell, D. R. (2013). Promoting school success through mentor families. In B. Gerrard & M. Soriano (Eds.), School-based family counseling: Transforming family-school relationships (pp. 571–578). San Francisco: Institute for School-Based Family Counseling.

Gerrard, B., & Soriano, M. (2013). School-based family counseling: An overview. In B. Gerrard & M. Soriano (Eds.), School-based family counseling: Transforming family-school relationships (pp. 2–15). San Francisco: Institute for School-Based Family Counseling.

McGovern, F., & Devine, D. (2016). The care worlds of migrant children – Exploring inter-generational dynamics of love, care and solidarity across home and school. Childhood, 23(1), 37–52. https://doi.org/10.1177/0907568215579734

Menjivar, C., Leisy, J. A., & Schmalzbauer, L. C. (2016). Immigrant families. Polity Press.

Selimos, E. D. (2017). Young immigrant lives: A study of the migration and settlement experiences of immigrant and refugee youth in windsor, Ontario [Dissertation]. University of Windsor.

Taylor, A., & Krahn, H. (2013). Living through our children: Exploring the education and career 'choices' of racialized immigrant youth in Canada. Journal of Youth Studies, 16(8), 1000–1021. https://doi.org/10.1080/13676261.2013.772575

Thomas, W. I., & Znaniecki, F. (1918). The polish peasant in Europe and America: Monograph of an immigrant group. Richard G. Badger and the gorham press. Received. https://web.archive.org/web/20110927161055/http://chla. http://library. cornell.edu/c/chla/browse/title/3074959.html

Tyyska, V. (2008). Parents and teens in immigrant families: Cultural influences and material pressures. Canadian diversity/diversité Canadienne, 6 (2). http://canada. metropolis.net/pdfs/Pgs_ can_ diversity_ parents_ spring08_ e.pdf

13 How to Provide a Parent Education

Workshop for Refugees and Immigrants

Nancy Rosenbledt

This chapter describes the process in developing and implementing parent education for school-based family counseling (SBFC) practitioners to provide family-preventive services for refugee and immigrant parents and guardians through psycho-educational trainings and workshops. Examples from parent education workshops within the SBFC model framework are included in PowerPoint slide format from actual presentations based on best practices from a positive parenting perspective.

Background

Immigrant and refugee parents play a critical role in developing their children and, therefore, can provide key components to effective intervention and prevention programs in the schools. Consequently, school-based family counseling (SBFC) professionals must work collaboratively with parents to target emotional, behavioral, and academic concerns to ensure children's home/school success. SBFC professionals are in an optimal position to form an alliance with families and help them access and develop interventions that will remediate problems. Parent education workshops and training represent a key intervention in addressing behavioral issues interfering with school success and overall well-being. Offering some type of programming for parents to learn effective parenting skills is paramount to the SBFC model.

Parent training is a preventive-family focus where SBFC professionals work with parents to reduce problematic behaviors that youth exhibit and increase positive, pro-social behaviors both in home and school. In this intervention, parents are instructed in a workshop format to use and apply behavioral principles and methods (positive parenting principles) that have been shown to be effective in reducing problematic child behaviors. Some such techniques include positive reinforcement of appropriate behaviors and mild discipline of inappropriate behaviors.

DOI: 10.4324/9781003097891-17

Procedure

This section outlines parent training in either a group workshop or an individual format. Common elements of effective principles when designing and presenting parent training are highlighted here. The presentation will demonstrate the effectiveness of an aspect of SBFC professionals modeling services through a parent training workshop.

Step 1: Theory and Research—Setting the Foundation

Read the research on prevention programs and identify existing prevention programs and resources for parent effectiveness training. Conduct a literature review and find significant professional/evidence-based research articles/resources that address prevention or intervention programs in SBFC regarding the topic.

Step 2: Assess Need

Assess the child's needs in view of the factors creating risk, problematic behaviors, and/or skill deficits. Providing culturally appropriate services by assessing the resiliency, strengths, and protective factors of families is critical. SBFC practitioners should use formal tools such as standardized tests, well-researched measurement instruments, transcripts, attendance records, discipline/behavior files, and informal assessments such as observations/interviews with students, family, staff, and community members to identify particular needs. (Center for Excellence in School Counseling and Leadership [CESCaL]). Interviews are frequently conducted as the first step in the assessment process. As discussed by Merrell et al. (2008), interviews should generally cover issues related to *intrapersonal functioning*, family relationships, *peer relationships*, *school adjustment*, and community involvement.

Observations are also commonly used in school settings to obtain a direct picture of the behaviors in question. The SBFC professional can conduct observations in the classroom setting. Gathering observational data from both home and school can provide useful information and a picture of the problem across settings. However, it is important to keep in mind that parents and teachers cannot always devote their full attention to the observational process and may need to be trained by the SBFC professional on remaining objective through functional behavioral analysis techniques. Comprehensive assessments can include self-report measures and rating scales in which the SBFC professional has achieved competency. By obtaining data about the problem behaviors and the function that these behaviors serve, the SBFC professional will be in a better position to develop the most effective parent training intervention that is most likely to reduce problematic behaviors children are exhibiting. Target the population, factors, and/or at-risk behaviors by using the needs assessment results. SBFC practitioners should research and implement best practices relative to similar populations, risk factors, or problems should be utilized.

Step 3: Planning and Implementation

Meet with appropriate staff and personnel to obtain input in planning for program support. The best prevention efforts have been based on collaborative, interdisciplinary teaming of the population members served. A description of the program should be presented to the administration and staff for further review, revision, and refinement. Plan for staff development to provide for opportunities for questions and concerns to be addressed. Stakeholder collaboration is essential for strengths-based, culturally sensitive action plans to promote student developmental outcomes. Identify appropriate school and community resources-adjunct services and referral options. Illustrate your partnerships with students' families and community. Provide evidence of your development as a learner and leader/collaborator with other professionals. Finally, plan variations for diversity in prevention programming that shows sensitivity and respect. Use knowledge of counseling diverse populations to apply counseling skills, techniques, and interventions within the parent training program.

Step 4. Plan Program Evaluation

Plan evaluation procedures before program implementation. Examine how your prevention planning and intervention services measure the accountability and efficacy of the parent training program. Make appropriate recommendations for improving the family-preventive program based on the data (Center for School Counseling Outcome Research at University of Massachusetts at Amherst).

Step 5: Workshop Model

SBFC professionals may want to use a packaged program or create their parents' workshop based on the needs assessment. The following training program format offers a diverse approach, yet provides for personalizing the material presented and for transfer of learning (Brigman et al., 2021):

> Warm-up: Begin the training session with an activity or brief sharing of something positive tied to the session's theme. Involve parents by having them think, write, and share in dyads their ideas, which is a safe way to get them into the topic. Ask for two or three volunteers to share their ideas with the larger group. This provides an opportunity

for the SBFC professional to tie experiences back into the session's theme, creating a rationale for parent involvement.

Ask before telling: Before offering information at any stage of the training, ask parents' ideas first. The more SBFC professionals use parents' input, the more it becomes their program.

Introduction of information and skills: It is best to use the "Model, Rehearse, and Practice" method when providing information or introducing new ideas or skills. This approach keeps parents involved and leads to the application of workshop skills and information.

Personalize and practice: After the information is presented, allow time for personalizing and practice by asking parents to think, write, share, and practice in small groups. This kind of learning is essential for understanding to occur. Small groups then report their experience to the large group.

Process and summarize: Help parents summarize the workshop by providing time at the end to reflect on process questions:

How involved was I in the activities and discussions?
How did I feel during the activities and discussions?
What did I learn or relearn?
How can I use what I learned?

It is important to ask each parent to share with a partner or small group what s/he learned (goal). Allow volunteers to share ideas for application with the large group. This provides the SBFC professional an opportunity for encouragement, coaching, and reinforcement of key concepts.

Evaluate: Have simple written evaluations at the end of the workshop/ training session (see Appendix B and C). Use the results to improve your next parent training and/or for positive public relations.

Multicultural Considerations

One of the most critical challenges facing school-based professionals is gaining competency in addressing an increasingly diverse student population (Coleman, 1995; House & Martin, 1998; Lee, 1995; Lewis & Hayes, 1991). Multicultural counseling competence refers to the SBFC professionals' attitudes, beliefs, knowledge, and skills in working with people from different cultural groups, including racial, ethnic, gender, social class, and sexual orientation (Arrendono et al., 1996). Accordingly, due to the increasing ethnic, social, and racial diversity of the US school system, SBFC professionals need to possess appropriate knowledge and skills to work with diverse students and their families (Durodoye, 1998; Hobson & Kanitz, 1996; Johnson, 1995).

These issues must be integrated within a context of family involvement. SBFC professionals are accountable for understanding and generating awareness of specific cultural factors relevant to particular cultural groups. This includes the knowledge to assess particular factors such as acculturation, migration history, language proficiency, and sociocultural history that are critical concerns for children's development in the schools (Paniagua, 1994; Vasquez-Nuthall et al., 1990). Strategies that support multicultural competence within the context of family involvement consist of three components; parent education and support, school–family curriculum activities, and school staff–parent partnership efforts (Banks, 1993).

Finally, systematic work on ethnicity and culture as moderators of treatment is needed. Professionals cannot assume that treatment developed primarily with a couple of cultural or ethnic groups will be applicable to other groups without modification. Many parent-child interactions and child-rearing practices are deeply woven into religious teachings and cultural beliefs and customs, for example, type of punishment, how and what demands are made on children, and so on. Therefore, it is reasonable to expect ethnicity and culture to moderate intervention effects (Weisz & Kazdin, 2010).

Challenges and Solutions

Although parent training can be a very effective intervention, it is not uncommon to encounter certain obstacles in implementing this intervention. One of the first obstacles frequently observed involves parent expectations or unawareness of what to expect when they seek assistance for their children. Often, parents view the problem as the child's and do not understand the need for their involvement. Therefore, it is important to get parent acceptance and commitment as the most effective method in modifying child's behaviors. The best recommendation for SBFCs is to adopt a collaborative approach by emphasizing a need to solicit parents' help in creating behavior change, that is, "co-counselors" in the process. In other words, SBFC professionals have the expertise in behavioral interventions, and parents have the expertise on their children and their home situation with a focus on parents having a greater impact in their children's lives than clinicians.

Another obstacle encountered with parent training involves parents who view the training program as possibly negative and believe that regular discipline may negatively impact their relationship with their child. The SBFC professional emphasizes the importance and appreciation children have for consistency and structure. The parent training program is designed so that parents lay a positive foundation of interacting with their child before beginning the discipline component.

The SBFC professional needs to understand and appreciate real obstacles a parent may face before implementing the training program. As skills are being introduced, it is important to anticipate, prepare, and problem-solve with parents as much as possible. For example, when discussing "special time," parents should think about when they can commit to this quality time, what they will do with their other children, and what problems they may encounter. There are typically multiple solutions to any given situation, so SBFC professionals must be flexible in finding solutions that best fit for the family while still ensuring effective behavioral methods. SBFC professionals must emphasize the need for parents' help in creating change by becoming collaborative partners to overcome these obstacles. Let parents know that we may be the experts on behavioral change, but they have the expertise on their children and home situations. Also, SBFC professionals need to focus on how much more important parents are in children's lives than the clinicians. Although schools cannot usurp the parenting process, they can provide parent effectiveness training.

Although behavioral parent training has shown empirical support in effectiveness, it does not work for all families and can end up alienating parents who interpret this approach as authoritarian, imposition of the parent's will, and conducted through a rigid process. Researchers have evaluated other interventions that involve working with parents as partners on the school team. In particular, Greene and Ablon (2006) provide a collaborative problem-solving (CPS) model, which initially focuses on the antecedents of the child's problem behaviors. By learning what predicts the targeted behavior, parents, children, and school staff can engage in a CPS process to resolve the problem.

As mentioned in the previous section, a fundamental challenge for SBFC professionals is involving and engaging parents as key partners in their children's education. Therefore, SBFC professionals may need to be oriented to a positive psychology perspective and belief system (Wilde, 2005):

Belief #1: Parents love their kids in the best way they know-how. Most people raise their children how their parents raised them, and most challenging parents did not have good role models as children.

Belief #2: Parents' inability to believe negative behaviors attributed to their children is biologically/evolutionary rooted. That's how parents protect their progeny and keep their line of DNA moving forward in the next generation.

Belief #3: Carefully consider the requests made of parents as they have the skills, understanding, self-discipline, and organization to be successful in the implementation of plans.

Belief #4: Except for parents who have mental health issues, most of their behaviors would be predictable if professionals had access to the complex patterns that have been ingrained in their life histories. By keeping this in mind while unraveling these complex patterns will most likely engender successful engagement of challenging parents.

Belief #5: Imagining sitting in the parent's chair as if an SBFC professional were talking about your child will dramatically increase your empathic understanding of parents.

Finally, in keeping with best practices supported by efficacious effects of evidence-based programs, PowerPoint slides are included in this chapter as examples of simple strategies that parents can implement to improve students' performance (see Appendix A).

Conclusion

In summary, parent training interventions for eliminating or reducing problematic behaviors in children have garnered significant empirical support in the research literature. Effective parent training components share a variety of common elements, including a social learning orientation/format, including modeling skills in session, role plays, or practice with feedback, and practice skills outside of sessions; a focus on changing existing environmental contingencies, frequently through a focus on creating changes in parents' behaviors; a dual focus on increasing adaptive behaviors and decreasing maladaptive/inappropriate behaviors; and the intervention techniques can be implemented by SBFC professionals in collaboration with school personnel and parents.

Resources

Arredondo, P., Toporek, R., Brown, S. P., Jones, J., Locke, D. C., Sanchez, J., & Stadler, H. (1996). Operationalization of the Multicultural Counseling Competencies. Journal of Multicultural Counseling and Development, 24(1), 42–78. https://doi.org/10.1002/j.2161-1912.1996.tb00288.x

Atkinson, D. R., & Juntunen, C. L. (1994). School counselors and school psychologists as school-home-community liaisons in ethically diverse schools. In P. Pederson & J. C. Carey (Eds.), Multicultural counseling in the schools: A practical handbook (pp. 103–119). Allyn & Bacon.

Banks, J. (1993). Multicultural education for young children: Racial and ethnic attitudes and their modifications. In B. Spodek (Ed.), Handbook of research on the education of young children (pp. 246–258). Macmillan.

Brigman, G., Villares, E., Mullis, F., Webb, L. D., & White, J. F. (2021). School counselor consultation: Skills for working effectively with parents, teachers, and other school personnel. John Wiley & Sons.

Capuzzi, D., & Gross, D. (Eds.). (2008). Youth at risk: A prevention resource for counselors, teachers, and parents (5th ed., p. 34). American Counseling Association.

Casas, M., & Furlong, M. J. (1994). School counselors as advocates for increased Hispanic parent participation in schools. In P. Pederson & J. C. Carey (Eds.), Multicultural counseling in the schools: A practical handbook (pp. 121–155). Allyn & Bacon.

Center for School Counseling Outcome Research at University of Massachusetts – Amherst. http://www.umass.edu/schoolcounseling

Research supporting school-based family counseling interventions.

Coleman, H. L. K. (1995). Cultural factors and the counseling process: Implications for school counselors. School Counselor, 42, 5–13.

Durodoye, B. A. (1998). Fostering multicultural awareness among teachers: A tripartite model. Professional School Counseling, 1(5), 9–13.

Eisenstadt, T. H., Eyberg, S., McNeil, C. B., Newcomb, K., & Funderburk, B. (1993). Parent–child interaction therapy with behavior problem children: Relative effectiveness of two stages and overall treatment outcome. Journal of Clinical Child Psychology, 22(1), 42–51. https://doi.org/10.1207/s15374424jccp2201_ 4

Gimpel-Peacock, G., & Collet, B. R. (2010). Collaborative home/school interventions: Evidence-based solutions for emotional, behavioral, and academic problems. Guilford Press.

Greene, R. W., & Ablon, J. S. (2006). Treating explosive kids. Guilford Press.

Hanf, C. (1969). A two stage program for modifying maternal controlling during mother–child (M-C) instruction. Paper presented at the meeting of the Western Psychological Association, Vancouver,British Columbia, Canada.

Hobson, S. M., & Kanitz, H. M. (1996). Multicultural counseling: An ethical issue for school counselors. School Counselor, 4(3), 45–55.

House, R., & Martin, P. J. (1998). Advocating for better futures for all students: A new vision for school counselors. Education, 119, 192–284.

Johnson, L. S. (1995). Enhancing multicultural relations: Intervention strategies for the school counselor. School Counselor, 43(2), 103–113.

Lee, C. C. (1995). Counseling for diversity: A guide for school counselors and related professionals. American Counseling Association.

Lewis, A. C., & Hayes, S. (1991). Multiculturalism and the School Counseling Curriculum. Journal of Counseling and Development, 70(1), 119–125. https://doi.org/10.1002/j.1556-6676.1991.tb01571.x

Merrell, K. W., Juskelis, M. P., Tran, O. K., & Buchanan, R. (2008). Social and emotional learning in the classroom: Evaluation of Strong Kids and Strong Teenson students' social-emotional knowledge and symptoms. Journal of Applied School Psychology, 24(2), 209–224. https://doi.org/10.1080/15377900802089981

Neugebauer, B. (Ed.). (1992). Alike and different: Exploring our humanity with young children. National Association for the Education of Young Children.

Paniagua, F. A. (1994). Assessing and treating culturally diverse clients: A practical guide. SAGE.

Prochaska, J. O., & DiClemente, C. C. (2005). The transtheroretical approach. In J. C. Norcross & M. R. Goldfried (Eds.), Handbook of psychotherapy integration (2nd ed., pp. 147–171). Oxford University Press.

Ramsey, P., & Derman-Sparks, L. (1992). Multicultural education reaffirmed. Young Children, 47(2), 10–11.

Thompson, R. A. (2002). School counseling: Best practices for working in the schools (2nd ed). Routledge-Taylor and Francis Group.

Vasquez-Nuthall, E., DeLeon, B., & Valle, M. (1990). Best practices in considering cultural factors. In A. Thomas & J. Grimes (Eds.), Best practices in school psychology II (pp. 219–235). National Association of School Psychologists.

Webster-Stratton, C. (1998). Preventing conduct problems in Head Start children: Strengthening parenting competencies. Journal of Consulting and Clinical Psychology, 66(5), 715–730. https://doi.org/10.1037//0022-006x.66.5.715

Weisz, J. R., & Kazdin, A. E. (Eds.). (2010). Evidence-based psychotherapies for children and Adolescents (2nd ed). Guilford Press.

Wilde, J. (2005). 80 Creative strategies for working with challenging parents: A resource for elementary, middle and high school professional educators. Youthlight, Inc.

Evidence-Based Parenting Programs

MegaSkills

Rich, D. (1992). MegaSkills. Houghton Mifflin.
Rich (1992) focused on ten values/traits presented to help parents with children aged 5–12 develop skills associated with school success:

Confidence	Perseverance
Motivation	Caring
Effort	Teamwork
Responsibility	Common sense
Initiative	Problem-solving

Roots and Wings: Raising Resilient Children

Rich, D. (1992). MegaSkills. Houghton Mifflin.
Wilmes (2000) is designed to help parents learn how to provide positive influences for their children in the following areas:

Risk and protective factors
    Standards about tobacco, alcohol, and drug use
    Teachable moments (improving communication skills)
    Setting boundaries, building bridges
    Feelings
    Rituals and traditions

Building Successful Partnerships: A Guide for Developing Parent and Family Involvement Programs

National PTA. (2000). Building successful partnerships: A guide for developing parent and family involvement programs. National Education Service.
National PTA (www.PTA.org.) is research based in showing the importance of high levels of parent involvement to outcomes such as academic performance and pro-social behavior. The standards for parent improving parent/school collaboration aimed at helping students succeed are the following:

Communicating
    Parenting
    Student learning
    Volunteering
    School decision-making
    Collaborating with the community

Systemic Training for Effective Parenting (Step)

Dinkmeyer, D. C., & McKay, G. D. (1997a). STEP (systematic training for effective parenting). American Guidance Service.
Dinkmeyer, D. C., & McKay, G. D. (1997b). STEP/TEEN (systematic training for effective parenting of teens). American Guidance Service.
Dinkmeyer and McKay (1997a) is a video-based parenting program for parents of elementary school children and an audio-based parenting program for parents of teens. STEP program consists of nine sessions:

Understanding children's behavior and misbehavior
Understanding how children use emotions to involve parents
Encouragement
Communication: Listening
Communication: Exploring alternatives and expressing your ideas and feelings to children
Developing responsibility
Decision-making for parents
The family meeting
Developing confidence and using your potential

The Next Step (Systemic Training for Effective Parenting Through Problem-Solving)

Dinkmeyer and McKay (1997b) is designed for parents who have participated in the previous mentioned program and want to gain additional practice in basic principles through a problem-solving group:

Taking a fresh look at your parenting
    Building self-esteem
    How lifestyle beliefs affect parenting
    Stress: Coping with changes and challenges
    Making decisions as a family
    Gentle strength and firm love

Active Parenting Now

Popkin, M. H. (2002). Active parenting now. Active parenting.
Popkin (2002) has two versions: a video-based parenting program for parents of children aged 5–12 and one for parents of teens

The active parent
    Winning cooperation

Responsibility and discipline
Understanding and redirecting behavior
Building courage, character, and self-esteem
The active family now

Family Talk (Popkin, 1998)

Family Talk *is designed to help families improve their communication skills using any of the following topics:*

Family decisions   Grandmother
Television   Mother's time
Okay to feel sad   Feeling alone
Money   Mom and Dad's time together
Stress   Minorities
What's a step mom?   Equality
Honesty   Choices
Teasing

Bowdoin Parent Education Program

Bowdoin, R.(1993, 1996). Webster 's international. Bowdoin Method of Parent Education,. & II.

Bowdoin (1993, 1996) is a research-based curriculum designed for "high-risk, low literacy" families who need simple and basic parenting skills. The video-based program is presented at parent meetings to help parents of children from ages 5 to 12 improve their self-concept and develop skills for school success:

How to develop values for responsible living

Help your child say "NO" to alcohol, tobacco, and drugs
Harmony at home
Healthy minds, healthy feelings
Expanding your child's reading ability
Expanding your child's math ability
The single parent

Appendix A

Sample Slides for a Parent Education Workshop

Slide 1

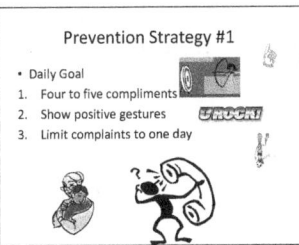

Parents need to create positive and upbeat home environments that are inviting and nurturing, and kids know that you are available for emotional connection and support when needed by them. Research show that a 5:1 ratio of compliments to complaints and criticisms keeps parent-child relationships intact.

Slide 2

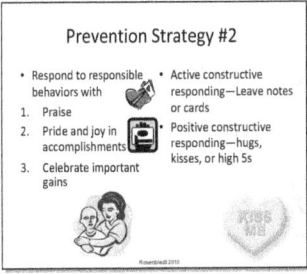

Set in motion purposeful positive relationships patterns that can strengthen and sustain connections.

Slide 3

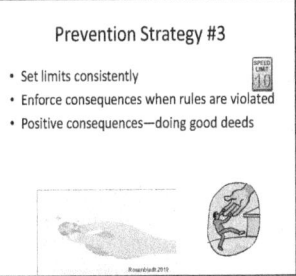

Experiment with positive consequences (time-limited) altruistic acts, which tend to raise socio emotional learning rather than always imposing taking away privileges or grounding.

Slide 4

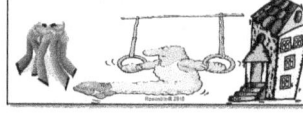

What do you do to manage your stress?

Slide 5

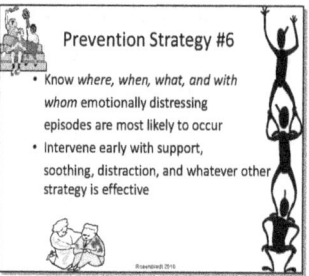

Monitor kids practicing using their coping strategies and tools at home. For example, if your daughter is experiencing emotional stress, you can ask her: "Which tool do you think can be most helpful to you right now?"

Slide 6

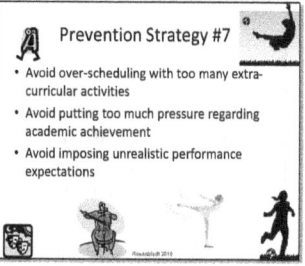

Slide 7

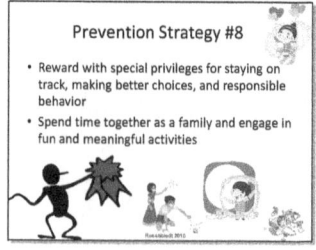

Slide 8

Research indicates that the second one is an important characteristic of strong families. The more parents and kids accrue positive experiences together, the more the relationship bonds will strengthen, which provides emotional insulation to better cope with their emotional distress and life stressors.

Slide 9

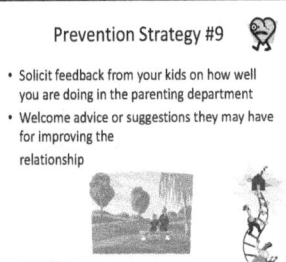

Prevention Strategy #9

- Solicit feedback from your kids on how well you are doing in the parenting department
- Welcome advice or suggestions they may have for improving the relationship

This shows kids how much you love and care about them and your willingness to go through great lengths to make the relationship better.

Slide 10

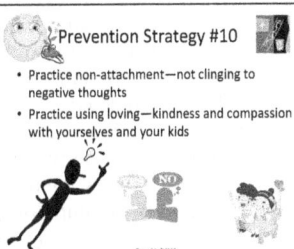

Prevention Strategy #10

- Practice non-attachment—not clinging to negative thoughts
- Practice using loving—kindness and compassion with yourselves and your kids

This will prevent parental burnout, and you will be better able to be more present with your kids. This will help strengthen your relationships.

Slide 11

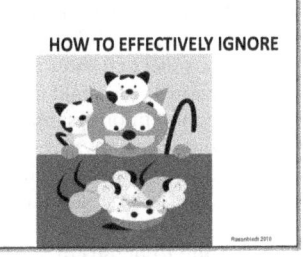

HOW TO EFFECTIVELY IGNORE

Here are the steps . . .

Slide 12

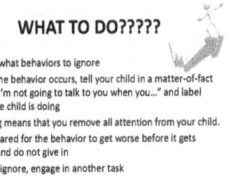

WHAT TO DO?????

- Decide what behaviors to ignore
- When the behavior occurs, tell your child in a matter-of-fact voice, "I'm not going to talk to you when you..." and label what the child is doing
- Ignoring means that you remove all attention from your child.
- Be prepared for the behavior to get worse before it gets better and do not give in
- To help ignore, engage in another task
- Once your child stops, be sure to reinforce/praise for appropriate behavior

Aggressive behaviors should not be ignored, but you will need to apply consequences. Ignoring is best used for minor misbehaviors especially involving crying, yelling, whining, pestering, and so on. Tell the child only once. Avoid lecturing because this typically reinforces the child's negative behavior. You should not communicate or talk with your child in any way. This means avoiding eye contact as well as not talking to your child at all. This sounds simple but is very hard to do. If you need to (and your child will be safe), you can leave the immediate area. If your child stops crying and begins doing a puzzle, you can say, "Great job putting that puzzle together. That looks like a lot of fun." Be sure to be genuine in your praise.

Slide 13

JOB CARD GROUNDING

- Alternative to time-out for older children
1. Create five to ten household jobs that your child can safely do
2. Write a detailed description of each job on a separate card
3. When breaks a rule, give one to three jobs to complete

4. Grounded until jobs are completed
5. Grounding ends when jobs are completed as determined by you
6. Grounding period lasts as long as it takes to correctly complete jobs

Rosenbledt 2012

Approximately 15–30 minutes. Jobs should not have to be completed immediately.

Steps should be specific enough that your child knows what to do without asking you for additional guidance.

Draws card randomly from a container.

If jobs are not completed correctly, you should review the steps with your child and have them redo the job. This should not be viewed as negotiation. Important to stick to grounding until job cards have been completed.

If child does job card immediately, grounding time will be very short or if s/he stalls, then grounding time may be quite long. Do not nag or remind your child about the jobs.

Slide 14

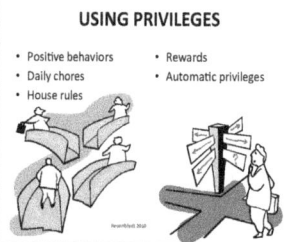

USING PRIVILEGES

- Positive behaviors
- Daily chores
- House rules

- Rewards
- Automatic privileges

Rosenbledt 2012

Providing privileges for positive behaviors: Generate a list of positive behaviors or extra chores your child can do to earn reinforcers/rewards. These should be rewards your child does not normally have access to or additional time in an activity your child has access to. Make sure to praise child w/reinforcer. Automatic privileges: Expected daily chores are tied to privileges children automatically have access to. Give one warning and time frame by which the chore should be started. If s/he fails to begin by specified time, take away one or more privileges. Generally best not to take away privileges for more than day. This way your child starts over with a "clean slate" each morning, and you don't have to worry about running out of privileges to take away. House rules: Whenever your child breaks one of the house rules, s/he should immediately lose 1 or more of the automatic privileges.

Slide 15

> **IMPLEMENTING PROBLEM-SOLVING STEPS**
>
> - Think ahead
> - Take a breath and make a plan
> - Think about solutions
> - Evaluate your solutions
> - Pick the best option and give it a try
> - How did it work?
> - Decide what went wrong and what else you could try

Sometimes you can guess when a problem might be coming and prevent it. You don't have to come up with a solution right away. Give yourself a chance to relax and think. We usually make better decisions when we're not mad, scared, or embarrassed. You have to get to the real problem before you can solve it. Think about all the possibilities, even ones that don't seem practical. Go through each solution you came up with and think about what would happen (good and bad) if you used that solution. There will likely be one or two that seem best. Pick the very best and give it a try. If you're satisfied, congratulate yourself. Maybe another option would work better and could be used.

Slide 16

> **SANITY SAVER—FIVE RULES FOR HW COMPLIANCE**
>
> 1. HW done in 1 place
> 2. Workspace equipped with appropriate materials
> 3. Limiting access to study area during HW
> 4. Keeping noise to a minimum
> 5. Starting HW at same time every day

Sanity savers home program is a homework compliance and behavioral program for reinforcement implemented in the home setting. Students and parents together determine most appropriate homework time and place.

Parents check planner/assignment sheet for assignments and confirm that students has begun working on each. Praise if child is already working.

After 10 minutes of work time, check for on-task behavior. Assist with homework tasks if needed and appropriate. Homework probably should not be done in the bedroom. Background music may be soothing and a focusing tool for some children. Prompt student to organize homework materials to bring to school the next day.

Slide 17

WHAT TO SAY AND DO

- Check with teacher about what will be expected and ask to be informed of assignments
- HW time is for learning, even if no HW is due
- Avoid power struggles
- Give limited choices
- Encourage daily!
- Show interest in child's work and help work through a problem
- Participate in classroom and school functions
- Consequences for not doing HW should be between your child and teacher and handled at school

For example, every Friday is spelling test and every month a book is to be read; you can reinforce it at home.

1. "Ashley, as soon as you finish 30 minutes of reading you may watch a ½ hour of TV. If you argue there will be no TV this eve."
2. "Megan, I know you are upset about having to do HW. Let's see what you need to do before TV time."
3. "Maria, your HW is to read for 30 minutes tonight. Do you want to read to me or read by yourself."
4. "Jose, this has been a week of great effort on your part! You have done a lot of work! Let's spend time together building with the Lego set that you got for your birthday over the weekend."
5. Do not do the work for your child. "Marnie, I love you, and I will be happy to help you. I know you will feel good when you accomplish this. I don't want to do the work for you and rob you of the opportunity to learn how to do it yourself."

Research shows children do better in school when parents take an interest and participate.

Slide 18

STEADY WARMTH

- Availability
- Comfort and reassurance
- Set warm emotional tone

Availability—Parents who are there when child wants to talk. Comfort and reassurance: Keep up family traditions and identities. Parents who set the emotional tone make a conscious decision on how they treat and react to children. Parents can decide how to act to have the kind of home they desire when they set a warm emotional tone that feels safe, steady, and welcoming.

Appendix B

Workshop Evaluation

Today's workshop was:
Check one: ____ Very helpful   ____ Helpful   ____ Not at all helpful

Some of my ideas that were supported were:

_____

_____

_____

Some new ideas that I can use are:

_____

_____

_____

I liked: _____

_____

_____

To make this workshop even better, I would:

_____

_____

_____

Additional comments:

_____

_____

_____

_____

THANK YOU!

Appendix C
Feedback to Workshop Facilitators

Title of workshop: _____

Name of workshop facilitator: _____

Please provide the following information with regard to your experience.

Warm-up: How did the "warm-up" help you get into the topic and ready to get involved?
Example/Comments:

Ask Before Telling: What about your own ideas were you asked to share before information was presented?
Example/Comments:

Personalize and Practice: As information was shared, what were you asked to think about, write, or share of your own experiences as related to the topic at hand? How were you given an opportunity to practice what you were learning?
Example/Comments:

Process and Summarize: At the end of the session, what were you asked to reflect on regarding your involvement in the workshop and how will you use what you have learned or relearned?
Example/Comments:

Evaluate: Please give feedback about the effectiveness of the workshop in reaching targeted outcomes. Example/Comments:

The most effective workshop strategy I experienced today was:
Something I might suggest for next time:

14 The role of information communication technologies in strengthening extended family connections with migrants and refugees

Maria C. Marchetti-Mercer

There is a growing need worldwide for appropriate therapeutic approaches to work with migrant/refugee children and their families, so the role of Information Communication Technologies (ICTs) in maintaining and strengthening ties in such families is attracting increasing attention in migration and family therapy literature. "ICTs" is an umbrella term for communication devices such as mobile phones, computers, television, and various applications, as well as social media, including Facebook, Twitter, and Instagram, and Zoom, and Google Meet. Given the separation and potential isolation of migrant families in a new host country, it is crucial to explore how ICTs and available social media platforms can support extended family relationships. This chapter discusses advantages and challenges of using ICTs in migrant and refugee families. It also considers how ITC use can be combined effectively with school-based family counseling (SBFC), as a culturally sensitive, innovative way to conceptualize the relationship between communities, schools, and families and propose new ways of engaging with these different role players in a therapeutic context, to assist clients to strengthen extended family connections. An ecological perspective is adopted, employing multicultural genograms.

Background

Transnational theoretical understanding of migrant families' experiences recognizes that today's migrant populations are able to maintain connections across the migratory spectrum, to both their host country and country of origin, as migrant families increasingly use and depend on technology. Migration no longer implies that family relationships end upon departure from one's country of origin. On the contrary, family and social relationships can be maintained and even strengthened through access to today's technological and social media platforms—today, "once migrants travel

DOI: 10.4324/9781003097891-18

across the border, their families do not cease to be active influences in their lives" (Silver, 2011, p. 213).

To describe this new type of migrating population with access to networks, activities, and ways of life that reflect their host countries and countries of origin, Glick Schiller et al. (1992) adopted the concept of transnationalism. Falicov (2007), writing from a family therapy perspective, also favors a transnational perspective because it describes how migrants can become part of a new culture while retaining their cultural roots and identity. Achieving transnationalism is important because mental health in families who retain aspects of their original culture seems to be better (Marchetti-Mercer & Roos, 2006), perhaps because having access to the strengths inherent to both cultures helps people not to experience feelings of isolation and ostracization in different social settings. It may also give them access to multiple support systems.

The motivations and lived experiences of every person who decides to leave his/her country of origin differ. A large body of work in the social and therapeutic sciences has focused on trying to understand what motivates people to move from their country of origin and identify specific stresses experienced by emigrants. Different countries have different examples and experiences of migration: migrants, refugees, and asylum seekers have radically different motivations and experiences. People also move to new countries as individuals leaving family members behind or as part of a family unit or social group.

Even if only one person migrates, migration is never an individual event: the ramifications of this decision are far-reaching, going beyond the individual and even the specific family that emigrates. The decision affects other members of emigrants' families, as well as friends and work colleagues left behind in the country of origin. These decisions have ramifications for generations to come (Falicov, 2007). This is particularly relevant to the experiences of second- and third-generation migrants and their challenges regarding their sense of identity and relationship with their ancestors' mother tongue. From this perspective, a systemic and ecological lens on the phenomenon of migration is particularly relevant. These are all important considerations for school-based family counseling (SBFC) practitioners, who work with the complex interface of child/family/school.

Key theoretical definitions related to the topic are discussed later, but there are too many vastly different groups of mobile populations (all with different experiences) across the world, and too much literature on those groups, to cover in detail in one chapter. I therefore focus only on migrants, with some reference to refugee populations. Equally, there are many different family forms, but I acknowledge writing from the perspective of Western "traditional" nuclear families (parents with their children) who move to a new host country.

Motivations underlying the decision to migrate

Many theories explain reasons underlying migrant and refugee populations' decisions to move. I focus on the seminal pull-and-push factor theory by Lee (1966), which remains relevant. Pull factors refer to the perceived attractiveness of the destination country (e.g., better living conditions, economic opportunities, or more educational opportunities for the children). Consequently, when migrants arrive in the host country, they may have high expectations and somewhat idealized views of what they will encounter. Conversely, people such as refugees and asylum seekers motivated by push factors feel forced to leave their country of origin because of negative and disadvantageous circumstances, fleeing economic, political, and social uncertainties, hoping to improve their living conditions in the destination country. People who feel forced to leave their country of origin often arrive with more potentially negative psychological experiences; their feelings of loss linked to migration may be more pronounced. They may be traumatized by political chaos or violence or volatile social and economic circumstances. Both groups may find that the host country does not match their expectations, adding to the challenges of adaptation. Some migrants are motivated by a combination of push and pull factors.

Differentiating between migrants and refugees

Underlying push or pull motivations (or combinations of these) may help to explain why different groups of migrants potentially have very diverse psychological experiences. Refugees are often dispersed mainly because of strong push factors, such as civil war or persecution, the expulsion of ethnic minorities, and conflict (Richmond, 1993). They leave their countries of origin non-voluntarily, often in the context of war and political upheaval, and may experience traumatic events in the process of moving (APA, 2012). Unsurprisingly, the emotional experience of refugees and asylum seekers differs from that of other migrants. Furthermore, ongoing separation from loved ones who may continue to be in danger may also be a predictor for future psychological symptoms (APA, 2012; Nickerson et al., 2010).

Migrants' experiences in a new country

The process of adaptation facing migrants entering a host country can be challenging. Berry (1992) suggests a continuum of the ways in which migrants engage with the culture of their host country, ranging from full integration to marginalization.

Other authors have favored an alternation model, which highlights connection to one's cultural roots and believing that a person can know and understand two different cultures (LaFromboise et al., 1993; Marchetti-Mercer,

2009). Thus, old cultural meanings are retained; simultaneously new cultural modes are acquired (Falicov, 1998). These ideas resonate with the transnational perspective discussed earlier and stress maintaining connections with non-migrant family members. Opportunities to remain connected with those left behind and maintain one's sense of cultural identity and roots are greatly facilitated by the present ease of international travel (at the time of writing, curtailed by the global Covid-19 pandemic), and advances in Information Communication Technologies (ICTs) (Wilding, 2006).

The emotional costs of transnationalism cannot be ignored (Falicov, 2007). Several studies have addressed challenges for those left behind, such as children or the elderly (e.g., Falicov, 2007; Gómez de León del Río & Guzmán, 2006; Marchetti-Mercer, 2012a, 2012b). Children may experience feelings of loneliness and abandonment, despite economic benefits associated with mothers' or parents' emigrating (Marchetti-Mercer, 2012b), and are profoundly affected by the emigration of parental figures (Glick, 2010). Some research has also considered negative psychological experiences of the elderly left behind by adult migrant children (e.g., Marchetti-Mercer, 2012b; Marchetti-Mercer et al., 2019). Again, ICTs can play a role in maintaining and strengthening these relationships, as discussed in the next section.

The use of ICTs in migrant/refugee families

Since the millennium, literature on the migration experience has increasingly considered how migrants negotiate the physical absence of loved ones by using different kinds of technology (e.g., Baldassar, 2007a, 2007b; Falicov, 2007; Horst, 2006; Panagakos & Horst, 2006; Wilding, 2006). Falicov (2007) believes that in today's globalized world, linked through technology, we can in fact speak of a "psychological family" or even a "virtual family" (p. 160).

I have previously (Marchetti-Mercer, 2017) outlined how technology has heralded what Baldassar (2007b) calls the "death of distance" (p. 401). Wilding (2006) comments: "The use of ICTs is important for some transnational families in constructing or imagining a 'connected relationship', and enabling them to overlook their physical separation by time and space— even if only temporarily" (p. 132). Bacigalupe and Lambe (2011) share this positive perspective; they see ICTs as offering "a splendid opportunity to maintain legacies, create new memories, and establish a coherent identity and continuity for family members" (p. 22). Baldassar (2007b) regards these new connections as constructing a "virtual co-presence" between migrants and those staying behind (Baldassar, 2008, p. 252) making mutually supporting relationships possible despite distance (Baldassar, 2007b). Borcsa and Hille (2016) describe virtual co-presence "as a social space in which people have an ongoing awareness of others" (p. 220).

Bacigalupe and Camara (2012) emphasize the role of mobile phones and social media as a coping mechanism for the refugee population, especially during their transition process. Alencar (2018) also reported that social media networking sites were particularly relevant for refugee participants to acquire language and cultural competences and build bonding and bridging social capital. Her study stressed the relevance of social media among refugees for contacting family and friends in the home country to obtain social and emotional support. Komito (2011) shows that social media allows refugees to contact and stay updated on the lives of those left behind—it may help them receive the emotional support they need to address the challenges of living in a new country. Ultimately, technology may serve as a tool to stay in touch with family members and friends and maintain a sense of belonging to one's community of origin (Komito, 2011). He argues that electronic communication, and the consequent sense of solidarity arising from such communication, may be important for those who wish to continue their participation in communities and social groups back in their country of origin. This is relevant because, as Falicov (2007) argues, migration always involves a loss of social capital, so it is important to develop community connections as a way to rebuild this social capital in either real or virtual spaces over time (p. 164).

Migrant children and youth's experiences

From an SBFC perspective, it is important to highlight salient experiences of migrant children/youth and reported uses of ICTs in the literature.

The APA (2012) points out that, in the United States (U.S.), successfully incorporating immigrant children into the educational system is one of today's most essential challenges. Consequently, it is vital to be sensitive to the experiences and needs of migrant children. Usually, children are not consulted in the decision to migrate and depend on the adults in their lives, who may themselves experience great stress and may therefore be unable to provide the security and support needed (Grinberg & Grinberg, 1989). Once they arrive in the host country, children may feel unable to communicate their challenges and problems to their parents, doubting their proficiency in the culture of the host country and its conventions. They may even experience their own parents as psychologically unavailable because of the stresses associated with the migration process (Birman, 2006; Suárez-Orozco & Suárez-Orozco, 2001) When the needs and stressors of the adults take precedence, children's needs may be ignored in this process.

Developmentally, immigrant children face challenges in the school system. For adolescents, peers, and peer acceptance, "fitting in" and "belonging" are crucial. Entering a new school system, feeling "different," perhaps unable to speak the local language and not understanding accepted ways of behaving, may be very challenging (Marchetti-Mercer & Roos, 2006). Grinberg and Grinberg (1989) argue that the effects of migration are most prominent in the school environment. If children originate from a more collectivist culture, with well-defined hierarchical relationships, moving to a host country with a more individualistic culture may increase the potential for intergenerational conflict at home (Hynie et al., 2006; Marchetti-Mercer, 2009, 2013), as the children absorb new values, especially in the school and peer context. Families may want to encourage their children to acculturate quickly, perceiving this as the road to greater success (better academic performance, successful peer relationships, quick acquisition of the new language), even though the parents may anticipate a loss of their original culture (especially their mother tongue) (Hynie et al., 2006; Marchetti-Mercer, 2009, 2013).

The literature on ICTs and migrant children has focused on three main topics: (a) technology use by children whose parental figures migrate to work in more developed countries and who stay behind in the country of origin (Hondagneu-Sotelo & Avila, 1997); (b) technology use to advance migrant students' education (Meyertholen et al., 2004); and (c) experiences of migrant students in foreign countries (Lim & Pham, 2016), when mobile phones/social media platforms allow young people opportunities to maintain a sense of belonging and emotional anchoring with their country of origin.

One noteworthy exception is Green and Kabir's (2012) study of experiences of migrant children in Australia and their use of ICTs in retaining some links with their original cultural context. They consider this process as a way to reproduce the social fields at the core of the transnational experience highlighted in the work of Glick Schiller et al. (1992). They found that, by using the internet, children who were older when they migrated to Australia were able to stay in touch with their friends back home. It was also a way to retain a sense of connection to their home country and feel a part of it. Therefore, using ICTs

> allows them to seek refuge in the familiarity of the old language and friendship system, whereas for others it provides an opportunity . . . of exercising their rights as global citizens with opinions on political activity at home and abroad.
>
> (Green & Kabir, 2012, p. 101)

Procedure

In looking at the role of ICTs in migrant families, we cannot identify a single specific procedure or intervention. What is essential is a conceptual lens in line with the APA's (2012) recommendation that, to increase accessibility and efficacy of services to migrant populations, clinicians should employ more ecological perspectives. Falicov (2007) suggests that family therapists become proficient at thinking in terms of "virtual and actual communities of concern for immigrants." This may include extended family members and other significant social relationships in both the country of origin and the host country.

SBFC practitioners work at the interface of individual/family/school/ community and therefore benefit from using such a conceptual framework. However, while the focus of this chapter is SBFC, these considerations and therapeutic applications are relevant to any mental health professionals working in various contexts with migrant populations.

I therefore propose that an effective way to identify such relational networks is using a multicultural genogram (Thomas, 1998). Genograms are based on the theoretical assumption that functioning of family members on different levels is interdependent and that changes in one part of the system affect the rest (Marchetti-Mercer & Cleaver, 2000). Consequently, genograms may be useful tools in identifying the impact of migration on an individual and on different interlinking systems, generating the information required. Falicov (1998) emphasizes the value of eliciting the migration narrative as a frame of reference for therapy with migrant families and as a way to explore the pre-migration experience, the migration process, and challenges related to cultural transition.

Traditionally, genograms are associated with the work of Murray Bowen (1993), McGoldrick and Gerson (1985) and McGoldrick (1995). It was devised as a visual map or family tree, depicting relational patterns in a family and identifying significant family life cycle events such as births, deaths, partnerships, and divorces (Yznaga, 2008). More recent variations of the genogram take a more "cultural" lens (see Hardy & Laszloffy, 1995; Thomas, 1998) to include questions about race or ethnicity, immigration, gender, socioeconomic status, spirituality, and worldviews (Yznaga, 2008). A more multiculturally focused genogram is therefore appropriate to identify the client/family's migration history and members of the extended family/community still residing in the country of origin.

A genogram can be compiled by an individual and/or a family group to elicit various narratives around the client(s) migration experiences. The therapist should explain that the genogram is essentially a family tree and guide the client through the different basic symbols used to depict the different family members and relationships (see Resources). There are several computer applications (see Resources), but a genogram can be compiled with nothing more than a piece of paper and a pencil. Yznaga (2008) suggests that clients should be invited to add as many members of the extended family as they wish in their genograms, including close friends and other members of their support network who may not be blood relatives, but still affect their lives.

Step 1: Developing a multicultural genogram

Identifying the family members

Borcsa and Hille (2016) suggest starting with what they call a "structural genogram" (p. 227). During this phase, the therapist collects demographic information about the family to draw up a basic genogram: education status, profession, relationship (marriage, divorce), medical histories; who lives in the household; and where other family members live (McGoldrick & Gerson, 1985).

Learning the family migration history

Thomas (1998) suggests asking some questions specifically related to the immigration experience, for example:

> What is the family's history of immigration?
> When did individual members migrate to the present host country and what were the reasons for the move?
> Are there any plans to return to the country of origin?
> What difficulties did they face during the process of immigration?
> How has each member of the family acculturated to the majority culture?
> Is there conflict between members who retain the culture of origin and [other]
> members of the family? (p. 28, cited verbatim)

Learning the relationship with the family members staying behind

Useful questions to explore with clients are related to their relationships with those staying behind, for example.

> Who are the family members left behind in the country of origin?
> Were elderly parents/children/siblings left behind?
> Are there other significant people in their lives whom they have left behind?
> How did their family members/significant others react to their decision to leave their country of origin?
> Are they in contact with those they have left behind?

Step 2: Exploring the family members' relationship with ICTs

> Do they stay in contact with those staying behind?
> Which forms of ICTs do they use?
> How do they feel about using ICTs?
> What do they find useful/challenging with regard to ICT use?
> Do they get a chance to visit? Are visits a viable option?
> If there are elderly people left behind and children who take care of them?
> What is their relationship with these caregivers?

Step 3: Discussing with the family ways ICT could be used to strengthen family relationships

During this part of the intervention SBFC practitioners can explore specific challenges the family experienced when using ICT. It is appropriate to share examples of how migrant families can use ICTs to maintain links with distant family members. Areas to explore are appropriate ways of connecting, which applications may be most useful, and how to navigate practical challenges such as time differences and access to connectivity. Searching for ways in which ICTs may be helpful in setting up relationships of care for older family members and creative ways to interact with younger children may also be valuable.

Case study: The Wilson Family

Jack (age 10) was referred to Janice, the SBFC practitioner at Meadow Middle School. His teacher said Jack was frequently tearful in class. When Janice met with Jack he reported that his grandmother wanted him to go and live with her in South Africa, but he did not want to leave his father and friends. Janice then invited Jack's parents to meet at the school to discuss how best to help Jack.

She learned that Jack's mother, Thabile, is a 35-year old Black South African woman who had been living in the U.S. for 15 years. Thabile entered the U.S. on a student visa and was placed with a host family, where she provided Au pairing services. She procured a scholarship and was able to go to college. She admits that she finds life in the U.S. difficult, but she is not ready to go back to South Africa, as she has a good career and a family. She works as a PR consultant at a hospital and is married to an African American, Jerry. They have two young sons, Jack (10) and Thomas (8). Her mother Dorothy lives in Soweto, South Africa, with Thabile's grandmother Agnes, and Thabile's cousins. Dorothy was very young when she had Thabile, so Thabile's grandmother raised Thabile (it is common for grandparents to take on this role in South African Black families). When Thabile first moved to the U.S., she did not call home very regularly because international calls were expensive. Now she finds WhatsApp a useful and cost-effective platform. Recently she became very concerned about Agnes's health and general well-being, as Agnes is getting older. Thabile is also concerned that her children do not have a close relationship with her own mother, Dorothy. Thabile only visited South Africa 5 years after moving to the U.S. and now tries to visit every second year but goes alone because of the cost. Dorothy first visited Thabile in the U.S. when the grandchildren were born and also tries to visit every second year, depending on finances. She does not get on well with her son-in-law and is frustrated by her grandchildren's American accent. On her last visit to the U.S., Dorothy announced that she would like Thabile and the children to come and live with her in South Africa, as their home. Jerry was angered when he heard this, resulting in a big argument, which the children witnessed. From this information, Janice deduced that family stress was affecting Jack.

Janice could use the following steps to develop a multicultural genogram and explore ways ICTs could be used to reduce family stress to help Jack.

Step 1: Developing the multicultural genogram

Identifying the family members

Using the genogram, identify relevant family members and where they live and ascertain the nature of the different relationships. Ascertain whether there are any other significant people in the family who are not necessarily blood relatives. Please refer to Figure 14.1.

Learning the family migration history

Identify when Thabile came to the U.S. and her motivation for moving there. Did she plan to move temporarily or permanently? Was her family part of the decision to move? What challenges did she face in adapting to the U.S.? Have any other family members migrated either to other countries outside South Africa or from rural to urban areas in South Africa? How much does Jack know about his mother's family in South Africa? Has he ever visited South Africa? Does he feel some connection with his mother's land of birth?

Learning the relationship with the family members staying behind

What is Thabile's relationship with her mother and grandmother? Are there any other important people in her family with whom she has significant relationships? How did her mother and grandmother react to her decision to move? Is there pressure from her family for her to return to South

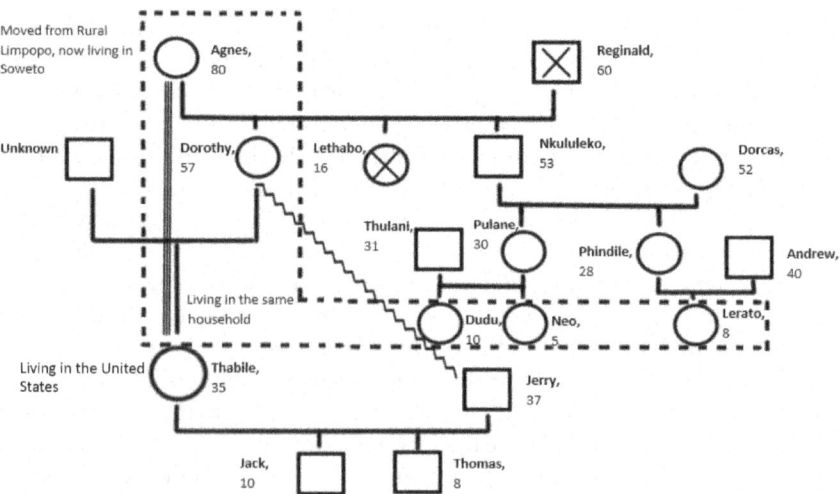

Figure 14.1 Genogram for Thabile

Africa? Does she send money back home? How did her family react to her marrying a U.S. citizen? What is the relationship between her mother/grandmother with her children and her husband? Explore Jack's relationship with his grandmother—are they close? Has he ever visited her in South Africa? Does he enjoy her visits to the U.S.?

Step 2: Exploring the family members' relationship with ICTs

Explore how over the years Thabile's ability to stay in touch with her family has changed. What means did she use when she first came to the U.S.? What was challenging then and what has changed? Does she visit her family regularly? Has her mother or another family members come to visit? Are there financial restrictions/limitations that her family in South Africa experience in using ICTs? As her mother and grandmother are becoming older, are they in need of additional care? If yes, who provides that care? Does Jack communicate regularly with his grandmother? What kind of technology does he use? Does he find it easy to communicate with her?

Step 3: Discussing with the family ways ICT could be used to strengthen family relationships

Explore Thabile's and Jack's use of ICTs with different family members. Is there a difference between Thabile's communication with her nieces/mother and grandmother? What kind of apps does she use? What apps do the older members in her family prefer? Do they prefer audio or visual interactions? How do they navigate the time differences between the U.S. and South Africa? Do they have specific times and/or days when they communicate? How do her children communicate with her mother and grandmother? Do they experience any linguistic difficulties when communicating? If her mother and grandmother require additional care is she able to communicate with caregivers through the use of ICTs? Explore how Jack's staying in touch with his grandmother more regularly through the use of ICT's could make her feel more connected to him.

After exploring these areas it would be useful to address any of challenges identified and explore strategies to address these, such as agreeing on applications that are suitable to everyone, how to set regular times for communication, respecting boundaries and maintaining ties across different generations.

In summary, the SBFC practitioner may want to highlight how distance and her advancing years are affecting Dorothy. If Thabile and Jack stay more closely in touch with her through regular and effective use of ICTs, this could alleviate her sense of isolation as well as make them more connected with their family in South Africa. By exploring the nature of the relationships with those left behind, the genogram may enable assessing clients' extended family networks and migration narratives and identifying the extended family's resources and strengths (Yznaga, 2008, p. 162). It may also allow clients to reconnect to their families and social support networks left behind in the migration process. Metaphorically bringing extended family members into the new culture may help migrants feel less alone and mitigate some of the stress associated with the loss and grief of migration (Yznaga, 2008, p. 163).

Importantly, therapists may explore ways in which clients could stay connected with those important figures by using ICTs. Having considered what means clients are already using to stay connected, questions can unpack what clients experience as useful and effective and, conversely, potential challenges related to these platforms (financial, psychological, and/or educational). The primary aim of therapeutic intervention is assisting clients to address how these opportunities may positively impact their relationship with those staying behind and how to negotiate potential challenges.

Multicultural considerations

The APA (2012) argues that there are several barriers to culturally sensitive and appropriate mental health services for immigrant populations. It may indeed be challenging for therapists to gain a comprehensive understanding of the cultural experiences of such clients. One particular difficulty in working with migrant families is that we may not be fully familiar with these clients' understanding of what constitutes a "family." Earlier work with multicultural groups in the South African context (Marchetti-Mercer & Cleaver, 2000) indicated that clients' definitions of a family differs across cultures and often includes more than blood relatives. It is therefore important to be guided by clients' understanding of their meaningful relationships and extended networks. Using the approaches outlined earlier and in studies by Hardy and Laszloffy (1995), Thomas (1998) and Yznaga (2008) offer ways to acknowledge various cultural experiences around what constitutes a client's family. Although the chapter is based on research I conducted in the South African context, these interventions may be applicable in other cultural contexts and several therapeutic contexts. What is required is an ecological perspective, which can be practically applied by using the multicultural genogram as a tool to connect with clients' experiences of family and migration. Thus, SBFC practitioners could apply the principles outlined earlier, whether working with children or families in school or other therapeutic settings.

Challenges and solutions

SBFC practitioners working in the context of ICTs and families need to note the important role ICTs can play but must also acknowledge some limitations and challenges.

Borcsa and Hille (2016) argue that ICTs have introduced qualitative changes in family functioning, creating new interaction scenarios and rearranging current family relational patterns (p. 219). They point out that studies show mixed results: some report a positive impact on family bonds and communication; others report a reduction in family time and intimacy and increased isolation of members living in the same household.

When it comes to the use of ICTs in transnational families, not everyone is equally enthusiastic about its uses, and some stress the importance of physical contact in maintaining relationships, something not easily replaced by technology (Marchetti-Mercer, 2012b, 2017; Mulder & Cooke, 2009). The question arises whether relationships can indeed be maintained over a distance or whether there is merely an "illusion of intimacy" (Marchetti-Mercer, 2012b; Wilding, 2006). In recent research (Marchetti-Mercer & Swartz, 2020) on South African migrant families, we note the ambivalence of migrant families regarding technology: families appreciate the access ICTs give separated families to connect with loved ones, but there is also a strong sense of the limitations arising from the lack of physical availability and close interpersonal interactions.

Even within the same family, different levels of competence regarding ICT usage must be taken into consideration. Prensky (2001) distinguishes between "digital natives" (those who grow up with technology and are familiar and comfortable with the different platforms) and "digital immigrants" (the older generation who remember a world without mobile phones and the internet). Using mobile devices and applications may be challenging for older people, and physical limitations such as poor vision are possible impediments to using mobile phones.

The "digital divide" is another important social and political factor therapist must consider: not everyone has equal access to these technologies, which may impinge on migrant families' ability to remain connected. Madianou (2015, p. 141) draws on a definition of digital inequality by Hargittai and Hsieh (2013)—it is "how existing social inequalities shape the adoption and uses of communication technologies as well as to how different uses of these technologies can influence social stratification." On the basis of this definition, she argues that socioeconomic status and education are strong predictors for the type of online activities that people pursue. Consequently, disparities in people's online uses can compound social inequalities rather than alleviate them.

In the era of Covid-19, we have all become more cognizant of the advantages, but also of the limitations, of ICT use. Falicov et al. (2020), who work with migrant families, warn that "[e]lectronic technology limitations intensify the perils of inequality and require focused attention to reduce it" (p. 874). SBFC should therefore consider disparities in the knowledge of, level of comfort with, and accessibility of ICTs in their work with migrant families. They should be mindful that even with ICT use, the pain and loss associated with migration may never be completely erased.

Conclusion

ICTs can play a very important role in maintaining and even strengthening migrant families' connections with loved ones left behind. By using ICTs families can feel supported in their host countries, support their own loved ones far away, and sustain a sense of transnational identity. SBFC practitioners can foster and bolster these relational connections, while remaining mindful of the continuous challenges that migrant families encounter daily.

Resources

Genograms

https://familytherapybasics.com/blog/2016/11/26/family-of-origin-exploration-for-the-therapist-create-your-genogram.

https://genopro.com/genogram/how-to-create/.

http://www.psychotherapy.net/data/uploads/5113c7cf41d4d.pdf. (Harnessing the power of genograms in psychotherapy—instructor's manual).

http://www.therapistaid.com/worksheets/genogram-symbols.pdf. (Useful sheet with the most relevant symbols).

https://genopro.com/ and. (Specific software that can be downloaded to draw a genogram). https://genopro.com/genogram/how-to-create/

Bibliography

Alencar, A. (2018). Refugee integration and social media: A local and experiential perspective. Information, Communication and Society, 21(11), 1588–1603. https://doi.org/10.1080/1369118X.2017.1340500

American Psychological Association (APA). (2012). Crossroads: The psychology of immigration in the new century. Report of the APA presidential task force on immigration. American Psychological Association.

Bacigalupe, G., & Cámara, M. (2012). Transnational families and social technologies: Reassessing immigration psychology. Journal of Ethnic and Migration Studies, 38(9), 1425–1438. https://doi.org/10.1080/1369183X.2012.698211

Bacigalupe, G., & Lambe, S. (2011). Virtualizing intimacy: Information communication technologies and transnational families in therapy. Family Process, 50(1), 12–26. https://doi.org/10.1111/j.1545-5300.2010.01343.x

Baldassar, L. (2007a). Transnational families and aged care: The mobility of care and the migrancy of ageing. Journal of Ethnic and Migration Studies, 33(2), 275–297. https://doi.org/10.1080/13691830601154252

Baldassar, L. (2007b). Transnational families and the provision of moral and emotional support: The relationship between truth and distance. Identities, 14(4), 385–409. https://doi.org/10.1080/10702890701578423

Baldassar, L. (2008). Missing kin and longing to be together: Emotions and the construction of co-presence in transnational relationships. Journal of Intercultural Studies, 29(3), 247–266. https://doi.org/10.1080/07256860802169196

Berry, J. W. (1992). Acculturation and adaptation in a new society. International Migration, 30, 69–85. https://doi.org/10.1111/j.1468-2435.1992.tb00776.x

Birman, D. (2006). Acculturation Gap And Family Adjustment: Findings With Soviet Jewish Refugees in the United States and Implications for Measurement. Journal of Cross-Cultural Psychology, 37(5), 568–589. https://doi.org/10.1177/0022022106290479

Borcsa, M., & Hille, J. (2016). Virtual relations and globalized families: The genogram 4.0 interview. In M. Borcsa & P. Stratton (Eds.), Origins and originality in family therapy and systemic practice. European Family Therapy Association Series (pp. 215–234). https://doi.org/10.1007/978-3-319-39061-1_ 13. Springer.

Bowen, M. (1993). Family therapy in clinical practice. Jason Aronson.

Falicov, C. J. (1998). Latino families in therapy. Guilford Press.

Falicov, C. J. (2007). Working with transnational immigrants: Expanding meanings of family, community, and culture. Family Process, 46(2), 157–171. https://doi.org/10.1111/j.1545-5300.2007.00201.x

Falicov, C., Niño, A., & D'Urso, S. (2020). Expanding possibilities: Flexibility and solidarity with under-resourced immigrant families during the COVID-19 pandemic. Family Process, 59(3), 865–882. https://doi.org/10.1111/famp.12578

Glick, J. E. (2010). Connecting complex processes: A decade of research on immigrant families. Journal of Marriage and Family, 72(3), 498–515. https://doi.org/10.1111/j.1741-3737.2010.00715.x

Schiller, N. G., Basch, L., & Blanc-Szanton, C. (1992). Towards a definition of transnationalism. Introductory remarks and research questions. Annals of the New York Academy of Sciences, 645, ix–xiv. https://doi.org/10.1111/j.1749-6632.1992.tb33482.x

Gómez de León del Río, J., & Guzmán, J. V. (2006). The impact of absence: Families, migration, and family therapy in Ocotepec, Mexico [Monograph] (pp. 34–43). American Family Therapy Academy, 2(1).

Green, L., & Kabir, N. A. (2012. (2013). Australian migrant children: ICT use and the construction of future lives. In L. Fortunati, R. Pertierra & J. Vincent (Eds.), Migration, diaspora and information technology in global societies. Routledge.

Grinberg, L., & Grinberg, R. (1989). Psychoanalytic perspectives on migration and exile. Yale University Press.

Hardy, K. V., & Laszloffy, T. A. (1995). The cultural genogram: Key to training culturally competent family therapists. Journal of Marital and Family Therapy, 21(3), 227–237. https://doi.org/10.1111/j.1752-0606.1995.tb00158.x

Hargittai, E., & Hsieh, Y. P. (2013). Digital inequality (Vol. 1, W. H. Dutton, Ed.). https://doi.org/10.1093/oxfordhb/9780199589074.013.0007. Oxford University Press.

Hondagneu-Sotelo, P., & Avila, E. (1997). 'I'm here, but I'm there': The meanings of Latina transnational motherhood. Gender and Society, 11(5), 548–571. https://doi.org/10.1177/089124397011005003

Horst, H. A. (2006). The blessings and burdens of communication: Cell phones in Jamaican transnational social fields. Global Networks, 6(2), 143–159. https://doi.org/10.1111/j.1471-0374.2006.00138.x

Hynie, M., Lalonde, R. N., & Lee, N. S. (2006). Parent–child value transmission among Chinese immigrants to North America: The case of traditional mate preferences. Cultural Diversity and Ethnic Minority Psychology, 12(2), 230–244. https://doi.org/10.1037/1099-9809.12.2.230

Komito, L. (2011). Social media and migration: Virtual community 2.0. Journal of the American Society for Information Science and Technology, 62(6), 1075–1086. https://doi.org/10.1002/asi.21517

Lafromboise, T., Coleman, H. L. K., & Gerton, J. (1993). Psychological impact of biculturalism: Evidence and theory. Psychological Bulletin, 114(3), 395–412. https://doi.org/10.1037/0033-2909.114.3.395

Lee, E. S. (1966). A theory of migration. Demography, 3(1), 47–57. https://doi.org/10.2307/2060063

Lim, S. S., & Pham, B. (2016). 'If you are a foreigner in a foreign country, you stick together': Technologically mediated communication and acculturation of migrant students. New Media and Society, 18(10), 2171–2188. https://doi.org/10.1177/1461444816655612

Madianou, M. (2015). Digital inequality and second-order disasters: Social media in the Typhoon Haiyan recovery. Social Media + Society, 1(2). https://doi.org/10.1177/2056305115603386

Marchetti-Mercer, M. C. (2009). South Africans in flux: Exploring the mental health impact of migration on family life. African Journal of Psychiatry, 12(2), 129–134. https://doi.org/10.4314/ajpsy.v12i2.43730

Marchetti-Mercer, M. C. (2012a). Is it just about the crime? A psychological perspective on South African emigration. South African Journal of Psychology, 42(2), 243–254. https://doi.org/10.1177/008124631204200211

Marchetti-Mercer, M. C. (2012b). Those easily forgotten: The impact of emigration on those left behind. Family Process, 51(3), 376–390. https://doi.org/10.1111/j.1545-5300.2012.01407.x

Marchetti-Mercer, M. C. (2013) (Chapter 46. Looking for "home" in a transnational world: Migration and school-based family counseling. In B. Gerrard & M. Soriano (Eds.), School-based family counseling: Transforming family-school relationships (pp. 382–394). San Francisco, CA: Institute for School-based Family Counseling.

Marchetti-Mercer, M. C. (2017). "The screen has such sharp edges to hug": The relational consequences of emigration in transnational South African emigrant families. Transnational Social Review, 7(1), 73–89. https://doi.org/10.1080/21931674.2016.1277650

Marchetti-Mercer, M. C., & Cleaver, G. (2000). Genograms and family sculpting: An aid to cross-cultural understanding in the training of Psychology students in South Africa. Counseling Psychologist, 28(1), 61–80. https://doi.org/10.1177/0011000000281004

Marchetti-Mercer, M. C., & Roos, J. L. (2006). Migration and exile—Some implications for mental health in post-apartheid South Africa. South African Journal of Psychiatry, 12(3), 53–64. https://doi.org/10.4102/sajpsychiatry.v12i3.67

Marchetti-Mercer, M. C., & Swartz, L. (2020). Familiarity and separation in the use of communication technologies in South African migrant families. Journal of Family Issues, 41(10), 1859–1884. https://doi.org/10.1177/0192513X19894367

Marchetti-Mercer, M. C., Swartz, L., Jithoo, V., Mabandla, N., Briguglio, A., & Wolfe, M. (2020). South African international migration and its impact on older family members. Family Process, 59(4), 1737–1754. https://doi.org/10.1111/famp.12493

McGoldrick, M. (1995). You can go home again. W.W. Norton & Company.

McGoldrick, M., & Gerson, R. (1985). Genograms in family assessment. W.W. Norton & Company.

Meyertholen, P., Castro, S., & Salinas, C. (2004). Project SMART: Using technology to provide educational continuity for migrant children. In C. Salinas & M. E. Fránquiz (Eds.), Scholars in the field: The challenges of migrant education (pp. 181–196). Educational Resources Information Center Clearinghouse on Rural Education and Small Schools.

Mulder, C. H., & Cooke, T. J. (2009). Family ties and residential locations. Population, Space and Place, 15(4), 299–304. https://doi.org/10.1002/psp.556

Nickerson, A., Bryant, R. A., Steel, Z., Silove, D., & Brooks, R. (2010). The impact of fear for family on mental health in a resettled Iraqi refugee community. Journal of Psychiatric Research, 44(4), 229–235. https://doi.org/10.1016/j.jpsychires.2009.08.006

Panagakos, A. N., & Horst, H. A. (2006). Return to Cyberia: Technology and the social worlds of transnational migrants. Global Networks, 6(2), 109–124. https://doi.org/10.1111/j.1471-0374.2006.00136.x

Prensky, M. (2001). Digital Natives, Digital Immigrants Part. On the Horizon, 9(5), 1–6. https://doi.org/10.1108/10748120110424816

Richmond, A. H. (1993). Reactive migration: Sociological perspectives on refugee movements. Journal of Refugee Studies, 6(1), 7–24. https://doi.org/10.1093/jrs/6.1.7

Silver, A. (2014). Families Across Borders: The Emotional Impacts of Migration on Origin Families. International Migration, 52(3), 194–220. https://doi.org/10.1111/j.1468-2435.2010.00672.x

Suárez-Orozco, C., & Suárez-Orozco, M. (2001). Children of immigration. Harvard University Press.

Thomas, A. J. (1998). Understanding Culture and Worldview in Family Systems: Use of the Multicultural Genogram. Family Journal, 6(1), 24–32. https://doi.org/10.1177/1066480798061005

Wilding, R. (2006). 'Virtual' intimacies? Families communicating across transnational contexts. Global Networks, 6(2), 125–142. https://doi.org/10.1111/j.1471-0374.2006.00137.x

Yznaga, Sd. (2008). Using the genogram to facilitate the intercultural competence of Mexican immigrants. Family Journal, 16(2), 159–165. https://doi.org/10.1177/1066480707313801

Part 5
School Prevention

15 Developing a Culture of Dialogue Among Students and Schools

A Proposal for Developing Newcomer Youth Advisory Councils

Erwin D. Selimos

This chapter discusses how SBFC practitioners can develop norms of dialogue between immigrant and refugee students and school faculty. The chapter assumes that students and teachers often have competing "definitions of the situation," which cause misunderstanding and conflict that interferes with student success. To overcome these differences and the problems they produce, we need interventions that promote schools that talk and listen. This chapter proposes the formation of Newcomer Youth Advisory Councils.

Background

The Curious Case of Course Placements

From 2012 to 2017, I was involved in several research projects exploring the migration and settlement experiences of immigrants and refugees living in a mid-sized, immigrant-receiving city in Canada (George et al., 2017; George & Selimos, 2018; Selimos & George, 2018). Through these experiences, I explored complexities of young immigrant and refugee lives and, not surprisingly, how schools were key institutions that helped and hindered them in pursuing their aspirations and goals (Selimos & Daniel, 2017). When speaking about their school experiences, young immigrants and refugees were exceptionally complimentary of their schools and teachers. They reported that their schools provided them with guidance in navigating their settlement and equipped them with knowledge and skills to build their lives. Teachers, especially English as Second Language teachers, were crucial sources of positive social supports. Young immigrants often referred to their teachers in familial terms: as parents, mothers, and fathers.

Despite these positive evaluations, I observed consistent and persistent disjunctures between how immigrant and refugee youth viewed their situation and defined their problems and how teachers and principals thought of

DOI: 10.4324/9781003097891-20

the problem. These differing perspectives were often a source of frustration among immigrant and refugee youth and represented underlying tensions between the school and immigrant and refugee youth.

Let me provide a case in point. The young immigrants and refugees who participated in my study were typically enrolled in two high schools. For various reasons, these high schools had become the de facto "newcomer schools," serving the majority of newcomer youth in the city. These schools had developed robust social and education supports for newcomer youth, including two academic streams for young newcomers: English Language Development (ELD) and English as a Second Language (ESL). The ELD programs targeted students with significant gaps in their previous education and spoke very little English. The ESL program was for students who have received a consistent education but required English language instruction. Both ELD and ESL programs had five levels, A through E. Levels A and B used sheltered classrooms and a combination of regular non-academic classes such as art, physical education, and drama. The sheltered classes allowed for intensive targeting remedial education and language instruction. Participation in the select mainstream classes offered social engagement opportunities. Students were placed into ESL and ELD streams after receiving a thorough educational evaluation by a specially trained teacher.

From the perspective of school officials, this was best practice, and I was astonished by the depth of care that teachers and school officials put into assessing their students' educational needs and designing educational supports to meet these needs. They were committed to the success of newcomer youth, and it showed in the system that was created. When students enter the C, D, and E levels, they begin to take more regular academic or non-academic classes. Level E students usually took only one ELD or ESL course and were enrolled mostly in regular course streams.

A curious thing occurred when listening to the perspectives of immigrant and refugee youth. I began to detect growing frustration with what young people viewed as unfair course placements. I noted these findings in an earlier research report:

> Some participants reported feeling that they were unfairly placed by school officials into course streams below their perceived abilities and in contrast to their academic and career goals. . . . Analysis of interview and focus group data suggests that racialized youth were more likely to remark on issues of course placement.
>
> (Selimos & Daniel, 2017, pp. 103–104)

What focused my attention on this frustration was a comment made by one young and exceptionally articulate refugee from Ethiopia who observed that "all the people who come from Africa, they put them in ELD. The people who come from European countries who don't speak English goes to ESL" (p. 104).

Differing Definitions of the Situation Produce Misunderstanding

What emerged from my research was a gap in understanding between the immigrant youth and school officials. On the one hand, teachers and other school officials defined the situation based on their roles in a bureaucratic system. The purpose of the in-take assessment was to identify the students' educational needs and place them into the appropriate learning streams. The process was rational, drawing upon the techno-bureaucratic norms of modern school systems. It made sense that many ELD students were from African countries. Many of these young people arrived in Canada as refugees and told heartening stories of displacement and trauma. Many *did have* significant disruptions in their education and *did need* intensive remedial intervention. By all estimates, the "system" was supportive and did what it was defined to do.

On the other hand, young immigrants and refugees defined the situation differently. These students drew on their own life experiences to make sense of their course placements. They had high aspirations, as their life and career dreams were deeply connected to their pre-migration experience and their sense of duty to their parents and families. However, racialized immigrants and refugees in my study were increasingly coming to understand that their local communities were somewhat segregated in terms of race, class, and immigrant status. Participants spoke of experiencing xenophobic and racist interaction in public. They also realized that their schools—the so-called "Newcomer Schools"—were stigmatized as "ghetto," "Welfare High," "Little Mogadishu," and "Terrorist High." Given such life experiences, it is no wonder that some immigrant and refugee youth would look upon the distribution of course placements as indicative of discrimination (Selimos & Daniel, 2017)

The story of course placements illustrates a fundamental tension in modern schooling. Teachers, principals, and other school officials develop definitions of a situation mainly based on their roles within a highly formalized professional bureaucracy. Students defined their problems through their social worlds. Given their different roles, it is predictable that school officials and students will have different definitions of the situation. The implications here are significant. Suppose school and student definitions of the situations become too incongruent. The necessary cooperative action required for learning is disrupted. Students will become distant from the school, perceiving it as an alienating place, unresponsive to their concerns. As a result, there will most likely be increasing school disengagement, interpersonal conflict between teachers and students, and academic problems.

To support immigrant and refugee youth in our schools, we must create opportunities for teachers and school officials to talk and listen to their students. Suppose we can develop specific ways to bring various definitions of the situation into more congruence. In such a case, schools will develop innovative and effective programs that increase immigrant youth engagement and address their concrete problems and concerns.

The SBFC practitioner occupies an ideal role to shepherd this process. Firstly, the SBFC practitioner understands that the problems and pressures children face are caused by micro, meso, and macro factors and are uniquely equipped to intervene at all three levels, including interventions that address norms underpinning school and peer culture (see School Prevention in the SBFC Counseling Meta-Model). Secondly, SBFC practitioners gain intimate knowledge of young immigrants' lives in ways different from teachers and principals. Because the SBFC practitioner is not a teacher, they occupy an important mediating role between teacher/school officials and immigrant and refugee students. They can use this unique position to broker cooperation and understanding. The following section discusses one potential strategy that SBFC practitioners and school staff can use to account for students' social worlds more deeply: a Newcomer Youth Advisory Council.

Creating Schools That Talk and Listen: Youth Advisory Councils as a Potential Tool

Youth Advisory Councils (YACs) are defined as "a body of young people who provide counsel and support to organizations and governing bodies and create and participate in a variety of projects and community initiatives" (generationOn, 2012, p. 9). As such, YACs provide a mechanism by which youth-serving organizations can support young people's socialization—namely by offering opportunities for leadership and skill development—and generate creative ideas from young people themselves to enhance the delivery of services and programs.

YACs represent one specific manifestation of a larger youth development model that has emerged in a variety of human service and social work fields, often under the term "positive youth development." The positive youth development framework takes a strength-based approach to children and youth. It places a high value on the role of positive adult-youth partnership and collaborative problem-solving in young people's socialization (National Research Council and Institute of Medicine, 2002). The values underpinning the positive youth development framework align with broader child-centered social planning efforts most clearly articulated by the Convention on the Rights of the Child, which famously declares that children and youth have the right to the 'Three Ps': provision, protection, and participation. The right to participation asserts that children and youth have the right to meaningfully contribute in ways corresponding to their developmental readiness to decisions in their families, schools, communities, and societies. This view places a normative demand on adults—they have the duty to include children and youth in the decision-making processes that impact their lives.

Even though young people spend a significant amount of their time in schools, schools have been slow to adopt YACs, most likely because school practices tend to emphasize adult control of time, space, and the social environment (Devine, 2003). However, YACs have been utilized by "third sector" youth-serving organizations to provide vital social services to their communities. I contend that when developed and implemented well, YACs can offer an excellent mechanism to creating norms of dialogue between teachers and students and generating effective school programming. More specifically, Newcomer YACs offer schools an opportunity to listen to their immigrant and refugee students' perspectives and design educational and social interventions to address their needs.

Procedures: Developing a Newcomer YACs

Step 1: Laying the Groundwork

The process for creating and sustaining a Newcomer YAC will take a lot of work, dedication, and additional training. In their manual "Creating and Sustaining a Thriving Youth Advisory Council," the Adolescent Health Initiative (2014) of the University of Michigan specifies five core components of successful YACs:

- They must be youth-led.
- They must have consistent and structured meetings.
- They must attend to community building within the group.
- They must offer a safe space for students.
- Their activities must include the planning, implementation, and reflection on meaningful projects.

The first step of creating and sustaining a Newcomer YAC includes reaching out to teachers or other staff members who you believe share the values underlying YACs and discuss the possibilities of such a school program.

Step 2: Recruiting Newcomer Youth

Once the organizational groundwork is laid, the next step is to begin recruiting young people. Who should participate in such a group? What can be done to recruit young people? In their manual "Creating and Sustaining a Thriving Youth Advisory Council," the Adolescent Health Initiative (2014) suggest that two primary criteria should be used to determine who should join: (a) any person who demonstrates passion, commitment, and excitement and (b) young people with varied backgrounds and viewpoints. In other words, participation should be relatively open and especially not determined by a persons' academic level of achievement.

Furthermore, the commitment to a varied viewpoint emphasizes the democratic values that underpin such groups. What is essential in recruitment is to ensure those who participate value the group's goals and are committed to participating regularly. The SBFC practitioner and other staff members could consider holding an interactive informational meeting to generate excitement about the group or giving classroom presentations to inform students of the opportunity.

Step 3: Developing Group Identity and Cohesion

After successfully recruiting participants, the time has come to dedicate a lot of energy to cultivating the newly formed Newcomer YAC's group identity and cohesion. Sociologists identify how rituals reaffirm people's membership in groups and help maintain group solidarity. In this way, the initial goal after recruiting members must be to establish the rituals that underpin group cohesion and identity. This is an essential step. More concretely, the Newcomer YAC must

- become knowledgeable of the other people in the group and form positive interpersonal relationships;
- develop a name for the group and other material objects that signify its identity (T-shirts, hats, emblems, and so on);
- create a mission and vision statement for the group;
- develop a routine for each meeting;
- set up consistent meeting times, dates, and locations; and
- negotiate rules of participation.

It is vital that developing group identity and cohesion be a collaborative process. A lot of care has to be taken to facilitate this process. Creating a group identity and mission in which the members want to belong and contribute often determines the group's ability to carry out its projects.

Step 4: Selecting Issues

Once group norms and identity have been established, and rituals developed to maintain cohesion, the next step is to undertake a process to identify engagement projects. The youth decided to join the group for various reasons; ultimately, most joined because of a desire to help others and solve the problems they see in their lives, among their peers, and in their community. A Newcomer YAC's primary purpose is for the young people to identify and address problems they see in their lives collectively. At this point, I think it is helpful to engage in structured group conversations about the types of issues newcomer youth face. There are many ways to create interactive discussions, and I encourage creativity. Ultimately, these conversations' goal is to generate a list of near and dear issues to the young people's hearts. If structured correctly, the list will probably be quite extensive and include challenges across various life domains, including family struggles, educational problems, difficulty with peer relations, mental health, and dissatisfaction with employment and leisure opportunities.

Once a good list of issues is identified, the task is for the group to decide which problem to focus on. A three-stage vote might be a helpful decision-making process. From the list, ask the youth to pick the top three issues they would like to address. The top three most voted issues would then be tabulated, followed by another vote to select from the list of three the top two issues. At this point, the group would have narrowed their focus to two issues. Here, I would suggest having an open discussion about the pros and cons of selecting either issue, followed by a final vote. By this point in the decision-making process, some consensus will emerge regarding which topic to focus on.

Step 5: Designing and Implementing a Project

The next step is to design and implement a project aimed to address the identified issue of concern. Because identifying a problem emerges from the discussions carried out in Step 4, it is challenging to specify concrete ideas for how a project should be implemented. The type of problem will vary depending on the interests of the group. For example, one Newcomer YAC may want to address bullying issues, while others may wish to address the stress that newcomer youth face during the first few weeks of arriving at school. In general, when designing and implementing a project, the Newcomer YAC should consider the following issues:

*   Is the project manageable? Don't commit to too large a project. In fact, choosing smaller projects that can be implemented in a shorter time-frame represents an excellent strategy to increase group cohesion and motivation. I recommend a project be no longer than 5 months.
*   Does the project need additional support? The desired project may need extra support, including money or personnel. For example, the New-comer YAC may wish to survey other immigrant students about their needs for extracurricular opportunities. Do you need to bring someone in to help construct the survey and help analyze its results? Sometimes the success of a project needs the support of the school administration. So it is essential to keep them informed and up-to-date about the project.
*   How will you distribute the workload? When implementing any project, who will do the work, when, and how are important questions. It is essential that the group discuss these issues and that there is a reasonable commitment on behalf of the group to work together to implement the project. When a clear division of labor is specified, it increases the chances of success and reduces intragroup tensions.

Step 6: Concluding the Project—Reflect!

After a project is complete, the final step is to reflect on it. This is an important step in the process, as it is in the reflection where the learning occurs! Ultimately, these project reflections should focus on what went well, what did not go well, and what might be done differently in future projects. This step must not be rushed, as it provides the base upon which the group can discuss how their involvement in the project led to their personal growth. In other words, concluding the project with reflection exercises is a wonderful way to celebrate achievement, share memorable experiences, build group cohesion, and identify essential skills that group members developed. The final reflection stage also allows the group to reflect on areas of improvement as a YAC. In these ways, it cultivates within the group members' dispositions toward continuous improvement. Even if the project was not successful, which can happen, this stage provides an opportunity to consider why. Reflecting on a failed project represents an excellent opportunity to move forward with the practical knowledge to make future projects a success.

Step 7: Selecting an Issue Again—Onward!

At this point, the cycle returns to Step 4. The Newcomer YAC must decide on what issue they wish to focus on. Because the group has just implemented a project, the group will have to discuss whether they want to start a new project or build on their previous one. However, the processes outlined in Step 4 remain a good starting point for the generation of new issues and potential projects.

Multicultural Considerations

Immigrant and refugee youth face specific problems related to their status as newcomers and share some common challenges faced by young people more generally. The Newcomer YAC model describes a way to develop a youth-focused problem-identification process. Because the Newcomer YAC employs a somewhat open approach, the issues that young people may choose to confront will also be open-ended. However, the democratic process it utilizes allows for identifying multiple issues germane to newcomer youth themselves in all their complexity and diversities.

Challenges and Solutions

Several challenges exist when attempting to implement a Newcomer YAC and will require some elegant negotiations on behalf of the SBFC practitioner.

Challenge 1: Finding Key Staff. Identifying key adult members is critical because sustaining YACs requires a lot of organizational support from adults. I would focus on recruiting ESL teachers because they often develop very positive relationships with immigrant and newcomer youth and are usually quite passionate about supporting this demographic group.

Challenge 2: Building Adult Knowledge of YAC Best Practices. Once key personnel are identified, the next step is building the knowledge and capacity of these adults about best practices in YACs. YACs are adequate to the extent that the adult partners understand the purpose and values that drive them. Thus, an essential step is to build the capacity and knowledge of adult participants. One way to do this is to organize a book study and discussion groups about YACs. The effective use of YACs requires that the adult partners understand their role, the values underpinning these councils, and the details of how to sustain them. Another option may be to bring an outside expert in to help with the Newcomer YAC's development. If your school is located in a city with a university, I recommend contacting their School of Social Work. There may be faculty members and graduate students who specialize in Positive Youth Development, and I imagine that they would jump at the opportunity to be involved in such a project. They would also bring the expertise, which would reduce the SBFC practitioner's burden in independently developing the necessary knowledge to organize a YAC successfully.

Challenge 3: Time and Commitment. The SBFC practitioner and the school staff should genuinely consider whether they are willing to implement such a program. While I believe the payoff is big, sustaining YACs requires a lot of energy. I caution moving forward on such a project if adult partners cannot make the necessary commitments. While I believe that YACs are excellent tools to develop young people's competencies and bridge the gap between schools and their students' needs, they require a lot of work. Other strategies promise to reduce the gaps between school and student definitions of the situation. For example, teachers could consider developing a yearly newcomer youth needs assessment.

Challenge 4: Getting Administrative Buy-In. If the school staff is interested in implementing such a program, the next step is to approach the administration to discuss such a group's formation. There are two reasons for this. Firstly, a Newcomer YAC program will be more successful if there is general support from administrators. YACs provide excellent opportunities to build social skills and reinforce learning already happening within a school. These are essential talking points when trying to elicit the support of the administration. The other reason for getting administrative support is to advocate for financial support from the school. While YACs operate on varied budgets, some funds will be needed for supplies and group cohesion-building activities. Even a $500 commitment would go a long way. Financial commitment on behalf of the school also demonstrates that the activity is meaningful and supports its efforts.

Challenge 5: Adult Takeover. Key values of YACs are that they are democratic, participatory, and youth-driven. Furthermore, the purpose of Newcomer YACs, as I articulated earlier in this chapter, is to bridge the gap between school and student definitions of situations. Adult takeover subverts the purpose of such groups and undermines the efforts to empower young people. The young people themselves should decide the projects that the group works on. Granted, the adult members play a vital organizational role, but they must not overstep their role and start dictating the group's direction. Adults may believe there are issues with one thing, but this may not be the youth members' primary concerns. Therefore, the critical challenge is to prevent adult takeover of the YAC's processes and projects. This can only be done if the adult members are thoroughly trained in YACs and commit to the values of being democratic, participatory, and youth-driven. The adult member's job is to support and guide but not to decide.

Conclusion

In this chapter, I emphasized that the SBFC practitioners must think of their role as broader than clinical practice and as mediators of school and community solutions. My research with immigrants and refugees suggests that a significant issue facing schools is competing definitions of situations between teachers and school staff and their immigrant and refugee students. I contended that bringing these definitions of the situation into better alignment represents a valuable way of creating innovative programming that promises to enhance immigrant and refugee youth's success and well-being. While certainly not the only solution, and certainly not without its challenges, I suggested that SBFC practitioners are well placed to lead these efforts. Newcomer YACs represent a possible way of creating schools that talk and listen to their immigrant and refugee students.

Resources

Neutral Zone's Youth–Driven Spaces

Neutral Zone is youth-driven teen center located in Ypsalanti, Michgan, USA. A key feature of this organization is the deliberate care it has taken in developing youth-adult partnerships in its activities and organizational design. Most interesting to SBFC practitioners is that the organization provides trainings on how to create youth-driven spaces. Participating in these trainings would be an excellent step in expanding the SBFC practitioner's skill set needed to implement YACs. Neutral Zone's website also has many resources on YACs. Neutral Zone's website can be accessed here: www.neutral-zone.org/

Sabo-Flores, K. (2008). Youth participatory evaluation. Jossey-Bass.
This book is an easily accessible "how-to" on participatory youth evaluation. Invariably, a youth advisory council will want to conduct some type of research project on young people's lives to inform their projects and activities. This book teaches the reader how to do it in a way that aligns with principles of positive youth development and SBFC's focus on a strength-based approach to children and youth.

Adolescent Health initiative. (2014). Creating and sustaining a thriving youth advisory youth council: A collection of youth experiences and recommendations. Adolescent Health Initiative.
Referenced in this chapter, the Adolescent Health Initiative is a nationally recognized leader in adolescent health. This toolkit is an accessible guide to implementing a YAC. The toolkit can be accessed here: www.umhs-adolescenthealth.org/wp-content/uploads/2017/02/manual-for-website.pdf

Bibliography

Adolescent Health initiative. (2014). Creating and sustaining a thriving youth advisory youth council: A collection of youth experiences and recommendations compiled by the Adolescent Health Initiative. http://www.umhs-adolescenthealth.org/wp-content/uploads/2017/02/manual-for-website.pdf

Devine, D. (2003). Children, power, and schooling. Trentham Books.

George, G., & Selimos, E. D. (2018). Using narrative research to explore the welcoming of newcomer immigrants: A methodological reflection on a community-based research project. Forum Qualitative Sozialforschung. Forum: Qualitative Social Research, 19(2), Art. 9. http://doi.org/10.17169/fqs-19.2.2907

George, G., Selimos, E. D., & Ku, J. (2017). Welcoming initiatives and immigrant attachment: The case of Windsor. Journal of International Migration and Integration, 18(1), 29–45. https://doi.org/10.1007/s12134-015-0463-8

GenerationOn. (2012). Game changers toolkit: Establishing a youth advisory council. https://static.globalinnovationexchange.org/s3fs-public/asset/document/game_changers_ yac_ toolkit.pdf?QHrlUeKPp_ vpvSObQ8NKwhcg0_ t_ huJm

National Research Council, & Institute of Medicine. (2002) J. Eccles & J. A. Gootman (Eds.). Community programs to promote youth development. Committee on community-level programs for youth. Board on Children, Youth, and Families, Division of Behavioral and Social Sciences and Education. National Academy Press.

Selimos, E. D., & Daniel, Y. (2017). The role of schools in shaping the settlement experiences of newcomer immigrant and refugee youth. International Journal of Child, Youth and Family Studies, 8(2). https://doi.org/10.18357/ijcyfs82201717878

Selimos, E. D., & George, G. (2018). Welcoming initiatives and the social inclusion of newcomer youth: The case of Windsor, Ontario. Canadian Ethnic Studies, 50(3), 69–89. https://doi.org/10.1353/ces.2018.0023

16 School-Based Suicide Prevention With Immigrant and Refugee Communities

Shashank V. Joshi and Andrea C. Tabuenca

This chapter describes the importance of school-based suicide prevention approaches for immigrant or refugee origin youth populations. Factors affecting suicidality in these students are reviewed. Several school-based suicide prevention programs that promote connectedness are described. A detailed description of the Stoplight Safety Plan approach to preventing youth suicide is provided with handouts that school-based family counseling practitioners can use with youth and their parents/guardians.

Background

For those clinicians who care for immigrant or refugee origin youth (IROY) populations, educational settings are crucial to engage with and to understand as fully as possible. Teachers and other school staff interact with youth on an almost daily basis, and they are key partners to help both clinicians, and parents comprehend the social, educational, and cultural context where mental health symptoms in IROY populations may interfere with learning, a feeling of safety, and overall access to the educational curriculum. *Mental health is part of overall health*, and our schools are charged with ensuring that students are *healthy enough to learn* and access the curriculum.

During the COVID19 pandemic when classes were taught virtually, school buildings and campuses continued to represent a very important, secure, predictable, and safe place for IROY populations and their families to receive medical care, mental health support, food and water, or social services. And while schools may not be designed as community mental health centers, they are places where interactions in the learning and psychosocial environment ought to be at least helpful and ideally therapeutic.

Several interventions have been developed to help affected youth gain better access to the school curriculum, despite their mental health symptoms. Many of these focus on trauma and post-traumatic stress disorder (PTSD), anxiety spectrum symptoms, and mood symptoms/disorders. A few of these will be described in this chapter, and there are several annotated resources for more information on evidence-supported interventions at the end of

DOI: 10.4324/9781003097891-21

this chapter. Careful attention should be paid to the supporting alliance among parents, teachers, and clinicians (Feinstein et al., 2009), such that members of each of these groups can be resources for one another to best support youth affected by mental health conditions (Joshi & Jassim, 2019).

As highlighted in a recent comprehensive review by Areba et al. (2021), suicide and suicide attempts (SA) among young people continue to be a public health concern in the United States (U.S.) and worldwide. In 2017, roughly 17% of 9th–12th graders seriously considered attempting suicide, and 7% made a suicide attempt during the preceding year (Kann et al., 2018). There is considerable variability in youth suicide rates by sex and race/ethnicity. For example, Black youth tend to be more vulnerable to, and die by, suicide at much younger ages, compared to White adolescents (Bridge et al., 2015; Garlow et al., 2005; Areba et al., 2021). Although not previously considered high risk for suicidal behaviors, SA among Black high school students increased substantially between 1991 and 2017 (Lindsey et al., 2019). Additionally, compared to males, females have consistently higher rates of suicidal ideation (SI) and SA, with the highest rates among Latino youth (females SI: 22.2%, SA: 10.5% versus males SI: 10.8%, SA: 5.8%), followed by Black and non-Hispanic (NH) White youth (Kann et al., 2018). Researchers have examined rates of suicidality among Latinx, Black, and Non-Hispanic White youth, but few cross-comparisons include ethnic sub-groups, such as Hmong or Somali youth.

Furthermore, the associations between robust predictors of suicidal behaviors over the life course—such as adverse childhood experiences (ACEs), defined as highly correlated, traumatic, and negative events experienced prior to age 18—remain understudied among ethnic minority youth (Ports et al., 2017; Areba et al., 2021). The literature focusing on risk and protective factors for suicidality among youth of color, especially among IROY populations is currently limited, highlighting the need for research that can inform suicide prevention efforts focused on ethnic minority youth with unique needs. Other important factors to be considered when conducting preventive and culturally responsive interventions with IROY populations have been described in both Europe and the United States (Montgomery, 2010; Nickerson et al., 2011; Tyrer & Fazel, 2014; Fazel & Betancourt, 2018).

Positive peer relationships, strong family bonds, and civic engagement are often used as some of the markers for positive youth development (Areba et al., 2021). However, significant language and acculturation issues unique to IROY populations require balancing the norms and expectations of their heritage culture and the majority (host) culture, and these can challenge psychosocial adjustment (Juang et al., 2018; Suarez-Orozco et al., 2018; Areba et al., 2021). Recent data has highlighted that the ethnocultural group at particular risk for fatal suicide attempts are Asian-American youth, where suicide is the leading cause of death in the 15–24 age group (CDC, 2018).

School Connectedness and Belongingness as Protective Factors

As Areba et al. (2021) have highlighted, the integrative model for the study of developmental competencies in minority youth (Coll et al., 1996) is one that places ethnic and racial minority youth development in a resiliency framework, which emphasizes strengths and assets, while acknowledging challenges within domains such as school environments, where IROY populations may experience marginalization (e.g., racism, prejudice, discrimination, xenophobia, Islamophobia). Intersecting social positions—ethnicity, gender, religion, and economic status—can shape youth development. IROY communities are subject to U.S. racialization experiences, which differ across ethnic groups and physical attributes, and risks associated with these experiences can contribute negatively to physical and mental health outcomes (Suarez-Orozco et al., 2018; Areba et al., 2021). This perspective highlights that resilience can be fostered even within deficient systems. Nurturing school environments (i.e., those with culturally relevant pedagogy, multiracial/ethnic integration, family and community involvement, teachers perceived as fair and attuned, and schools where students feel safe) can facilitate positive IROY developmental trajectories and adaptation (Areba et al., 2021).

According to Blum (2005), school connectedness can be thought of as "students' perceptions that adults care about their learning and about them as individuals" (p. 16). Evidence suggests that relationships with adults at school represent an important protective factor against suicidality for many youth (Wyman et al., 2010), including high-risk groups such as sexual and gender minority youth as discussed later (Eisenberg & Resnick, 2006; Taliaferro & Muehlenkamp, 2017; Areba et al., 2021).

However, the buffering effect of the school environment in the context of ACEs remains understudied (Eisenberg et al., 2007), and studies examining ACEs and suicidality in large non-clinical samples either aggregate racial/ethnic groups or do not address racial/ethnic differences in these associations (Areba et al., 2021). Thus, more research is needed using large samples that include adequate numbers of ethnic minority youth and IROY populations specifically. This will help facilitate comparisons to clarify these relationships and inform the development of interventions aimed at benefiting ethnically diverse youth (Areba et al., 2021). School belonging/belongingness is adapted from theories of belonging and refers to a student's need to form and maintain at least a minimum quantity of lasting, positive, and significant interpersonal relationships (Baumeister & Leary, 1995, p. 497). Belonging is defined as "an individual's sense of being accepted, valued, included, and encouraged by others" (Baumeister & Leary, 1995).

Though it is only now getting studied in ethnoculturally diverse youth, an important theory worth considering for suicide prevention among IROY populations is the Interpersonal Theory of Suicide (IPTS) (Van Orden et al., 2005). It provides a theoretical model of suicide behavior that explains the emergence of SI and SA. In a study that tested the full IPTS model in a non-clinical community-based sample of adolescents, Calear and colleagues recently completed the Sources of Strength Australia Project, which included 1,382 adolescents aged 12–17 years (Calear et al., 2021). Participants completed measures of perceived burdensomeness, thwarted belongingness, capability for suicide (fearlessness about death), and SI and behavior. Their findings support the predictions of the IPTS in relation to SI in adolescents. Given the clear associations between perceived burdensomeness and thwarted belongingness with suicide risk in adolescents, there may be value in targeting these factors in the assessment and prevention of suicide in IROY populations (Calear et al., 2021).

The authors proposed that future research should examine whether other protective factors, such as positive ethnic identity, religion and spirituality, and cultural beliefs and norms, mitigate the negative effects of multiple ACEs on suicide risk among ethnic minority youth. In a study which included IROY populations in the Midwestern United States, rates of SI among male youth were similar to national estimates, except for Somali boys who had slightly higher (8.5%) prevalence compared to Black males (6.6%) nationwide (Kann et al., 2018; Areba et al., 2021). Additionally, although students in higher grades exhibit more suicidal behaviors, ethnic minority youth, especially Black boys, have been found to be more vulnerable to suicide at younger ages (Bridge et al., 2015; Garlow et al., 2005). Thus, risk prevention and health promotion efforts should target youth in lower grades to address and potentially mitigate the effects of interacting factors within the community, family, and schools including, but not limited to poverty, exposure to violence, and humanitarian emergencies (Areba et al., 2021).

Furthermore, the authors emphasized the recently issued CDC guidelines on suicide prevention, highlighting a need to focus on violence prevention and the promotion of protective factors such as school connectedness (Ports et al., 2017; Areba et al., 2021). Experts advocate for targeted, comprehensive suicide prevention efforts that involve schools, families, governments, and communities for at-risk adolescents (Stone et al., 2017). As a school-based family counseling (SBFC) community, we must ensure suicide prevention programs and the contexts within which they are delivered, are effective for all youth, both those of majority cultures and those from IROY communities. The authors conclude with this reminder (Areba et al., 2021):

> Similar to many problems that require societal change and institutional investments to improve household and community environments, primary prevention of ACEs is challenging, and screening can be complex and controversial. However, it is imperative to understand the role

of early adversity in health outcomes and screen for ACEs effectively among ethnic minority youth who are also IROY to help reduce suicidal behavior.

(p. 8)

Sexual and Gender Minority Youth

Suicide attempts are over three times more likely in queer youth compared to straight peers (Johns et al., 2020), with the risk of increasing by 20% in unsupportive environments (Hatzenbuehler, 2011). Family rejection poses the greatest risk to youth safety (Ryan et al., 2010) and is unfortunately notable in many immigrant communities where cultural views are less congruent with LGBTQ acceptance (Hafeez et al., 2017). By establishing specific spaces for queer students, schools can buffer these risks by providing safety through acceptance and affirmation. Programs such as a Gay-Straight Alliance (GSA) can reduce suicidality and offset numerous risk factors that impact mental health among queer youth (Heck et al., 2011). Furthermore, teachers at schools with a GSA and LGBTQ youth-specific training are more likely to engage in supportive behaviors on behalf of students being bullied, further promoting a sense of safety and belonging (Swanson & Gettinger, 2016). However, teachers must remain aware that students of color and immigrant youth may benefit less directly from GSAs, due to a sense of racial and ethnic isolation within the group or risk of rejection from their own communities if GSA membership is detected (Baams et al., 2020). While some students may be "out" in certain settings, their capacity to safely be "out" more publicly may be limited. It is imperative that teachers also create an inclusive environment offering opportunities for individualized support and assure students confidentiality with regard to sexual and gender identity.

School-Based Suicide Prevention Programs That Promote Connectedness

Sources of Strength is a Tier 1 universal prevention program that seeks to understand the role of peers and peer leader influences in school settings (Wyman et al., 2010; Joshi et al., 2015). It is both a school-wide health promotion program and suicide prevention program that provides training for both peer leaders and adult advisors. These students then conduct focused peer-to-peer prevention and messaging activities on campus, designed to build social and ecological protective influences across the full student population. In an 18-school randomized clinical trial (RCT), Wyman et al. (2010) demonstrated that the training of peer leaders with this program led to changes in norms across the full population of high school students after 4 months of school-wide messaging. Youth opinion leaders from diverse social cliques, including at-risk adolescents, were trained to change the norms and behaviors of their peers by conducting well-defined social messaging activities with close adult guidance. The two social norms most strongly enhanced through the intervention were (a) students' perceptions that adults in their school can provide help to suicidal students and (b) the acceptability of seeking help from adults. The largest, most positive increases in perceptions of adult help for suicidal youths occurred among students with a history of SI. In the larger high schools studied, sources of strength training also increased peer leaders' referrals of friends to adults because of concerns about suicide. By training a diverse group of peer leaders within each school, the program was able to provide well-adapted students with opportunities to influence at-risk students, thereby reducing possible iatrogenic effects that may occur by grouping at-risk adolescents (Wyman et a., 2010; Joshi et al., 2015). The investigators proposed that because adolescents are far more likely to be aware of suicidal behavior in their friends than adults are, increasing students' partnering with adults to help suicidal peers may be a key process for reducing adolescent suicidal behavior. They also highlight that the protective factors pertaining to help seeking, connectedness with adults, and school engagement not only lowers the risk for suicidal behavior, but these factors are also associated with a reduced risk for school dropout, depression, and substance use problems. The overlap of suicide prevention objectives with other school-based educational and health promotion goals, such as keeping students enrolled in school and increased academic achievement, can increase the attractiveness and feasibility of disseminating this peer leader intervention (Wyman et al., 2010; Joshi et al., 2015).

Programs That Focus on Trauma in Schools

Cognitive behavioral interventions for trauma in schools (CBITS) is an established group skills-based treatment approach to addressing trauma in the school setting utilizing a treatment model with elements similar to, but distinct from, Trauma-Focused Cognitive Behavioral Therapy. Because the program is administered in schools, teacher education about the effects of trauma is included, and there is a parent psycho-education component. Advantages of CBITS are that school-based treatment can be made available to children who may not otherwise have access to treatment, and participating in a group at school may reduce stigma associated with obtaining mental health services outside this naturalistic environment. In addition, peer support and modeling are facilitated through the group format. The most significant disadvantage is that treatment cannot be tailored to individual children's symptoms, and certain kinds of trauma (e.g., sexual abuse) may not be appropriate for a school-based group format. CBITS is most suited for addressing PTSD and other symptoms associated with exposure to domestic or community violence in underserved youth who are unlikely to access clinic-based mental health services. CBITS was developed through a collaborative partnership with schools and community members (including parents), and it has been supported in randomized clinical trials and a quasi-experimental trial. These studies found reductions in PTSD and depressive symptoms in elementary and middle school children participating in the treatment compared to a control group. The developers report success in implementing CBITS in numerous communities with students from diverse racial, ethnic, and socioeconomic backgrounds (Kataoka et al., 2012; Wilson & Joshi, 2018).

Cue-Centered Treatment (CCT) was first developed with diverse, mostly immigrant populations to address PTSD and other trauma-related symptoms in children who have experienced chronic, ongoing trauma and other adversities and has been delivered in school settings successfully. CCT recognizes that children with multiple traumatic experiences (or "complex trauma") may gain limited benefits from processing a focal trauma. This treatment helps the child to become their own agent of change through increased awareness of trauma-related experiences and symptoms, development of skills for coping with trauma symptoms, and increased insight into relationships among traumatic experiences, emotional reactions, and behavioral responses. Although CCT remains an emerging treatment, the first randomized controlled trial with 65 youth with histories of interpersonal violence exposure found that compared to a waitlist control condition, CCT was associated with greater reduction of PTSD and anxiety symptoms and improvement in overall functioning. These gains were maintained over a 3-month period following treatment (Carrion et al., 2013; Wilson & Joshi, 2018).

Procedure

Regarding suicide prevention specifically, clinicians must become facile with safety planning. A safety plan can be conducted as a brief yet comprehensive intervention that emphasizes both crisis prevention and effective crisis management. It is a list of coping strategies and social supports that people can use when they are in a suicidal crisis or very distressed. Stanley and Brown (2012) describe the basic components of a safety plan created through their "Safety Planning Intervention" deemed a best practice by the American Foundation for Suicide Prevention (also available as a free app for smart phones titled "Safety Net"). These components include

> (a) recognizing warning signs of an impending suicidal crisis; (b) employing internal coping strategies; (c) utilizing social contacts and social settings as a means of distraction from suicidal thoughts; (d) utilizing family members or friends to help resolve the crisis; (e) contacting mental health professionals or agencies; (f) restricting access to lethal means.; and g) identifying the most important thing(s) to live for.

(p. 258)

Tabuenca and colleagues have adapted the Safety Plan template by Stanley and Brown (2012) and utilized tools from evidence-based psychotherapy (CBT) such as the feelings/fear thermometer in creating the Stoplight Safety Plan (SSP; Tabuenca et al., [2021]). This plan is created with the patient and reviewed in detail with the custodial parents/guardians and is a critical component of discharge planning from an emergency department or inpatient unit. It can also be part of outpatient treatment planning for IROY and other youth populations at risk for suicide. This not only gives agency and responsibility to the child/teen but helps them regain their sense of agency and self-efficacy so crucial to their psychosocial development. Figures 16.1–16.3 provide specific examples of how an SSP is developed and utilized.

Table 16.1. Stoplight Safety Plan, Example 1

10	**Describe the RED ZONE**
	Thoughts: Prompt for specific thoughts that contribute directly to SI such as thoughts about self/others and the future. Facilitate patient in identifying any distortions that could benefit from therapeutic support.
	Feelings: Prompt for specific emotional reactions that could benefit from adaptive coping strategies that patients can learn during hospitalization such as DBT skills for distress tolerance.
9	**Actions:** Prompt for any maladaptive actions that serve to link distressing emotions with suicidal behaviors (e.g., isolating/shutting others out, continuing to engage in unproductive discussions, seeking immediate relief in ways that exacerbate the issue at hand).
	Coping plan
	—I communicate that I am in this zone by (what words will you use?)
	Ensure that specific words so that parents can distinguish this zone from others. If verbal communication is too difficult, explore nonverbal strategies for communicating unsafe urges.
	—Others can respond to me by (what can they say and do?).
8	Support patient in considering the types of behaviors they might expect from parents after communicating unsafe urges. Identify which of these contribute to communication avoidance and help the patient explore appropriate alternatives that parents can be coached in. If the plan includes taking space, identify the specifics of where and for how long. Establish a check-in frequency and define what check-ins will look like (verbal/nonverbal, numerical). Establish a threshold for calling 911 or going to ED.
	—I can use the following coping skills
	Support the patient in exploring coping skills that target distressed feelings described earlier. Ensure all coping strategies selected are safe for this patient (e.g., going for a walk alone may be high risk and require supervision for some patients). Consider coping tools that may cause family conflict (e.g., using screens, isolating from family in room) and plan concretely to balance patient coping and limit setting for the parents.
7	**—I can show others that I am safe by** Establish check-ins from parents, keeping doors open/unlocked, continuing to verbalize safety/zone number from family. Review threshold for calling 911 or going to ED.

(Continued)

Table 16.1 (Continued)

Describe the YELLOW ZONE

Thoughts: Prompt for thinking patterns that place patient at risk for continuing to escalate toward the red zone.

6   **Feelings:** Prompt for feelings that can serve as cues/alerts that they are in the yellow zone and need to take action.

Actions: Prompt for actions that can increase exposure to triggers toward the red zone.

Coping plan

—I communicate that I am in this zone by (what words will you use?)

5   Explore communication with anyone in the social support network who can facilitate problem-solving or help the patient avoid trigger exposure (e.g., parents, school staff, peers).

—Others can respond to me by (what can they say and do?)

Identify common triggers that link patient from yellow zone to red zone. Support patient in identifying how others can help them avoid these and support problem-solving to return to green.

4   **—I can use the following coping skills**

Coping should focus on reducing trigger exposure and increasing problem-solving or self-care.

Describe the GREEN ZONE

Thoughts

Feelings

3   **Actions**

Coping plan

Things I can do to stay in the green zone

Consider strategies for targeting any issues that made patient vulnerable to crisis and hospitalization. Examples include plans for targeting school challenges, sleep hygiene, medication adherence, therapy adherence, and

2   family communication. Most plans include goals for re-entry/504 meetings, increasing family check-ins, increasing structure and routine, and increasing regular self-care activities.

Things others can help me do to stay in the green zone

Support patient (and family in meeting) with identifying how to concretely support anything patient listed earlier. Consider providing family with any psycho-education handouts to facilitate their support (e.g., parent validation

1   sheet or behavioral management sheet).

National Suicide Prevention Lifeline 1–800–273–8255

Text: CONNECT to 741741

(Clinicians to put other [local] resources, warm lines here)

Ref: This *Stoplight Safety Plan* template is taken from
Tabuenca, Kim, and Gipson (2021): "When time is tight and stakes are high: Pharmacotherapy, alliances, and the inpatient unit," *in* Joshi S. V. and Martin A. (eds.) *Thinking About Prescribing: The Psychology of Psychopharmacology with Diverse Youth & Families*; Washington, DC, American Psychiatric Association Press, 315 pages, 2021.

Table 16.2. Spotlight Safety Plan, Example 2

Describe the RED ZONE
Cues that define this zone have been identified thoughts/feelings/actions.
Frequency and length of time typically spent in this zone have been included.
Coping plan
—**I communicate that I am in this zone by (what words will you use?)**
—Language agreed upon is specific enough that family will understand the severity
  of patient's distress and be able to distinguish this communication from how the
  patient might communicate distress in other zones.
—Backup plans are in place if needed, including access to other trusted adults,
  therapist if appropriate, and/or contact for suicide hotlines.
—**Others can respond to me by (what can they say and do?).**
—Specific behaviors for parent/family responses that are deemed supportive were
  identified.
—Specific behaviors that could exacerbate patient's distress in this zone were
  explored and alternatives identified.
—If patient plan includes taking space, a plan for safe space is established
  (i.e., location, line of sight, proximity to parent, and so on). If plan includes no
  verbal communication about stressors, ensure plan is in place for other verbal or
  written communication about safety, such as use of color codes or numbers on
  scale to be able to disclose severity of safety concern.
—**I can use the following coping skills**
—Specific coping strategies are identified with barriers to accessing these strategies.
—Coping skills explored have included somatic skills (ice, hot shower, breathing,
  scents, food), cognitive skills (challenging between thinking, accessing wise mind,
  using comparisons, positive journaling), behavioral skills (distraction via activities,
  accessing pets, physical activity, and so on).
—Psycho-education was provided regarding any maladaptive coping skills that
  patient included, and plan for ways to avoid these has been included
  (e.g., avoiding excessive isolation, avoiding accessing social media if deemed to
  be triggering in the past).
—Included PRN ('when required') plan if appropriate.
—**I can show others that I am safe by**
—Supervision plan is established, including frequency and nature of parental visual/
  verbal check-in while in red
—Threshold for establishing need to call 911 or visit ED is established (through
  either planned communication or agreed-upon behavioral observations).

Describe the YELLOW ZONE
—Cues that define this zone have been identified thoughts/feelings/actions.
—Frequency and length of time typically spent in this zone has been included.
Coping plan
—**I communicate that I am in this zone by (what words will you use?)**
—Language agreed upon is specific enough that family will understand the severity
  of patient's distress and be able to distinguish this communication from how the
  patient might communicate distress in other zones.
—**Others can respond to me by (what can they say and do?)**
—Specific behaviors for parent/family responses that are deemed supportive were
  identified.
—Specific behaviors that could exacerbate patient's distress in this zone were
  explored and alternatives identified.

(Continued)

Table 16.2 (Continued)

—If behaviors that parents are asked to avoid are of eventual necessity (e.g., discussing school progress) then plan has been made to identify when/how these conversations can occur in a more controlled setting, for example, scheduling time-limited conversations in the home and/or postponing discussions until therapy sessions.
—Potential triggers for red zone escalation have been identified, and plan was made for how family can help patient minimize exposure to these triggers.
—**I can use the following coping skills.**
—Specific coping strategies were identified with barriers to accessing these strategies problem solved.
—Coping skills include a patient plan to address the issues that have resulted in yellow zone escalation to prevent ongoing escalation and return to green (i.e., a plan for problem-solving is included).

Describe the GREEN ZONE
—Cues that define this zone have been identified thoughts/feelings/actions.
—Frequency and length of time typically spent in this zone has been included.
Coping plan
Things I can do to stay in the green zone
Plan addresses all aspects of chain analysis vulnerabilities that team deemed contributory to hospitalization. Examples include the following:
—Explored need for sleep hygiene plan
—Explored need for medication adherence plan
—Explored need for commitment to change in level of care or style of therapy
—Explored plan for patient to address school stressors
—Explored plan for patient to address social stressors (i.e., modify communication with triggering individuals or increase communication with helpful individuals)
—Explored plan for behavioral activation by increasing physical and recreational activities available
—Explored need for substance use plan (i.e., plan for reduced access to substances and/or toxicology monitoring by parents or providers)
—Explored need for further consultations/supports from other providers (e.g., if patient needs additional support for eating disorder, gender dysphoria, Autism Spectrum Disorder supports, among others).
—Established patient commitment to frequency and type of communication that will happen daily with family regarding level of distress until this plan is further modified by outpatient team (e.g., twice daily check ins? verbal/written? number scale/zone/emotion labels?)
Things others can help me do to stay in the green zone
—Explored commitment that family is willing to make to daily family routine to reduce triggers/stressors
—Explored parental commitment to frequency and type of patient daily communication about distress
—Explored ways in which parents can facilitate any of the items that patient is committing to in the green zone (e.g., facilitate enrollment in activities, provide transportation, plan supervision for patient to spend time with friends, and so on)
—Explored parent role in reducing school-related stressors by working with school to establish accommodations.

National Suicide Prevention Lifeline 1-800-273-8255
Text: CONNECT to 741741
(Clinicians to put other [local] resources, warm lines here)

Ref: This *Stoplight Safety Plan* template is taken from
Tabuenca, Kim, and Gipson (2021): When time is tight and stakes are high: Pharmacotherapy, alliances, and the inpatient unit, *in* Joshi S. V. and Martin A (eds.) *Thinking about Prescribing: The Psychology of Psychopharmacology with Diverse Youth & Families*; Washington, DC, American Psychiatric Association Press, 315 pages, 2021 in press.

Table 16.3 Stoplight Safety Plan, Example 3

10   **Describe the <u>RED ZONE</u>** (typical duration: 1–2 days monthly)
      Thoughts: I hate life, everything is my fault; it'd be better if I wasn't here anymore.
      Feelings: Sad, low, anxious, more sensitive to parent's negative feedback
      Actions: Self-isolation (in room-hard share my thoughts and feelings clearly), crying, bottling up emotions, cutting (9), making plans to kill myself, or trying to kill myself (10)
      Coping plan
      —I communicate that I am in this zone by (what words will you use?)
      I can tell/text my parents "I'm really low right now" and give number (preferably mom). If only dad is available, I can say or text code word: "red." If at 9 and unable to reach others, will call suicide hotline
9   **—Others can respond to me by (what can they say and do?)**
      —Ask "How are you feeling right now?"
      —If I don't want to talk, respect that and give me physical and verbal space until I'm lower on the scale.
      —If I do want to talk, listen and avoid problem-solving. Tell me that you hear me. Wait until I'm in yellow to pick a time to problem-solve.
      —Offer me my Hope box If I don't already have it.
      —Let me FaceTime my girlfriend.
      —During a meal, bring it up to me so I don't have to go get it.
      —Put my pet in my room.
      —Supervision
8   —If 10, parents will be with me physically.
      —If 9, parents/sister can watch me from their room or in common area downstairs.
      —If 7–8, visual check-ins every 60 minutes.
      —I will provide texts with my number and short description every 30 minutes.
      —Bedroom door to stay open when in red zone; leaving the house must be with supervision
      Triggers to be avoided
      —Yelling/fighting with me
      —When someone tells me I have to tell them exactly what is going on (hard for me to think clearly)
      —Trying to solve my problems
      —Blind affirmations
      —Constantly checking social media or posting about my feelings and waiting for responses
7   **—I can use the following coping skills**
      —Share my feelings with my girlfriend, sister, or friend
      —Writing thoughts down through lyrics and poetry
      —Listening to music while drawing
      —Watching TV
      —Skateboarding (in front of house where parents can keep track of my location)
      It is important to go to the hospital or call 911 when
      I want to kill myself (10), when I show I'm not able to follow the supervision plan in this zone, if parents notice I'm looking for or hiding means to hurt myself, if I'm taking any actions that show I'm trying to kill myself.

(Continued)

Table 16.3 (Continued)

6	**Describe the YELLOW ZONE** (typical duration: about a week or two) **Thoughts:** Life sucks right now, I'm stuck, questioning whether I'm stupid, questioning whether my friends actually care **Feelings:** Switching between apathy and sadness, anxiety, and self-doubt.
5	**Actions:** pushing friends away, procrastinating on work, skipping skating days to avoid friends, snapping at my parents and sister, less effort to do things I like, skipping meals *Coping plan* **—I communicate that I am in this zone by (what words will you use?)** —I can tell my mom my zone number during evening check in (usually right after dinner). —Tell my school counselor my yellow zone number during weekly check-in (if going up, get an appointment sooner)
4	**—Others can respond to me by (what can they say and do?)** —Ask me if I want to talk about it. If I say no, we can pick a time to talk about it later within 48 hours. —Help me make a plan to see my girlfriend or friends more. —Send my teachers/school counselor a note to check in with me so I can make a work plan or get support to avoid falling behind. —Work with me to avoid arguments when I'm irritable. If I snap at you, remind me: "I know things are hard for you right now, and we need to keep an effort to be kind to each other." —Use validation statements when we do talk about feelings. —Make a coping recommendation or hand me the coping menu and ask me to pick one for the day. **—I can use the following coping skills** —Hanging out with friends, playing guitar, watching a movie, going skating, or getting one assignment done to feel productive, going for ice cream with the family, sitting with my planner to map out the week, write in my CBT journal, make a list of things I'm looking forward to. Spend time on TikTok (30 minutes max in one sitting). —When parents make a recommendation for coping I will accept at least one out of every three suggestions.
3	**Describe the GREEN ZONE** **Thoughts:** Life is going better; I'm doing better **Feelings**: Happy, hopeful, motivated, encouraged **Actions:** Doing more activities, hanging out with friends, talking more to my parents, keeping on top of my work
2	*Coping plan* **Things I can do to stay in the green zone** —Keep activities in my life (hanging with friends/girlfriend, skating, music, kickboxing, walking dog, spending time with mom). Schedule one per day. —Attend my Individualized Education Plan (IEP) meetings so I can help decide the best way to get support from my teachers and counselor. —Avoid all substances.
1	—Use my sleep hygiene tips (avoid screen time before bed, family phones all plugged in downstairs by 10 p.m.). —Eat 2.5–3 meals per day plus snacks.

Things others can help me do to stay in the green zone
—Create a family activity menu for fun things we can do as a family (learning to cook, museums, skiing, movies). Schedule one per week.
—Work on validation skills.
—Work on understanding that time with friends and girlfriend are important to my mental health and not just taking time away from studies.
—Reserve homework check-ins for designated check-in times (twice a week). If something school-related comes up and needs to be addressed sooner, ask me to pick a time to talk about it rather than springing it on me.
—Keep up with my IEP meetings.

National Suicide Prevention Lifeline 1-800-273-8255
Text: CONNECT to 741741
(Clinicians to put other [local] resources, warm lines here)

Ref: This *Stoplight Safety Plan* template is taken from
Tabuenca, Kim, and Gipson (2021): When time is tight and stakes are high: pharmacotherapy, alliances, and the inpatient unit, *in* Joshi S. V. and Martin A (eds.) *Thinking about Prescribing: The Psychology of Psychopharmacology with Diverse Youth & Families*; Washington, DC, American Psychiatric Association Press, 315 pages, 2021 in press.

During a collaborative process of safety planning, clinicians should remain attentive to the potential vulnerabilities and lack of supports in place to make the plan realistic and reliable. For example, adolescents may plan to communicate SI to parents while not accounting for relationship dynamics that may impede communication in times of acute distress. IROY populations may have specific challenges in having these conversations with their parents/caretakers due to stigma, discomfort with describing distress to their parents, a feeling of "not wanting to burden" their parents/caregivers, or previous negative experiences of sharing their feelings of distress. Thus, clinicians can address modifiable barriers by conducting brief interventions with the patient and family, during which concrete communication and support plans are outlined. By defining specific parental behaviors that would be perceived by the patient as effectively supportive (and also identifying those behaviors that would be triggering or unhelpful), providers can coach families to respond to crises in a manner that optimizes communication. For some teens, this may mean coaching parents to emphasize supportive validation and avoid problem-solving recommendations until distress is reduced. For others, it may involve reducing all verbal communication and relying on visual supervision of the teen to ensure safety, while the patient agrees to use distress tolerance skills independently. A parent's contract with this plan is equally important to a patient's safety plan because it may impact an adolescent's willingness to follow through on safety communication (Tabuenca et al., 2021).

Multicultural Considerations

As Staudenmeyer and her colleagues have highlighted in their very thorough review (2016), environmental and other stressors have been found to predict negative psychosocial outcomes in youth, but this relationship has been studied less often in IROY populations. These youth often face additional stressors compared to their non-IROY peers. Socioeconomic status may contribute to existing stressors for IROY students in addition to expected adolescent challenges. For example, in 2014 approximately 28% of first-generation immigrant youth and 25% of second-generation immigrant youth in the U.S. lived below the federal poverty threshold, compared to 19% of non-immigrant youth.

Acculturation represents a normative process of immigrants navigating and negotiating between familiar, native cultural values and new norms within a host country. "Acculturative stress" is a term characterizing the challenges and conflicts that may result when immigrants are faced with cultural differences between their native and host cultures (Berry, 1997). Aspects of acculturative stress for immigrant youth include learning new cultural norms and expectations, balancing new host values with heritage cultural values, and dealing with covert and/or overt instances of discrimination by the host culture (Berry, 2006). Over the past decade, more focus has been given to the parallel and distinct process of enculturation, or the extent to which immigrants retain the dominant values, practices, and language of their culture of origin (Ramirez Garcia et al., 2010). High levels of acculturation and enculturation, also discussed in terms of biculturalism, have been studied as protective factors against negative psychosocial adaptation in immigrant youth (Smokowski et al., 2010; Ramirez Garcia et al., 2010; Staudenmeyer et al., 2016).

Gaps in levels of acculturation and enculturation between immigrant youth and their parents have been investigated as predictors of poor mental health outcomes and engagement in risk behaviors, and this concept is known as acculturative family distancing (AFD). Hwang and colleagues (2010) describe AFD as

> the distancing that occurs between immigrant parents and their children and is caused by breakdowns in communication and cultural value differences. It is a more proximal and problem-focused formulation of the acculturation gap and is hypothesized to increase depression via family conflict.
>
> (p. 655)

In the U.S., students affected by specific disorders that may place them at risk for suicide are entitled to educational interventions through both formal (legal) and informal mechanisms (Joshi & Jassim, 2019). Unfortunately, IROY populations with mood disorders specifically are at high risk for school problems, including poor attendance, underachievement, and dropping out and are also at risk for suicide if the mood disorders are severe and untreated. During a depressive, manic, or other severe mood episode, these students can find it especially hard to pay attention, think clearly, solve problems, recall information, engage in group learning activities, and sit still—let alone follow classroom rules (Joshi & Jassim, 2019).

Extending beyond symptom-based outcomes to account for functioning in school, family, and peer contexts allows research on immigrant youth to be unbound by its traditional focus on psychopathology (Suárez-Orozco et al., 2010) and calls attention to the multiple domains in which immigrant youth face challenges that can be effectively targeted by intervention. Addressing depression, anxiety, and PTSD symptoms among immigrant youth would be incomplete and misinformed without a thorough inventory of sociocultural stressors faced by the youth, such as poverty, neighborhood violence, discrimination, intergenerational conflict, family separation, legal status, and language acquisition. Psychological interventions for immigrant youth must involve collaboration between the various systems and contexts to which the youth belongs (p. 4).

Mood disorders can cause at least three types of problems for any student, but IROY populations may be at particular risk in school settings. These problems include those caused by the core symptoms themselves (e.g., difficulty concentrating), those caused by secondary factors (e.g., peer issues), and those associated with the treatment itself (e.g. medication side effects or life inconveniences associated with treatment). IROY populations with mood conditions may struggle with learning and acculturation issues, and educators would do well to be aware of the additional layers of impaired concentration, reduced motivation, and emotional upheavals that a mood disorder or social and environmental stressors can create (Joshi & Jassim, 2019).

Challenges and Solutions

Interventions must emphasize cultural competence and humility. Parent behaviors identified by teens as communication barriers may be rooted within parental cultural norms. This may pose challenges for parents navigating differences in what discipline and communication styles are considered acceptable by a new culture. Thus, asking parents to modify certain behaviors could be perceived as intrusiveness from an unsupportive and permissive culture (Fleck & Fleck, 2013). Exploring and understanding the cultural foundation of certain parenting behaviors allow school-based family counseling practitioners to align the intervention with parental goals underpinning these behaviors. The family can then agree on alternative behaviors that meet these goals in a manner that also promotes parent–child communication about safety. For example, teens may avoid communicating crisis feelings to a parent that responds by asking them to control their feelings, get off social media, and focus on their studies. This response may be experienced as invalidating, isolating, and shifting focus toward their primary stressor. Conversely, the parent's goal may include having the teen take agency over their experience, reduce negative influences, and focus the teen on a path toward success. Clinicians can align themselves with the family unit by focusing the intervention on identifying behaviors that promote these goals, while also increasing the likelihood of crisis communication from the teen. For IROY populations, it may be necessary to have a cultural broker (friend, relative, teacher, coach, spiritual, religious or community leader, or someone else that both the youth and parent feel comfortable with) in the room to assist the process and facilitate the planning conversation.

At times, students may be admitted to the inpatient psychiatric unit after challenges in enacting previously created safety plans. In these circumstances, the specific barriers to safety plan adherence should be explored because they can inform both pharmacological and nonpharmacological interventions needed to increase adherence and promote favorable outcomes in the future. For example, certain safety plans may have been effective when crises occurred in the home but were unable to be implemented in the school context. In these situations, collaboration with school staff is essential (e.g., a re-entry meeting prior to starting school, after discharge from an inpatient or residential treatment setting) to ensure that the patient/student has adequate outlets for support in different environments. In other situations, lack of adherence to safety planning may bring to light the potential need for fast acting as-needed (PRN) medication that should be made accessible to patients who are still struggling to apply distress tolerance skills rapidly enough to remain safe (Tabuenca et al., 2021).

Conclusion

Suicide accounts for more deaths among youth and young adults in the U.S. than do all natural causes combined. IROY populations (Immigrant and Refugee Origin Youth) may have special risks, given their very diverse life circumstances. Most deaths by suicide occur in people who have had mental health conditions such as PTSD, depression, or severe anxiety. Thus, school efforts must focus on stigma reduction, implementation of evidence-supported approaches, parent/student education about mental health conditions, and help-seeking from peers or trusted adults on campus. Prevention efforts must focus on school-based mental health education and promotion. The IPTS highlights the importance of belonging and connectedness as potential protective factors in suicide prevention with IROY populations in particular and needs to be studied further. Safety planning and school re-entry/planning can be adapted easily for diverse youth, including those from IROY communities, and must be used regularly as part of best practices in school-based suicide prevention.

Resources

Promising Practices Network. (PPN) on children, families and communities. http://www.promisingpractices.net/programs.asp

   The PPN site features summaries of programs and practices that improve outcomes for children.

National Center for Youth Law: (https://youthlaw.org)

The National Center for Youth Law (NCYL) leads high-impact campaigns that weave together litigation, research, public awareness, policy development, and technical assistance. The center's goal is not to reform one particular system but to transform the multiple public systems serving vulnerable children—including education, child welfare, public health, behavioral health, juvenile justice, and workforce development—such that they receive the supports they need to advance and thrive.

The Collaborative for Academic, Social, and Emotional Learning (CASEL)
(www.casel.org/programs/selecting.php)

   "CASEL Select" programs provide outstanding coverage in five essential SEL skill areas; have at least one well-designed evaluation study demonstrating their effectiveness; and offer professional development supports beyond the initial training.

The National Registry of Evidence-Based Programs & Practices (NREPP)
(www.nrepp.samhsa.gov)

   Intervention summaries are provided to help determine whether a particular intervention may meet identified needs.

Suicide Prevention Resource Center: Best Practices Registry (BPR) for Suicide Prevention
(www.sprc.org/featured_ resources/bpr/index.asp)

www.schoolpsychiatry.org

   Mental health information for school staff, parents, and clinicians; interventions for psychiatric disorders and symptoms; rating scales to assess disorders and monitor treatments

http://csmh.umaryland.edu

   Up-to-date information about national school mental health training, practice, research and policy has numerous resources for IROY populations as well

www.schoolmentalhealth.org

   A repository of useful resources for school clinicians, educators, families, and students on school mental health

http://smhp.psych.ucla.edu

   Clearinghouse of important mental health, school, and education materials

http://ies.ed.gov/ncee/wwc/

   Information on broad categories of findings of "what works" in schools including academics and mental health

www.ldonline.org

   Information on classroom changes for students with learning disabilities, including ADHD

www.ideapartnership.org

   Up-to-date information on changes in the IDEA parameters

www.wrightslaw.com

   Information about legal aspects of education, including IDEA 504 Plans

www.r14success.org

Response to Intervention school programming across academic and emotional areas

www.heardalliance.org

A collaborative website that features resources for suicide prevention and mental health promotion and also features a best practice K12 Toolkit for Mental Health Promotion and Suicide Prevention

www.nctsn.org

The National Child Traumatic Stress Network

Contains very useful resources for educators to reach and teach students with trauma, loss, and anxiety; it also has useful tips for speaking with parents, children, and the media about the consequences of human-caused and natural disasters and has resources for preventing burnout in educators.

www.thetrevorproject.org/education/

Contains resources to help educators implement suicide prevention policies with emphasis on LGBTQ youth

https://genderspectrum.org/articles/educator-resources

Contains educator-specific resources on creating a gender-affirming environment

Bibliography

Appleton, J. J., Christenson, S. L., Kim, D., & Reschly, A. L. (2006). Measuring cognitive and psychological engagement: Validation of the Student Engagement Instrument. Journal of School Psychology, 44(5), 427–445. https://doi.org/10.1016/j.jsp.2006.04.002

Areba, E. M., Taliaferro, L. A., Forster, M., McMorris, B. J., Mathiason, M. A., & Eisenberg, M. E. (2021). Adverse childhood experiences and suicidality: School connectedness as a protective factor for ethnic minority adolescents. Children and Youth Services Review, 120. ISSN 0190-7409. https://doi.org/10.1016/j.childyouth.2020.105637

Baams, L., Pollitt, A. M., Laub, C., & Russell, S. T. (2020). Characteristics of Schools With and Without Gay-Straight Alliances. Applied Developmental Science, 24(4), 354–359. https://doi.org/10.1080/10888691.2018.1510778

Baumeister, R. F., & Leary, M. R. (1995). The need to belong: Desire for interpersonal attachments as a fundamental human motivation. Psychological Bulletin, 117(3), 497–529. https://doi.org/10.1037/0033-2909.117.3.497

Berry, J. W. (1997). Immigration, acculturation, and adaptation. Applied Psychology, 46(1), 5–34. https://doi.org/10.1111/j.1464-0597.1997.tb01087.x

Berry, J. W., Phinney, J. S., Sam, D. L., & Vedder, P. (2006). Immigrant youth: Acculturation, identity, and adaptation. Applied Psychology, 55(3), 303–332. https://doi.org/10.1111/j.1464-0597.2006.00256.x

Blum, R. (2005). A case for school connectedness. Educational Leadership, 62(7), 16–20.

Bridge, J., Asti, L., Horowitz, L., Greenhouse, J., Fontanella, C., Sheftall, A., Kelleher, K., & Campo, J. (2015). Suicide trends among elementary schoolaged children in the United States from 1993 to 2012. JAMA Pediatrics, 169(7), 673–677. https://doi. https://doi.org/10.1001/jamapediatrics.2015.0465 Erratum in: JAMA Pediatrics. (2015 July), 169(7), 699. PubMed: 25984947.

Calear, A. L., McCallum, S., Kazan, D., Werner-Seidler, A., Christensen, H., & Batterham, P. J. (2021). Application of the interpersonal psychological theory of suicide in a non-clinical community-based adolescent population. Journal of Affective Disorders, 294, (235–240). https://doi.org/10.1016/j.jad.2021.07.011

Carrion, V. G., Kletter, H., Weems, C. F., Berry, R. R., & Rettger, J. P. (2013). Cue-centered treatment for youth exposed to interpersonal violence: A randomized controlled trial. Journal of Traumatic Stress, 26(6), 654–662. https://doi.org/10.1002/jts.21870

Center for Disease Control (CDC). (2018). Deaths, percent of total deaths, and death rates for the 15 leading causes of death in 5-year age groups, by race and Hispanic origin, and sex: United States, 2017. Retrieved July 31, 2021. http://www.cdc.gov/nchs/data/dvs/lcwk/lcwk1_ hr_ 2017-a.pdf (pp. 167–168).

García Coll, C., Lamberty, G., Jenkins, R., McAdoo, H. P., Crnic, K., Wasik, B. H., & Vázquez García, H. (1996). An integrative model for the study of developmental competencies in minority children. Child Development, 67(5), 1891–1914. https://doi.org/10.1111/j.1467-8624.1996.tb01834.x

Eisenberg, M. E., Ackard, D. M., & Resnick, M. D. (2007). Protective factors and suicide risk in adolescents with a history of sexual abuse. Journal of Pediatrics, 151(5), 482–487. https://doi.org/10.1016/j.jpeds.2007.04.033

Eisenberg, M. E., & Resnick, M. D. (2006). Suicidality among gay, lesbian and bisexual youth: The role of protective factors. Journal of Adolescent Health, 39(5), 662–668. https://doi.org/10.1016/j.jadohealth.2006.04.024

Fazel, M., & Betancourt, T. S. (2018, February). Preventive mental health interventions for refugee children and adolescents in high-income settings. Lancet. Child and Adolescent Health, 2(2), 121–132. https://doi.org/10.1016/S2352-4642(17)30147-5. Epub November 21 2017. PubMed: 30169234

Fazel, M., Wheeler, J., & Danesh, J. (2005). Prevalence of serious mental disorder in 7000 refugees resettled in western countries: A systematic review. Lancet, 365(9467), 1309–1314. https://doi.org/10.1016/S0140-6736(05)61027-6

Feinstein, N. R., Fielding, K., Udvari-Solner, A., & Joshi, S. V. (2009). The supporting alliance in child and adolescent treatment: Enhancing collaboration among therapists, parents, and teachers. American Journal of Psychotherapy, 63(4), 319–344. https://doi.org/10.1176/appi.psychotherapy.2009.63.4.319

Fleck, J. R., & Fleck, D. T. (2013). The immigrant family: Parent–child dilemmas and therapy considerations. American International Journal of Contemporary Research, 3(8), 13–17.

Garlow, S. J., Purselle, D., & Heninger, M. (2005). Ethnic differences in patterns of suicide across the life cycle. American Journal of Psychiatry, 162(2), 319–323. https://doi.org/10.1176/appi.ajp.162.2.319

Hafeez, H., Zeshan, M., Tahir, M. A., Jahan, N., & Naveed, S. (2017). Health care disparities among lesbian, gay, bisexual, and transgender youth: A literature review. Cureus, 9(4), e1184. https://doi.org/10.7759/cureus.1184

Hatzenbuehler, M. L. (2011). The social environment and suicide attempts in lesbian, gay, and bisexual youth. Pediatrics, 127(5), 896–903. https://doi.org/10.1542/peds.2010-3020

Heck, N. C., Flentje, A., & Cochran, B. N. (2011). Offsetting risks: High school gay-straight alliances and lesbian, gay, bisexual, and transgender (LGBT) youth. School Psychology Quarterly, 26(2), 161–174. https://doi.org/10.1037/a0023226

Hjern, A., & Angel, B. (2000). Organized violence and mental health of refugee children in exile: A six-year follow-up. Acta Paediatrica, 89(6), 722–727. https://doi.org/10.1080/080352500750044089

Hwang, W. C., Wood, J. J., & Fujimoto, K. (2010). Acculturative family distancing (AFD) and depression in Chinese American families. Journal of Consulting and Clinical Psychology, 78(5), 655–667. https://doi.org/10.1037/a0020542

Johns, M. M., Lowry, R., Haderxhanaj, L. T., Rasberry, C. N., Robin, L., Scales, L., Stone, D., & Suarez, N. A., . . . Suarez. (2020). Trends in Violence Victimization and Suicide Risk by Sexual Identity among High School Students – Youth Risk Behavior Survey, United States, 2015–2019. MMWR Supplements, 69(1), 19–27. https://doi.org/10.15585/mmwr.su6901a3

Joshi, S. V., & Jassim, N. (2019). School-based Interventions for mood disorders. In M. K. Singh (Ed.), A clinical handbook for the diagnosis and treatment of pediatric onset mood disorders. Am. Psychiatric Association Press.

Joshi, S. V., Hartley, S. N., Kessler, M., & Barstead, M. (2015). School-based suicide prevention: Content, process, and the role of trusted adults and peers. Child and Adolescent Psychiatric Clinics of North America, 24(2), 353–370. https://doi.org/10.1016/j.chc.2014.12.003

Juang, L. P., Simpson, J. A., Lee, R. M., Rothman, A. J., Titzmann, P. F., Schachner, M. K., Korn, L., Heinemeier, D., & Betsch, C., . . . Betsch. (2018). Using attachment and relational perspectives to understand adaptation and resilience among immigrant and refugee youth. American Psychologist, 73(6), 797–811. https://doi.org/10.1037/amp0000286

Kann, L., McManus, T., Harris, W. A., Shanklin, S. L., Fiint, K. H., & Queen, B., . . . Ethier, K. (2018). Morbidity and mortality weekly report: Youth risk behavior surveillance—_ United States, 2017. http://www.cdc.gov/healthyyouth/data/yrbs/pdf/2017/ss6708.pdf

Kataoka, S., Langley, A. K., Wong, M., Baweja, S., & Stein, B. D. (2012). Responding to students with posttraumatic stress disorder in schools. Child and Adolescent Psychiatric Clinics of North America, 21(1), 119–33, x. https://doi.org/10.1016/j.chc.2011.08.009

Korpershoek, H., Canrinus, E. T., Fokkens-Bruinsma, M., & de Boer, H. (2020). The relationships between school belonging and students' motivational, social-emotional, behavioural, and academic outcomes in secondary education: A meta-analytic review. Research Papers In Education, 35(6), 641–680. https://doi.org/10.1080/02671522.2019.1615116

Lindsey, M. A., Sheftall, A. H., Xiao, Y., & Joe, S. (2019). Trends of suicidal behaviors among high school students in the United States: 1991–2017. Pediatrics, 144(5). https://doi.org/10.1542/peds.2019-1187

Montgomery, E. (2010). Trauma and resilience in young refugees: A 9-year follow-up study. Development and Psychopathology, 22(2), 477–489. https://doi.org/10.1017/S0954579410000180

Nickerson, A., Bryant, R. A., Silove, D., & Steel, Z. (2011). A critical review of psychological treatments of posttraumatic stress disorder in refugees. Clinical Psychology Review, 31(3), 399–417. https://doi.org/10.1016/j.cpr.2010.10.004

Ports, K. A., Merrick, M. T., Stone, D. M., Wilkins, N. J., Reed, J., Ebin, J., & Ford, D. C. (2017). Adverse childhood experiences and suicide risk: Toward comprehensive prevention. American Journal of Preventive Medicine, 53(3), 400–403. https://doi.org/10.1016/j.amepre.2017.03.015

Ramírez García, J. I., Manongdo, J. A., & Cruz-Santiago, M. (2010). The family as mediator of the impact of parent-youth acculturation/enculturation and inner-city stressors on Mexican American youth substance use. Cultural Diversity and Ethnic Minority Psychology, 16(3), 404–412. https://doi.org/10.1037/a0019725

Ryan, C., Russell, S. T., Huebner, D., Diaz, R., & Sanchez, J. (2010). Family acceptance in adolescence and the health of LGBT young adults. Journal of Child and Adolescent Psychiatric Nursing, 23(4), 205–213. https://doi.org/10.1111/j.1744-6171.2010.00246.x

Sharma, N., & Pumariega, A. (2018). Culturally informed treatment of suicidality with diverse youth: General principles. In A. J. Pumariega & N. Sharma (Eds.), Suicide among diverse youth. Springer Int.'l.

Smokowski, P. R., Rose, R. A., & Bacallao, M. L. (2010). Influence of risk factors and cultural assets on Latino adolescents' trajectories of self-esteem and internalizing symptoms. Child Psychiatry and Human Development, 41(2), 133–155. https://doi.org/10.1007/s10578-009-0157-6

Stanley, B., & Brown, G. K. (2012). Safety planning intervention: A brief intervention to mitigate suicide risk. Cognitive and Behavioral Practice, 19(2), 256–264. https://doi.org/10.1016/j.cbpra.2011.01.001

Staudenmeyer, A., Macciomei, E., Del Cid, M., & Patel, S. (2016). Immigrant youth life stressors. In S. Patel & D. Reicherter (Eds.), Psychotherapy for immigrant youth (pp. 3–24). Springer International Publishing AG.

Stone, D. M., Holland, K. M., Bartholow, B., Crosby, A. E., Davis, S., & Wilkins, N. (2017). Preventing Suicide: A Technical Package of Policies, Programs. *National Center for Injury Prevention and Control*. Retrieved from https://www.cdc.gov/violenceprevention/pdf/suicidetechnicalpackage.pdf

Suárez-Orozco, C., Hee Jin Bang, & Ha Yeon Kim (2011). I Felt Like My Heart Was Staying Behind: Psychological Implications of Family Separations & Reunifications for Immigrant Youth. Journal of Adolescent Research, 26(2), 222–257. https://doi.org/10.1177/0743558410376830

Suárez-Orozco, C., Carhill, A., & Chuang, S. S. (2010). Immigrant children: Making a new life. In S. S. Chuang & R. P. Moreno (Eds.), Immigrant children: Change, adaptation, and cultural transformation (pp. 7–26). Lexington Books.

Suárez-Orozco, C., Motti-Stefanidi, F., Marks, A., & Katsiaficas, D. (2018). An integrative risk and resilience model for understanding the adaptation of immigrant-origin children and youth. American Psychologist, 73(6), 781–796. https://doi.org/10.1037/amp0000265

Suárez-Orozco, C., Todorova, I. L. G., & Louie, J. (2002). Making up for lost time: The experience of separation and reunification among immigrant families. Family Process, 41(4), 625–643. https://doi.org/10.1111/j.1545-5300.2002.00625.x

Swanson, K., & Gettinger, M. (2016). Teachers' knowledge, attitudes, and supportive behaviors toward LGBT students: Relationship to Gay-Straight Alliances, antibullying policy, and teacher training. Journal of LGBT Youth, 13(4), 326–351. https://doi.org/10.1080/19361653.2016.1185765

Tabuenca, A., Kim, J. W., & Gipson, S. (2021). When time is tight and stakes are high: Pharmacotherapy, alliances, and the inpatient unit. In S. V. Joshi & A. Martin (Eds.), Thinking about prescribing: The psychology of psychopharmacology with diverse youth and families. American Psychiatric Publishing Association Press.

Taliaferro, L. A., & Muehlenkamp, J. J. (2017). Nonsuicidal self-injury and suicidality among sexual minority youth: Risk factors and protective connectedness factors. Academic Pediatrics, 17(7), 715–722. https://doi.org/10.1016/j.acap.2016.11.002

Tyrer, R. A., & Fazel, M. (2014). School and community-based interventions for refugee and asylum seeking children: A systematic review. PLOS ONE, 9(2), e89359. https://doi.org/10.1371/journal.pone.0089359

Van Orden, K. A., Merrill, K. A., & Joiner, T. E. (2005). Interpersonal-psychological precursors to suicidal behavior: A theory of attempted and completed suicide. Current Psychiatry Reviews, 1(2), 187–196. https://doi.org/10.2174/1573400054065541

Wilson, H. W., & Joshi, S. V. (2018). Recognizing and referring children with posttraumatic stress disorder: Guidelines for pediatric providers. Pediatrics in Review, 39(2), 68–77. https://doi.org/10.1542/pir.2017-0036

Wyman, P. A., Brown, C. H., LoMurray, M., Schmeelk-Cone, K., Petrova, M., Yu, Q., Walsh, E., Tu, X., & Wang, W., . . . Wang. (2010). An outcome evaluation of the Sources of Strength suicide prevention program delivered by adolescent peer leaders in high schools. American Journal of Public Health, 100(9), 1653–1661. https://doi.org/10.2105/AJPH.2009.190025. Epub July 15 2010. PubMed: 20634440, PubMed Central: PMC2920978

17 Culturally responsive pedagogy and school-based family counseling

A pathway to equitable spaces for students from refugee backgrounds

Shirley Mthethwa-Sommers and Otieno Kisiara

This chapter draws from research on parents and students from refugee backgrounds in U.S. schools. It delineates pathways that school-based practitioners can apply to ensure that students from refugee backgrounds are developed holistically and have a sense of belonging in schools. Culturally responsive teaching and school-based family counseling frameworks provide a foundation for understanding how practitioners can actualize equitable schools. The chapter essentially provides recommendations on how practitioners can implement culturally responsive teaching and school-based family counseling frameworks to ensure refugee students' mental, cognitive, and physical safety in schools.

Background

The state of students from refugee backgrounds in the U.S.

The U.S. has been devastated by the Covid-19 pandemic. The pandemic has uncovered inequities in the health system as it has disproportionately impacted communities of color. The Covid-19 pandemic has also unveiled deep-rooted racialized inequities within the school system. Students who attend predominantly Black and Latinx schools have received disrupted and limited online educational opportunities. The expectation that parents take over some teaching responsibilities has left many students, particularly those from refugee backgrounds, without access to education. This situation occurred despite research demonstrating that recently arrived refugee families that have recently arrived in the U.S. do not interact with school personnel, as they are usually focused on the tasks of settling in a new country (Githembe, 2009; Han & Love, 2015). Studies also show that school personnel do not reach out to families unless students have transgressed from expectations. Even for many refugee families already established in the U.S., pivoting to online also proved to be an issue as they encounter linguistic

DOI: 10.4324/9781003097891-22

and cultural barriers when interacting with school personnel and end up not trying to interact with them (Tadesse, 2014). A study by Mthethwa-Sommers and Kisiara (2019) on parents from refugee backgrounds shows that these parents, like any other parents, are invested in their children's education and development; they want what is best for their children. Before the Covid-19 pandemic, the National Center for Education Statistics (2013) reported that students who speak English as a Second language, mainly students from refugee backgrounds, have high dropout rates. One can deduce that these high dropout rates have been exacerbated by online learning and learning complications concomitant to Covid-19. Doyle (2020) reported that students who Covid-19 has adversely impacted are students in urban areas, areas that serve many students from refugee backgrounds.

The complications, challenges, and disruptions engendered by Covid-19 on learning render this chapter salient as it shines a light on refugee students' and parents' experiences. Drawing on refugee parents' and students' experiences, we contend that culturally responsive teaching (CRT) coupled with the school-based family counseling (SBFC) framework meets refugee students' needs and actualizes the ideal of equity in schools. The chapter is organized as follows. Firstly, we provide a background review of CRT as a theoretical framework and its alignment with SBFC. Secondly, drawing on insights from our research, we specify SBFC- and CRT- informed recommendations for SBFC practitioners. We conclude the chapter with CRT and education resources for students from refugee backgrounds.

CRT and SBFC

CRT refers to a teaching method designed to reach students of color who are often systematically marginalized and failed by normative teaching practices (Gay, 2000). Gay (2000) identifies five essential attributes of CRT.

1. The first attribute requires a mindset shift from a deficit perspective of the students' cultural background to an informed perspective of students' cultural background. The mindset shift requires viewing students as having cultures worthy of inclusion in the curriculum.
2. The second attribute of CRT urges teachers to perceive students of color as knowledgeable beings possessing necessary "funds of knowledge" (Moll et al., 1992). Teachers see students of color not as tabula rasa but as individuals who live and thrive within cultured communities. Teachers must be researchers of their students' cultures. Understanding this will entail changing the curriculum, textbooks, and teaching materials to reflect the multicultural nature of the student body.
3. The third characteristic of CRT pertains to the learning environment. It essentially asks the question: what kind of environment is required for teachers to engage with students who have funds of knowledge and rich cultural backgrounds? The type of classroom and learning environment

required should be nurturing, caring, and academically demanding. Additionally, caring for students involves paying attention to the symbolic curriculum (Gay, 2002), the decorations and posters that teachers use in their classrooms, hallways, offices, and schools in general.

4. The fourth attribute of CRT deals with the delivery modes of lessons. Gay (2010) suggests that teaching delivery modes should reflect the different ways of knowing as exhibited by disparate cultural groups. For instance, some cultures encourage and rely on orality, which means oral delivery modes should also be incorporated into teaching. This also applies to assessment. Most assessments privilege text more than other evaluation methods, placing students who value orality at a disadvantage.

5. The last attribute of CRT is classroom instruction that draws from the previous four characteristics. Gay (2010) argues that education cannot be effective if the content and delivery modes do not reflect the different cultures in the classroom. In essence, CRT is anti-racist as it calls for equitable spaces in the classrooms, in the hallways, and how teachers interact with students. There is research that many educators can simultaneously use an ethnic additive model of teaching while engaging in White supremacist practices. This attribute avers that cultural inclusion is underpinned by critical consciousness and anti-racism.

As Soriano and Gerrard (2013) argue that the SBFC approach conceptualizes the child's problems within the interpersonal contexts of their family, peer group, school (teacher, principal, other students), and community setting. As such, the SBFC framework postulates that a student cannot be understood in a vacuum: students are part of families and communities, which require recognition and inclusion in the school setting. SBFC's systems approach aligns with CRT's insistence that school practitioners approach students as knowledgeable individuals and acknowledges that students bring funds of knowledge to which schools need to capitalize on developing as holistic individuals. Most importantly, like CRT, the SBFC approach calls on the practitioners to center the students' needs in redesigning their work. Both frameworks invite teachers to restructure the curriculum and pedagogical practices to acknowledge the student at the center of the learning process.

So how can SBFC practitioners use CRT to support refugee students in our schools? The following section specifies concrete steps to do so. The recommendations outlined draw from a study of students and parents of refugee backgrounds who were interviewed to ascertain what an equitable educational experience means. Eager to share their experiences, students and parents from refugee backgrounds articulated what they expected from schools. As you will see, they shared ideas demonstrating culturally responsive tenets. They pointed out that teachers lacked knowledge about people from refugee backgrounds and various countries, religions, and worldviews. Overall, their recommendations revealed a need to educate teachers and school personnel on making schools equitable spaces.

Procedures

Step 1: Mindset shift and embracing new knowledge

For CRT to be actualized, teachers must perceive their students as knowledgeable individuals with viable cultures that can contribute to their learning and development. Students should feel valued and affirmed by their teachers. One parent, Somali American, reported an experience that made her daughter feel valued and affirmed.

> I went to school to talk to my daughter's teacher. The teacher showed me on the computer that my daughter was doing well, that her behavior is fine. The teacher said that if all children behaved like Halima (pseudonym) and were respectful, it would be great. The teachers said, "I am very proud of Halima and will praise her all my life." Halima [13 years old] has moved to a different class, but the teacher said she wishes she could keep her in her class.

The teacher was intentional about affirming the student in front of her mother by pointing out that she was doing well in class and respectful. While the teacher, who is White, and the mother, a Black Somali American, had cultural and linguistic differences, the teacher made the parent feel welcome by pointing out the value that she had for her child. Parents from refugee backgrounds do not want to interact with teachers only when their child has transgressed. They want to have positive interactions with teachers when students are behaving appropriately. Using a positive, strength-based mindset requires a fundamental mindset shift that focuses on assets rather than deficits.

- How am I honoring the dignity of the student in this conversation? Listening to students and showing empathy when listening is critical for the dignity and centering of students' voices.
- Am I reaching out to parents only to discuss negative issues? Reach out to parents when you have good news. The first interaction with a parent should never be a negative one.
- How is this discussion contributing to the healthy development of the student? Be mindful of the words you use; use words that are always affirming.
- Am I welcoming to the students and parents? You can learn how to say "hello" in the students' or parents' language; this may seem minor, but it is impactful when it comes to being welcoming and establishing a sense of belonging.

Both students and parents reported that schools propagated stereotypes about people of African descent and Muslim students. For instance, one student discussed a situation in which a teacher was leading a discussion on characteristics of a terrorist: "A girl in my class was talking about who was going to be terrorist, I was the only one in the class [to fit the stereotyped Muslim terrorist]." The student felt she was criminalized and labeled a terrorist because one characteristic of a terrorist was being a Muslim. Students also reported that some teachers try to move away from stereotypes by asking students from refugee backgrounds to present their cultures and experiences to their classmates. On the surface, this might look like a reasonable approach to teaching as it capitalizes on students' knowledge and centers student voice. However, students indicated that this approach does not work: "Other students don't really care, the students laugh, and it gets us bullied." In other instances, students shared traumatic experiences without any therapeutic and structural interventions in place, which leads to the retraumatization of students (Matthews, 2008).

In essence, students report that CRT needs to be done in a manner that is also mindful that we live in a racist world that values Whiteness and Western perspectives. Teachers must be cognizant of the impact of stereotypes as research shows that negative stereotypes directly impact student performance (Steele, 2003). When students are asked to share incongruous experiences with Whiteness and Western values, these students will be mocked and become a laughingstock.

CRT also demands that teachers are researchers of their students' cultures, as students alone cannot be the only conveyors of knowledge. A parent from Tanzania highlighted the significance of teachers as researchers of students' cultures when she shared the following:

> A teacher insisted that my daughter remove her headscarf. The teacher asked her, "are you Muslim?" My daughter said no, "then you have to remove your headscarf." My daughter refused, and the teacher sent her home. I went to school to talk to the principal because I also did not want my daughter to remove her scarf. They allowed my child to wear her scarf.

A Muslim student also shared a negative interaction with a teacher. She reported that "a teacher told me to remove my headscarf because it was hot. Are you kidding me! I cannot take off my headscarf, it is like taking off your clothes. And students joined in."

These incidences highlight the need for teachers to be informed about students' cultures. In a culturally responsive classroom, the teacher would not have made both of these requests, which ultimately allowed other students to engage in verbal taunting. While these experiences may seem minor, they have harmful psychological impacts on students. Schools ought to serve as "'sites of refuge' . . . places where immigrants and refugee students should be able to express religious identities and religious expressions in the absence of discrimination or persecution" (DeNicolo et al., 2017, p. 519).

Given these insights, it is recommended that SBFC practitioners encourage and assist school personnel in conducting background research on students in their classroom, office, and schools. The following questions are an excellent place to start in conducting individual research:

- What are the countries they come from?
- What are the religions practiced in the country?
- What are the languages spoken in the country?
- How can the epistemology of that country be incorporated into the curriculum?
- How am I using local refugee communities as reservoirs of knowledge?
- Am I interacting with students in a manner that honors their dignity, heritage, and humanity?

SBFC practitioners should advocate for periodic teacher and staff development workshops on topics specific to refugee histories, cultures, and experiences. For example, the second author of this chapter was invited by a local school district a few years ago to conduct a workshop funded by the National Endowment for the Humanities (NEH) for teachers and school administrators on refugee histories, cultures, and pedagogical approaches working with refugee-background students and families. The workshop centered around the structural barriers refugee-background students and their families face and called on teachers and school administrators to treat refugee trauma as an empirical question rather than a defining characteristic of displacement. The pathologizing of refugee experiences tends to lead to a greater focus on psychological interventions at the individual level, focused on individual refugees while ignoring broader structural issues, such as racism and xenophobia, that CRT seeks to address. Teachers and administrators must build pedagogical practices around the strengths and multidimensionality of refugee-background students and their families.

We recommend that school personnel who want to create equitable spaces for students from refugee backgrounds conduct outreach to refugee-background communities, where school administrators and teachers go out into the community to meet with parents and other community stakeholders. These community-based engagements provide great opportunities to learn about students' cultural backgrounds, their families' aspirations, assets, and challenges that can then be incorporated in developing, implementing, and evaluating effective CRT. The more common, school-based parent-teacher meetings engagements do not provide opportunities for meaningful conversations on concerns or viewpoints parents have. As a parent in our research shared, these parent-teacher meetings are always short and only focused on reviewing their children's performance on specific subjects/courses. Outreach to communities can be organized through community organizations such as refugee resettlement agencies and places of worship. For example, around our research site, a church serves refugees from Burma where church services are held in the Karen language. A local mosque serves many refugees from Somalia, Afghanistan, Yemen, and Syria. Additionally, school personnel can attend community events organized by refugee communities. For example, World Refugee Day, marked in many cities and towns in the U.S. and around the world annually in June, provides an opportunity for school personnel to participate in discussions and presentations that address local and global refugee issues, as well as refugee histories and cultures.

Step 2: Create a nurturing environment

The tenets of CRT include creating a nurturing environment that provides for caring and is academically demanding. Almost all the parents and students from refugee backgrounds reported an encounter with school personnel that made them believe schools were not nurturing environments. As one Somali American parent reported,

> My daughter asked her teacher for permission to go to the bathroom, and the teacher would not allow her. So, my child peed on herself. So, I went to school and complained to the principal. The principal said my child was lying and that I was also lying. I continued to complain, and the principal said if I persisted, I would be sent to jail.

In this case, the student was placed in a situation where she had to urinate on herself because her teacher told her she could not go to the restroom. Fear of being punished for disrespecting the teacher left her with no choice but to urinate on herself. When the mother advocated for her child, the principal told her she was lying and threatened to call police on her. The parent further reported that while she believed her child, she also started doubting her child's story. This is a prime example of what Wood and Harris (2021) call racelighting. Racelighting is defined as when the experiences of people of color are dismissed and invalidated through micro-aggressions, leading to people doubting themselves and their own reading of their experiences. The principal chose to weaponize the police and racelight the mother and the student. This student was no longer comfortable going to school because other children made fun of her for urinating on herself. These interactions between student and teacher, and parent and principal are instructive of how schools can be dehumanizing sites to people from refugee backgrounds.

When there is conflict among American-born students and students from refugee backgrounds, students reported that they are often not believed or even provided with an opportunity to present their side of the story, "[T]eachers they don't wait for you when you are thinking and translating into English in your head, they just say you are thinking of lies." Not being believed is another form of racist and xenophobic marginalization (Wood & Harris, 2020). Another student offered, "Teachers make fighting students shake hands, but this doesn't work if the grudge is not resolved."

This student is providing a blueprint on how teachers can resolve issues in a manner that builds community. The orthodox way of shaking hands after a fight is inadequate as it leaves issues unresolved and the class community fragmented.

Therefore, for schools to practice CRT, they must be hospitable and inviting to students. What can practitioners do to create nurturing environments in schools?

- Believe students from refugee backgrounds when they say they hurt or that they have a problem.
- When there is a conflict or a fight, seek restorative practices that center victims and resolve conflicts.
- Be patient with students who speak English as a second language and be cognizant of your own cultural lenses. For example, if a person speaks slowly, that does not mean they are formulating lies—that is a cultural lens that is not universally applicable.
- Ask for clarification before you make assumptions.

Using restorative justice practices that honor and center the harmed individual can resolve conflicts and hold the person who harms others accountable. The approach to dealing with conflict using restorative justice practices restores relationships and engenders respectful interaction among students.

Step 3: Reach out to the families

The SBFC theory locates students' mental health and success within schools and families (Soriano & Gerrard, 2013). Families are a critical part of understanding the essence of a student. SBFC and CRT practitioners need to have a relationship with family members.

A parent who speaks mainly Arabic and limited English reported that she had a neighbor write notes for her (in English) to send to the teacher, asking how her child was doing in school. She would place these notes in her child's school bag, and the child would give them to the teacher. The teacher would send notes back to her, putting the notes in the child's school bag. She could also message the teacher through Facebook, and the neighbor would translate for her. This is an example of a teacher who understood the significance of including families, despite a linguistic barrier.

What can SBFC practitioners do? Our suggestion is for school staff to adopt an approach that can enable school personnel to learn about refugee communities' cultures, for example, for schools to invite refugee-background parents and refugee community leaders into schools. Getting parents and community leaders engaged in school activities regularly enables schools to gain more significant insights into refugee histories, cultures, and perspectives that can be used to build CRT pedagogies.

School participation by refugee parents and community leaders can occur in several ways. They can be invited to join school boards, hence providing an opportunity to represent their communities' perspectives in developing school curriculum and school administration. Schools can also invite refugee-background parents to schools to observe classroom activities and participate in school events. For example, in our research area, the principal of a refugee-serving school has developed a program where parents come in and observe their children's classroom activities and provide feedback on how they can best serve the students. This school has also intentionally reached out to refugee-background to offer them employment in the school, further providing opportunities for these parents to engage with schools.

Multicultural considerations

The transition from one cultural lens to another, from one country to another, and from one language to another is an immense challenge. Students from refugee backgrounds are ready to embrace the challenge. School practitioners should be aware of the challenge and be willing to open spaces for students to adapt to their new environment healthily. CRT and SBFC are central to facilitating healthy adaptation to new environments. The interventions presented earlier have considered various cultural contexts, which are often marginalized and overlooked. The intervention strategies provided are a call to action for practitioners to move away from the notion of cultural "sensitivity" to embrace culturally responsive pedagogy, which is rooted in anti-racism.

Challenges and solutions

Applying CRT with SBFC requires that practitioners engage in introspection, reflection, and reflexivity.

1. **Lack of knowledge:** This is a challenge for many school practitioners. We all believe we are generally good people who do not intentionally engage in harmful behaviors toward students through lack of knowledge. Engaging in introspection is critical when one practices CRT and engages in SBFC. Educate yourself on students from refugee backgrounds represented at your school and avoid unwittingly inflicting harm.
2. **Reach out to local communities**: School practitioners need to reflect on the policies and practices that marginalize and make schools inhospitable to students from refugee backgrounds. To effectively do this, they must work in collaboration with local communities from refugee backgrounds. Invite them to plan meetings about the environment and welfare of their children. Ensure that you have interpreters where necessary so that people for whom English is a new language do not feel left out.

Conclusion

Students' and parents' experiences from refugee backgrounds presented in this chapter highlight the need and urgency for school practitioners to revise their policies and practices to make schools equitable spaces. The students and parents from refugee backgrounds located inhospitable treatment received in schools in lack of knowledge and understanding of complexities of being a refugee. We contend that using CRT and SBFC frameworks will provide a pathway to making schools fair and sites of refuge for students from refugee backgrounds. It is important that practitioners engage in self-education and do research about students' home countries and languages. It is equally vital to capitalize on the knowledge available in local communities of people refugee backgrounds. Extending the circle of practice to authentically engaging children, families and communities is fundamental to the effective implementation of CRT and SBFC.

Resources

Articles on engaging with refugee and immigrant families

Bridging refugee youth and Children's Services. (n.d.). Involving refugee parents in their children's education. https://brycs.org/schools/involving-refugee-parents-in-their-childrens-education/
This website has general information about the need to involve parents of students from refugee backgrounds and some of the challenges that school practitioners can circumvent.

Education Development Center. (2011). Strategies for engaging immigrant and refugee families. http://www.promoteprevent.org/sites/www.promoteprevent.org/files/resources/strategies_ for_ engaging_ immigrant_ and_ refugee_ families_ 2.pdf
This website provides relevant information and strategies on how to reach out and engage families from refugee backgrounds.

Gichiru, W. (2012). Challenges and prospects of providing critical educational opportunities for Somali refugees in the United States. In M. Knoester (Ed.), International struggles for critical democratic education (pp. 49–68). Peter Lang Publishing.
This chapter provides details of experiences of Somali-born students from refugee backgrounds in the U.S. schools. It is a must-read for all practitioners who work with students from refugee backgrounds.

Keengwe, J., & Onchwari, G. (Eds.). (2019). Handbook of research on assessment practices and pedagogical models for immigrant students. IGI Global.
This edited volume provides a wealth of strategies in dealing with students from refugee backgrounds.

Mendenhall, M., Bartlett, L., & Ghaffar-Kucher, A. (2017). 'If you need help, they are always there for us': Education for refugees in an international high school in New York City. Urban Review, 49(1), 1–25. https://doi.org/10.1007/s11256-016-0379-4
This article contains effective strategies on how to develop schools that are caring and nurturing to students from refugee backgrounds.

Bibliography

Banks, J. (2006). Race, culture and education: The selected works of James A. Banks. Routledge.

Baugh, R. (2019). Refugees and asylees: 2019. http://www.dhs.gov/sites/default/files/publications/immigration-statistics/yearbook/2019/refugee_ and_ asylee_ 2019.pdf. United States Department of Homeland Security.

DeNicolo, C. P., Yu, M., Crowley, C. B., & Gabel, S. L. (2017). Reimagining critical care and problematizing sense of school belonging as a response to inequality for immigrants and children of immigrants. Review of Research in Education, 41(1), 500–530. https://doi.org/10.3102/0091732X17690498

Doyle, O. (2020). COVID-19: Exacerbating educational inequalities? https://public-policy.ie/papers/covid-19-exacerbating-educational-inequalities/?msclkid=28d1210 7a55511ec818bc9cd8ee1ceed

Freire, P. (1970). The pedagogy of the oppressed. Seabury Press.

Gay, G. (2000). Culturally responsive teaching: Theory, research and practice. Teacher's College Press.

Gay, G. (2002). Preparing for culturally responsive teaching. Journal of Teacher Education, 53(2), 106–116. https://doi.org/10.1177/0022487102053002003

Gay, G. (2010). Acting on beliefs in teacher education for cultural diversity. Journal of Teacher Education, 61(1–2), 143–152. https://doi.org/10.1177/0022487109347320

Githembe, P. K. (2009). African refugee parents' involvement in their children's schools: Barriers and recommendations for improvement [Doctoral Dissertation]. University of North Texas.

Gonzales, S. M. (2015). Abuelita epistemologies: Counteracting subtractive schools in American education. Journal of Latinos and Education, 14(1), 40–54. https://doi.org/10.1080/15348431.2014.944703

Han, Y. C., & Love, J. (2015). Stages of immigrant parent involvement—Survivors to leaders. Phi Delta Kappan, 97(4), 21–25. https://doi.org/10.1177/0031721715619913

Harushimana, I., & Awokoya, J. (2019). The Threat of Downward Assimilation Among Young African Immigrants in US Schools. In. Advances in educational technologies and instructional design. IGI Global, (330–354). https://doi.org/10.4018/978-1-5225-9348-5.ch018

Love, B. (2019). We want to do more than survive: Abolitionist teaching and the pursuit of educational freedom. Beacon Press.

Matthews, J. (2008). Schooling and settlement: Refugee education in Australia. International Studies in Sociology of Education, 18(1), 31–45. https://doi.org/10.1080/09620210802195947

Moll, L. C., Amanti, C., Neff, D., & Gonzalez, N. (1992). Funds of knowledge for teaching: Using a qualitative approach to connect homes and classrooms. Theory into Practice, 31(2), 132–141. https://doi.org/10.1080/00405849209543534

Mthethwa-Sommers, S., & Kisiara, O. (2019). Refugee parents' perceptions of bullying practices of their children in urban schools. In G. Onchwari & J. Keengwe (Eds.), Handbook of research on engaging immigrant families and promoting academic success for English language learners (pp. 378–392). IGI Global.

Nieto, S. (1996). Affirming diversity: The socio-political context of multicultural education. Longman.

Ogbu, J. U., & Simons, H. D. (1998). Voluntary and involuntary minorities: A cultural-ecological theory of school performance with some implications for education. Anthropology Education Quarterly, 29(2), 155–188. https://doi.org/10.1525/aeq.1998.29.2.155

Pallares, A. (2014). Latinidad: Transnational cultures in the United States: Family activism: Immigrant struggles and the politics of non-citizenship. Rutgers University Press.

Sleeter, C. E. (2010). Decolonizing curriculum. Curriculum Inquiry, 40(2), 193–204. https://doi.org/10.1111/j.1467-873X.2010.00477.x

Soriano, M., & Gerrard, B. (2013). School-based family counseling: An overview. In B. Gerrard & M. Soriano (Eds.), School-based family counseling: Transforming family-school relationships. San Francisco: Institute for School-Based Family Counseling.

Steele, C. (2003). Stereotype threat and African American student achievement. In D. B. Grusky & S. Szelenyi (Eds.), The inequality reader: Contemporary and foundational readings in race, class, and gender (pp. 276–281). Routledge.

Tadesse, S. (2014). Parent involvement: Perceived encouragement and barriers to African refugee parent and teacher relationships. Childhood Education, 90(4), 298–305. https://doi.org/10.1080/00094056.2014.937275

Teachman, G., & Gladstone, B. (2020). Guest editors' introduction: Special issue: Constructions of "Children's Voices" in qualitative research. International Journal of Qualitative Methods, 19, 1–5. https://doi.org/10.1177/1609406920980654

Wood, L., & Harris, F. (2020). Black minds matter [Webinar]. https://www.youtube.com/watch?v=9IXgbRMkJUk

Wood, L., & Harris, F. (2021). race lighting: A prevalent version of gaslighting facing people of color. Diverse: Issues in Higher Education. diverseeducation.com.

18 How to Increase Immigrant and Refugee Student Engagement

Emily J. Hernandez and Alia R. Elasmar

This chapter describes how school-based family counseling practitioners can increase student engagement in a school setting. While there are many aspects to student engagement, this chapter will focus on cultivating a positive school climate, establishing school organization and infrastructure, and fostering student interactions. These interventions, while structural in nature, can have a positive impact specifically when working with immigrant and refugee students in the educational system.

Background

Student Engagement

Student engagement has been widely studied in educational research and is a term that is used to measure a student's relationship to the school. While there are many terms used to describe student engagement, there are consistent themes found by Libbey (2004) that relate to student engagement: a sense of belonging and being a part of a school; whether or not students like school; level of teacher supportiveness and caring; the presence of good friends in school; engagement in current and future academic progress; fair and effective discipline; and participation in extracurricular activities (Libbey, 2004). Student engagement and the factors described earlier are highly associated with student outcomes.

Research repeatedly shows that student engagement is a robust predictor of school achievement and behavior (Appleton et al., 2008; Shernoff & Schmidt, 2008) and also enhances the probability of high school completion (Reschly et al., 2007). Student engagement is considered the primary theoretical model in understanding student dropout (Christenson et al., 2012; Finn, 1989; Reschly & Christenson, 2012). Hart et al. (2011) recommend that student engagement interventions be a key to promoting school completion and academic outcomes. Reschly and Christenson (2012) refer to student engagement as the "glue, or mediator" that links the various important contexts (life, home, school peers, and community) to students, which in turn affects the outcome of interest and connection

DOI: 10.4324/9781003097891-23

Box 18.1   Known Facts About Student Engagement

- Student engagement is crucial to understanding student dropout
- Engagement behavior is complex and much more than just attending school or doing well academically.
- Student engagement is associated positively with academic, social, and emotional learning outcomes.
- Student engagement is a multidimensional construct that requires an awareness and understanding of affective connections within the academic environment and student behavior.
- Context is important. Engagement is inextricably linked and influenced by the context of the student's life (school, peers, family, community). Therefore, focusing on the individual alone is not enough.
- Student engagement and motivation must be a component of effective instruction for positive learning outcomes.
- Measuring student engagement is a powerful tool to drive data-driven decision-making in schools.
- Some evidence-based practices and interventions are known to increase student engagement.

(Christenson et al., 2012)

---

to school (p. 3). Student engagement has become an important topic in the field of education. The Handbook of Research on Student Engagement is an excellent resource to review for a more comprehensive understanding of the research on student engagement. Some commonly known facts about student engagement are reviewed in Box 18.1.

Student engagement is an important topic to consider when working with immigrant and refugee student populations. The risks associated with school failure are more significant today than ever before (21st Century Workforce Commission, 2000), demanding we deepen our understanding of the processes that contribute to trajectories of academic success. Studies have found that immigrant students undergo many unique migration-related stresses while adapting to a new schooling environment (Suárez-Orozco & Suárez Orozco, 2001), placing them at particular educational risk. Immigrant students experience trauma, including exposure to violence, family separation, stays at detention centers, unstable living situations, living in a climate of fear, challenges of acculturation, and other types of disturbing events. Immigrant students also experience daily stressors that non-migrant students typically do not (Cleary et al., 2018). These traumatic experiences impact their social, mental, and physical well-being, leading to decreased engagement. Evaluating current systems and implementing best practices for student engagement with immigrant and refugee student populations will assist these student populations in feeling a sense of belonging and care, decreasing their disengagement and risk of school failure.

School-Based Family Counseling Meta-Model and Framework

Considering student engagement as it applies to immigrant and refugee students can be viewed through the school-based family counseling (SBFC) meta-model and framework. There are eight main strengths of the SBFC meta-model: school and family focus, systems orientation, educational focus, parent partnership, multicultural sensitivity, child advocacy, promotion of school transformation, interdisciplinary focus, and evidence-based support. Using the strength areas of the SBFC model provides a way for collaborative and systems-oriented approaches to prevention and intervention. The SBFC meta-model, as described by Soriano and Gerrard (2013), illustrates the primary focus of SBFC to be on the school and the family in the area of prevention and intervention. The model consists of four quadrants: school prevention, school intervention, family prevention, and family intervention. It provides a framework to help SBFC professionals stay focused on working systemically within a school structure at the heart of the SBFC approach.

Student engagement falls mainly in the area of the prevention quadrants. A specific focus on prevention within a systems perspective reduces the need for intervention-related services. The emphasis on prevention shifts the balance from a reactive model to a more proactive one. The development of a prevention-focused school system will allow for more time and intentional interventions for youth and families by SBFC professionals (Hernandez, 2016). Focusing on student engagement with a prevention focus is an effective solution for school-wide problems—including dropout prevention and bullying—and can mitigate barriers associated with the immigrant and refugee student experience.

Student Engagement and Student Dropout

Student engagement is a central construct in student dropout. Dropping out of school is a process of disengagement and is identifiable early on in the student's academic career. Disengagement from school is a critical element in this process. Dropping out is more of a process than an event (Rumberger & Rotermund, 2012). The eventual act of dropping out involves a slow process of disengagement that begins early on in a student's academic career. Signs of disengagement are prevalent and can be observed in students as early as elementary school. Warning signs include poor attendance, behavior problems, and low grades in middle and early high school. Attendance is often a key barometer of a student's connection with the school. Failing in school was also reported as a significant contributing factor (Balfanz et al., 2010). The long-term effects of school disengagement on problem behaviors have been identified (Henry et al., 2012), and student engagement is central to most theories of school dropout (Finn, 1989). The level of a student's engagement to school is an important precursor to student dropout, so our model emphasizes student engagement as a prevention initiative.

Student engagement should be prioritized when working with immigrant and refugee students. According to the National Center for Education Statistics, immigrant and refugee students in the U.S. are almost twice as likely to drop out than their native-born peers (2017). On the basis of the multicultural sensitivity of the SBFC meta-model, practicing inclusion to empower and elevate immigrant/refugee students and their families is significant for effective student engagement. Inclusivity and awareness around immigrant and refugee students ensure that student engagement initiatives are preventative. Often, these initiatives are stand-alone interventions instead of embedded in a school's culture of equity and belonging. Stand-alone initiatives can further harm and marginalize immigrant and refugee students because reactive initiatives tend to blame-based and ignore system-based issues. Therefore, immigrant and refugee students internalize this blame, which further increases their disengagement. As we continue to examine student engagement with immigrant students, it's important to note that dynamics in peer relationships are contributing factors.

Student Engagement and Bullying

Bullying has become a growing concern among students, parents, educators, and the community (Lederman, 2012). Robers et al. (2012) conducted a national study and found that 28% of students reported being bullied. Bullying is a common worldwide phenomenon, and students in multiple countries report being involved in bullying (Harris & Petrie, 2002; Smith et al., 1999). One in five children and adolescents are victims of bullying (Limber, 2002), and one in three are involved as a bully, victim, or both (Nansel et al., 2001). Bullying impacts a student's overall adjustment to school, which affects their level of engagement. Bullying negatively influences student engagement, attendance, behavior, academic outcomes, and increases dropout rates (Gastic, 2008; Morrison, 2002). Research has shown that victims of bullying exhibit poor social and emotional adjustment, lower social skills and abilities to make friends, poor relationships with classmates, and higher levels of loneliness and anxiety (Harris & Petrie, 2002). Further, even the perception of bullying in a school plays a role in disengagement. Students who perceive high levels of bullying in their school may become less engaged in school and, consequently, be less motivated to learn. This disengagement contributes to problems with school attendance, including truancy and dropout (Gastic, 2008; Klein et al., 2012). Students involved in bullying experience difficulty adjusting to the school environment, which further results in their disengagement from school.

Adjusting to new school climates can put immigrant students at higher risk for bullying. Research has found that immigrant students significantly experience more bullying than native students (Flores & Clares-López, 2014). The most repeated bullying behaviors that immigrant students experience are: exclusion, spreading lies, and teasing (Flores & Clares-López, 2014). Bullying can affect school performance, and the researchers noted that language barriers were also a significant factor (Flores & Clares-López, 2014). This study emphasized the importance of developing preventative school-wide interventions such as intercultural education in classrooms (Flores & Clares-López, 2014). In addition, research has revealed that the relevance of anti-immigrant prejudice was a driving factor in racial bullying (Caravita et al., 2019). Findings further indicated that prejudice also needs to be addressed in anti-bullying interventions (Caravita et al., 2019). The SBFC meta-model provides a lens that integrates knowledge and awareness around socio-emotional issues.

Evidence-Based Support

Dropout prevention and bullying are major educational issues at the center of school reform and contribute to school disengagement. Student engagement has repeatedly been demonstrated to be a robust predictor of achievement and behavior in schools (Appleton et al., 2008; Shernoff & Schmidt, 2008). Student engagement is linked to multiple educational outcomes such as achievement, attendance, behavior, and dropout/completion (Finn, 1989; Jimerson et al., 2003; Jimerson et al., 2009). Studies show that student engagement is considered the primary theoretical model in understanding student dropout (Christenson et al., 2012; Finn, 1989; Reschly & Christenson, 2012). Immigrant and refugee students are greatly at risk of disengaging from school due to multiple educational barriers. Immigrant and refugee students have greatly benefitted from schools that have adjusted their climates to include prevention and intervention efforts focused on student engagement. According to the U.S. Department of Education, policies, structures, and systems have been initiated to address gaps in academics and establish equity to build student engagement. However, research has shown that students need equitable support systemically with academic interventions and systemic interventions that address their mental health and well-being (Aldana & Martinez, 2018). This chapter focuses on systemic and direct service student engagement interventions that can be put in place by SBFC practitioners at a school site to increase the engagement of immigrant students to school, thereby improving opportunities for long-term educational outcomes for this student population. Following the procedures listed in the next section can help increase student engagement for immigrant and refugee school success outcomes.

The procedure presented is based on a research study of a model utilizing student engagement as a promising practice in dropout prevention and bullying (Hernandez, 2014). The procedure was adapted to address the needs and application for working with immigrant student populations for this chapter. Three prevalent themes with accompanying strategies emerged from the data. The themes are positive school climate, school organization and infrastructure, and student interactions. The various tables presented below show how the findings, consistent themes, and supporting strategies align with the prevention focus quadrants of the SBFC meta-model.

Procedure

Step 1. Positive School Climate

The first step in the process is to cultivate a positive school climate (see Table 18.1). While there are many aspects to cultivating a school climate, this section will focus on developing a positive school climate.

Leadership and Whole-School Approach

Leadership must be involved to build a positive school climate, and a whole-school approach must be utilized. The whole-school approach requires involving all stakeholders with the school vision, mission, and operations and involving parents and students. Consistent and transparent communication and engagement with stakeholders increase cohesiveness and positively affect school climate. The leadership style of the principal and administrative team transforms and empowers the entire school and community. School leadership is the integral component to developing, implementing, and sustaining a systems-level, whole-school approach. Having administrators, teachers, counselors, staff, and volunteers all share the same beliefs about the school, and students' potential becomes a powerful message to the community. Building a foundation for these shared beliefs is critical. In the *Cultural Proficiency* manual, Lindsey et al. suggest that school teams create an environment where staff feel safe to explore their implicit biases and deeply reflect on their perspectives and practices in the classroom and interactions with students (2019). The "inside-out approach" in the manual suggests that change starts with each staff member reflecting within to identify and address barriers to cultural proficiency. Lindsey et al. describe that

Table 18.1 Supporting Strategies for Positive School Climate

Theme	Supporting strategies	
Positive school climate	Leadership	Whole-school approach

a culturally proficient school leadership would foster policies and practices that are culturally inclusive and provide the opportunity for effective interactions among students, educators, and community members.

Further, examples of effective and culturally proficient school leadership and whole-school approach practices to foster a positive school climate for working with immigrant student populations include the following:

- Envision a plan for the school community together that is inclusive of all students.
- Build a school team around shared educational values and belief systems that include inclusion and cultural competency. The team should be supported, guided, and empowered to become change agents for students.
- Foster the belief system that all students can learn if they feel safe and cared about.
- Create a cohesive school team of educators that are committed and accountable to their mission.
- Internalizing the idea that "it all starts in the classroom," cultivate the sense that the students are "theirs" (teachers') and that the teachers have an essential role to play for students as human beings, with their learning, their behavior, and their social-emotional growth. This attitude can change the dynamics between students, teachers, and administrators.
- Stakeholders (students, parents, teachers, staff, and community members) should be viewed as "assets" and treated as partners, welcomed, respected, and given the message that they are necessary to the school family.
- Clear visual images and displays around the school should communicate inclusive and welcoming messages to all stakeholders.
- Teachers at the school should be highly regarded, celebrated, respected, and seen as important change agents.
- Teachers should be provided training and guidance toward the mission and vision of the school. Additional training should include contextual information (i.e., cultural norms), statistics, and reflection on the experiences of immigrant and refugee students. These trainings can include guest speakers, community circle practices, and rehearsing strategies that can be used in the classroom.
- The school should support and invest in a robust parent and community center representative of various students and families, including nontraditional students and immigrant and refugee students and families.

Step 2. School Organization and Infrastructure

The second step in the procedure is to focus on the organization and infrastructure of the school. While there are many aspects to school organization and infrastructure, this section will focus on student safety and learning, campus supervision, and student groupings/cohort model (see Table 18.2).

Table 18.2 Supporting Strategies for Facilitating School Organization and Infrastructure

Theme	Supporting strategies		
School organization and infrastructure	Student safety and learning	Campus supervision	Student groupings/ cohort model

Student Safety and Learning

The organization and infrastructure at a school have an indirect impact on the school climate. Developing internal school policies related to daily school operations and infrastructure creates a school system that flows well and creates a positive school climate. The flow and consistency of day-to-day school operations set the tone for the campus. School operations should be clear, consistent, and demonstrated by the administrators and leadership team. After focusing on step 1, this procedural step should be easier to implement as it requires buy-in from school staff and stakeholders. All school infrastructure must have an underlying focus on student safety and learning.

Physical Organization and Layout of the School

The main issue related to student safety and learning is focusing on key operational issues related to the physical organization and layout of the school. Safety and learning are critical issues when specifically working with immigrant student populations that often have struggled with compromised safe spaces, experiences of trauma, and interrupted schooling and opportunities for learning. The physical organization and layout of the school should be evaluated and incorporated into the school plan. This plan can include strategic but straightforward, logical solutions to common school problems that affect student safety and learning. These common problems include traffic in hallways, stairwells, lunch areas, entry and exit areas, and the routine trash and cleanliness problems many schools deal with. These problems are often seen as uncontrollable realities by schools that, in effect, contribute toward a chaotic feeling, especially in larger schools. Spending time gathering information and understanding the intricacies of the school plant and operational issues is key to making strategic improvements that will directly impact how the school "feels," which will impact school climate. Making changes in these areas will impact the "experience" of school for immigrant students. It will increase a sense of safety, facilitate learning, and help with the navigation of the school environment in a way that does not overwhelm immigrant students.

Examples of some school changes focused on the physical organization and layout of the school include the following:

- Gather information using observation, interviews, and surveys to understand the main issues related to safety at the school.
- Gather and analyze school data related to office referrals and begin tracking the location of incidents to gain a better understanding of where issues related to safety may frequently be occurring.
- Have a good understanding of traffic flow in the school during key transition times: school arrival, transition periods, nutrition, lunch, and school dismissal.
- Implement a stairwell system to control the flow of student traffic during transition times. The stairwell system should identify one stairwell for going up only and the opposite stairwell for going down. This arrangement could also be applied to directional traffic in hallways.
- Use line dividers to teach students where to stand in lines and use painted walk paths to follow when going to certain areas of the school.
- Implement specific entry and exit doors from the buildings.
- Develop school norms for lunch and nutrition-related breaks.
- Revitalize the physical look of the school and spaces. Make efforts to "beautify" the school campus. Examples may include murals, planted gardens, art, benches or gathering spaces, painted lines for sports areas, and so on. Adding color and green to spaces, classrooms, and hallways has a positive effect on school climate.

Campus Supervision

The second finding within the theme of school organization and infrastructure is an effective campus supervision protocol. Campus supervision is a simplified concept that all schools utilize. Campus supervision should be an organized, structured, and goal-directed form of supervision. Members of the team should be trained and held accountable for quality supervision of students. The campus supervision system at the school is a consistent daily function of the school staff, including the administrators. Everyone works together for the safety and structure of the whole. This "active" form of supervision requires staff to be visible regularly and provides consistency and ample opportunities for interactions with students. The campus supervision plan should have documented guidelines, norms, and regular meetings to monitor the effectiveness of supervision. Once the system is in place, it can become so embedded into the school culture that teachers may voluntarily supervise their hallways during transition periods without being asked because they want to do their part. Monitoring the hallways becomes an integral part of being visible and interacting with students. This active form of campus supervision directly supports immigrant and refugee students' inclusion, integration, and support. It makes school staff more available, visible, and accessible to these students who may need more support from school staff. Using campus supervision opportunities to be more intentional about connecting with students can serve as a great prevention and intervention effort on behalf of the school.

Some simple but effective guidelines and norms for schools to adopt when providing campus supervision are as follows:

- Be on "active" supervision and meet with the supervision team regularly.
- Move from group to group of students or spaces.
- Position yourself separate from other adults.
- Be on time and consistent with locations for coverage.
- Engage! Talk to students, greet them, and smile.

Student Groupings/Cohort Model

How students are grouped is a central component of the complex infrastructure of the school. Developing a grouping system, or cohort model, keeps students and teachers together in contiguous space areas. This grouping system allows a large school to feel like a relatively small school for a student, increasing opportunities for the development of friendships, which increases the cohesiveness of the groups. Secondly, it directly addresses safety in that students travel together from class to class in groups, albeit they do not travel very far as their classes are right next to each other in the same hallway. This, with the addition of their teachers outside in the halls during transition times, can create a safe and positive climate in the hallways. Due to the groupings, the teachers can have closer relationships with students, know them all by names, and, since teacher teams work together, have a sense of the needs of the different students. Lastly, implementing advisory periods can serve as a "school family," and teachers can take responsibility for a small group of students' academic and social/emotional well-being. This advisory period allows students and teachers to develop relationships together and focus on non-academic content such as life skills, character development, and growing together as a class community. This time is also used to provide guidance when struggling with academic or home issues. Implementing a grouping system at a school creates a sense of safety, community, equity, and access for all students.

This grouping system has great benefits for working with immigrant and refugee students because of the opportunities for relationships with educators and peers. Research on the in-group/cohort model approach increased immigrant students' sense of cohesiveness and well-being (Motti-Stefanidi et al., 2008). Further, through the cohort model, immigrant students were able to feel connected in that other students had similar histories and experiences due to trauma. Groups like this can build unity and a support system that makes students feel like they belong and are safe and understood. Most importantly, it allows for access to a supportive adult that is consistent.

Examples of how to implement a student grouping/cohort system can include the following:

- Review student data and create an academic program that includes a heterogeneous grouping of students.
- Student cohorts, or teams, are developed based on a balance of high- and low-performing students, inclusive of all students: English Language Learners, English Only, Gifted, and Students with Disabilities. The classes are equally balanced so that each class has students who represent all areas.
- Student groups are matched with a group, or team, of teachers that all work together with the same students. The classrooms for these teams are set up next to each other, so teachers are logistically close to each other to communicate frequently. In addition, this physical arrangement allows students not to have to travel much between their classes.
- The teacher teams work together to develop their curriculum uniformly and deliver the same content to all students. All teacher teams follow the same curriculum and content consistently from class to class and grade to grade.
- Implement a daily advisory that meets with students every morning to cover a multitude of topics and focus on developing relationships and engaging with students.
- The advisory teacher stays with the same group of students for the duration of their stay at the school, allowing multiple years of a consistent, stable relationship with students and families. This advisor period can become somewhat of a "school family" in that it is where the students develop strong and meaningful connections with each other and their teachers. The advisory teacher also serves as a case manager of sorts, reviewing their students' grades, attendance, behavior, and works with the teacher team in communicating regarding students.
- The SBFC team also can adopt a grouping model and travel with their students in the same way. They remain with their students until they leave the school and transition to the next school. This allows SBFC practitioners to develop strong bonds with their students and have enough time to work with students and families before the year is over, and they need to get to know an entirely new group of students.

Step 3. Student Interactions

The third step in the procedure is to focus on interactions with students (see Table 18.3). This step is developed last because there will be great difficulty implementing these components without the foundational pieces of positive school climate and school organization and infrastructure implemented. Focusing on

Table 18.3 Supporting Strategies for Facilitating Student Interactions

Theme	*Supporting strategies*	
Student interactions	Cooperative learning model	Character building and social skills

student interactions requires the shared educational belief that student engagement in school begins in the classroom. Immigrant and refugee students benefit significantly from having access to and support from an identified person (i.e., teacher, counselor) who they trust and who can serve as a mentor/advocate. Two main components can be focused on to increase student interaction in the classroom: (a) implementing a consistent cooperative learning model in every classroom focusing on student and teacher interactions and relationships and (b) teaching character building and social skills to all students.

Cooperative Learning Model

Cooperative learning is an effective instructional tool to use when focusing on how to increase student interaction in the classroom. Cooperative learning is a teaching method that refers to small, heterogeneous groups of students working together to achieve a common goal. The students work together to learn and are responsible for their teammates' learning and their own. Basic elements of cooperative learning include positive interdependence, individual accountability, equal participation, and simultaneous interaction between students (Murie, 2004). The various structures utilized in the cooperative learning model increase the interactions between students and teachers in the classroom, which has an overall positive effect on academic and social outcomes because students learn and practice communicating with each other positively (Murie, 2004). When students are exposed to this model all day, every day, consistently in every class, student engagement increases. Teaching and creating opportunities for students to interact and communicate with each other in appropriate ways foster this engagement. Once engagement in the classroom is established with their teachers, with the academic content, and with their class group, other aspects of engagement to the larger school, such as clubs and sports, are more likely to follow.

Examples of how to begin implementing cooperative learning methods in a classroom/school:

* Develop the belief among all school personnel that increasing positive interactions and communication among students will increase engagement to school.
* Research and invest in quality training and provide professional development time for school staff to learn and implement cooperative learning structures in the classroom.

- Encourage student talk time in the classroom. Adopt a goal that there should be "at least 50% student talking" in every classroom to normalize student verbal exchanges in the class.
- Physically organize classrooms into spaces that encourage cooperative learning, such as desks arranged in pods of four so that students could work collaboratively together.
- Encourage the development of relationships among students and teachers and staff in the classroom and during transition times.

Character Building and Social Skills

Teaching character and social skills is a necessary component that supports the theme of student interactions. These skills should be infused into the culture in multiple dimensions, beginning with the classroom, the daily school environment and culture, and specific programs used. Social skills are modeled and taught starting in the classroom and reinforced through cooperative learning structures. It is crucial to create opportunities for meaningful interaction between students, which allows for many teaching opportunities about "how" to interact with each other. Character building and social skills are taught on multiple levels, from indirect messaging to a direct curriculum in the classroom. It can also be infused into discipline and conflicts that may arise in the school. A variety of curricula are available that focus on integrating character building and social skills teaching into schools. Student clubs, student leadership, and partnerships are another way to incorporate character building and social skills training into school environments. Providing opportunities for students to increase their skills in character building and socialization increases positive student interactions and contributes toward academic and social/emotional engagement of students to school. Social-emotional learning was identified as the optimal theoretical framework to adapt when working with immigrant students because interventions that have followed this model have effectively improved participating students' academic and social outcomes (Olivo, 2007). Examples of other successful interventions using the framework mentioned earlier include affinity groups based on socio-emotional needs, school values visible on campus grounds and reinforced in conversations and restorative circles in classrooms, and professional development for staff to explore their implicit bias and broaden their knowledge of immigrant and refugee population strengths.

Examples of how to begin implementing character and social skills building into a classroom/school are the following:

- Research with your school team and agree on the main character-building traits and social skills to focus on.
- Develop school messaging regarding what you would like to focus on and how it will be taught and communicated to students.

- These concepts should be infused throughout the school through visual displays, posters, signage, bulletin boards, and so on in classrooms and hallways.
- Use other messaging such as newsletters, websites, social media, assemblies to communicate, teach, and remind students and families.
- Use school messaging whenever opportunities arise to teach these skills. Examples include in the classroom, during campus supervision, counseling office, discipline, and assemblies.
- Utilize student leadership to develop activities and engage students related to the character-building program.
- Research and invest in a social skills training curriculum for the school. Identify an administrator, an SBFC practitioner, and a teacher team responsible for the training and implementation.
- Utilize a course period, homeroom, advisor, or study period to implement social skills training curriculum by grade.
- Use technology to deliver the curriculum through the computer lab or through student discipline modules on relevant social skills training specific to the situation.
- Use a positive reinforcement method program to highlight positive social skills and character building.
- Integrate active school clubs onto campus that focus on character building and social skills training. Examples can include friendship clubs, peer mentoring and conflict resolution programs, peer leaders, student government, student ambassadors, mentoring, and so on.

Multicultural Considerations

Culture is a powerful and pervasive influence on students, families, stakeholders, and attitudes and behaviors. For that reason, multicultural counseling issues should be taken into consideration by the school as a whole. Being aware of issues related to the context and histories of the students and families that we serve as educators and SBFC practitioners is an ethical requirement of the profession. In order to increase student engagement for immigrant and refugee students, families must feel safe and trust their school environments. As previously mentioned, educators must be aware of multicultural education and relevant issues in the schools and communities that they serve. It is helpful for educators and practitioners to take a step back to listen and understand their immigrant/refugee students and families, where they are at, where they are coming from, and what they have to say before moving forward with an agenda. This form of presence in the classroom is an integral piece for immigrant/refugee students experiencing different acculturation levels. Acculturation is a challenging process, especially when developmentally students are already in the process of exploring their identities. It is important to note that a multicultural framework includes educators helping immigrant/refugee students maintain connections with their cultural identities. This means avoiding pressure or messages that would cause immigrant/refugee students to feel like they have to assimilate to feel safe or welcomed. The model presented in this chapter creates a safe place for community and learning that is inclusive of all students. It provides safety, learning, structure, and opportunities for meaningful communication, engagement, and sustained relationships between students and with students. The model works to create a school and community climate that embraces cultural diversity and helps to promote students' academic, career, and social/emotional success because it begins and ends with students.

Challenges and Solutions

The model described presents challenges that should be considered and anticipated before implementation. When examining immigrant/refugee student population and school engagement challenges, barriers include communication, language, navigating school environments, transiency, financial difficulties, problems obtaining housing, trust, and family engagement. If there aren't systemic interventions to address these challenges, immigrant/refugee students can become disengaged. Often, schools have engaged students with stand-alone interventions but then lose immigrant/refugee engagement due to not having a multicultural trauma-informed lens and framework. The solution is understanding the difficult decisions and challenges immigrant/refugee students make for their basic needs and their family's best interest. With this in consideration, a multicultural solution would be to address systemic issues and offer resources and school-wide interventions to address those challenges so that immigrant/refugee students can maintain their engagement and socio-emotional well-being. The biggest systemic challenges are related to time, buy-in, and funding. The model is focused mainly on prevention and macro-level systemic changes that will impact school climate. This type of work takes a considerable amount of time and does not happen overnight. The model does not offer a quick change, or packaged solution, with immediate effects frequently sought after by schools because of the time pressures and demands on them for immediate outcomes. In contrast, it requires time, buy-in, and effective leadership to steer the change. The solution is to focus on one aspect of the model, with leadership being first and most important. Without effective leadership in place and utilizing the whole school approach, achieving buy-in from the school community will be very difficult. This model's focus should be considered a part of a school transformation rather than as implementing a "program." This approach is key when working with immigrant/refugee students as often "programs" serve as stand-alone interventions with an unintentional foundation of savior complex and "othering" of marginalized groups. Being mindful of these mindsets is important when working with immigrant/refugee students because those mindsets stem from a deficit approach. A multicultural approach would highlight, support, and transform the immigrant/refugee strengths and encourage them to use those strengths to support a healthy adjustment to school.

Additionally, the maintenance and success of the stand-alone interventions aren't sustainable by school staff due to lack of buy-in and the limited value emphasized on the transformational process. Transformational processes take time and planning but frequently yield more positive and sustainable outcomes. Establishing the first step can take up to 1 year. Steps two and three will require planning by the leadership and school team to advance the beginning of the new school year. This work is frequently done in the summer while students are not in school. Implementing steps two and three will also require funding for school staff to receive training/professional development and/or attend school retreats throughout the year. Funding solutions can include streamlining resources allocated for staff professional development to focus on implementing the model and engaging in community partnerships to provide training. Also, additional funding sources can be used, such as grants, to supplement funding and be utilized solely for the model implementation. Fortunately, the model's core does not require substantial amounts of additional funding but a reorganization of existing financing, school structures, and operations.

Resources

Reschly, A. L., & Christenson, S. L. (2012). Jingle, jangle, and conceptual haziness: Evolution and future directions of the engagement construct. In *Handbook of research on student engagement* (pp. 3–19). New York, NY: Springer.
  This chapter provides an overview of the history of the concept student engagement, and would be useful for SBFC practitioners interested in how definitions of ideaas impact practices.
Hernandez, E. J. (2016). Reducing bullying and preventing dropout through student engagement: A prevention-focused lens for school-based family counselors. *International Journal for School-Based Family Counseling, 7,* 1–13.
  Student engagement is a key domain influencing many areas of academic achievement, including reducing bullying and preventing dropouts. This article is a must read for SBFC practitioners.

Bibliography

Aldana, U. S., & Martinez, D. C. (2018). The development of a community of practice for educators working with newcomer, Spanish-speaking Students, Spanish. Theory into Practice, 57(2), 137–146. https://doi.org/10.1080/00405841.2018.1425813
Appleton, J. J., Christenson, S. L., & Furlong, M. J. (2008). Student engagement with school: Critical conceptual and methodological issues of the construct. Psychology in the Schools, 45(5), 369–386. https://doi.org/10.1002/pits.20303
Balfanz, R., Bridgeland, J. M., Moore, L. A., & Fox, J. H. Enterprises, C, & center, E.G. (2010). Building a grad nation. Progress and Challenge in Ending the High School Dropout Epidemic: Civic Enterprises. LLC.
Caravita, S. C. S., Stefanelli, S., Mazzone, A., Cadei, L., Thornberg, R., & Ambrosini, B. (2020). When the bullied peer is native-born vs. immigrant: A mixed-method

study with a sample of native-born and immigrant adolescents. Scandinavian Journal of Psychology, 61(1), 97–107. https://doi.org/10.1111/sjop.12565

Christenson, S. L., Reschly, A. L., & Wylie, C. (Eds.). (2012). Handbook of research on student engagement. Springer Science+Business Media.

Cleary, S. D., Snead, R., Dietz-Chavez, D., Rivera, I., & Edberg, M. C. (2018). Immigrant trauma and mental health outcomes among Latino youth. Journal of Immigrant and Minority Health, 20(5), 1053–1059. https://doi.org/10.1007/s10903-017-0673-6

Finn, J. D. (1989). Withdrawing from school. Review of Educational Research, 59(2), 117–142. https://doi.org/10.3102/00346543059002117

Peskin, M. F., Tortolero, S. R., Markham, C. M., Addy, R. C., & Baumler, E. R. (2007). Bullying and victimization and internalizing symptoms among low-income Black and Hispanic students. Journal of Adolescent Health, 40(4), 372–375. https://doi.org/10.1016/j.jadohealth.2006.10.010

Flores, J. G., & Clares-López, J. (2014). Bullying in students belonging to immigrant families in primary schools. Procedia - Social and Behavioral Sciences, 132, 621–625. https://doi.org/10.1016/j.sbspro.2014.04.363

Gastic, B. (2008). School truancy and the disciplinary problems of bullying victims. Educational Review, 60(4), 391–404. https://doi.org/10.1080/00131910802393423

Gerrard, B., & Soriano, M. (Eds.). (2013). School-based family counseling: Transforming family-school relationships. Phoenix. Createspace.

Harris, S., & Petrie, G. (2002). A study of bullying in the middle school. National Association of Secondary School Principals Bulletin. NASSP Bulletin, 86(633), 42–53. https://doi.org/10.1177/019263650208663304

Hart, S. R., Stewart, K., & Jimerson, S. R. (2011). The student engagement in schools questionnaire (SESQ) and the teacher engagement report form-new (TERF-N): Examining the preliminary evidence. Contemporary School Psychology, 15, 67–79.

Henry, K. L., Knight, K. E., & Thornberry, T. P. (2012). School disengagement as a predictor of dropout, delinquency, and problem substance use during adolescence and early adulthood. Journal of Youth and Adolescence, 41(2), 156–166. https://doi.org/10.1007/s10964-011-9665-3

Hernandez, E. J. (2014). Promising practices for preventing bullying in K-12 schools: Student engagement. University of Southern California.

Hernandez, E. J. (2016). Reducing bullying and preventing dropout through student engagement: A prevention-focused lens for school-based family counselors. International Journal for School-Based Family Counseling, 7, 1–13.

Jimerson, S. R., Campos, E., & Greif, J. L. (2003). Toward an understanding of definitions and measures of school engagement and related terms. California School Psychologist, 8(1), 7–27. https://doi.org/10.1007/BF03340893

Jimerson, S. R., Renshaw, T. L., Stewart, K., Hart, S., & O'Malley, M. (2009). Promoting school completion through understanding school failure: A multi-factorial model of dropping out as a developmental process. Romanian Journal of School Psychology, 2, 12–29.

Klein, J., Cornell, D., & Konold, T. (2012). Relationships between bullying, school climate, and student risk behaviors. School Psychology Quarterly, 27(3), 154–169. https://doi.org/10.1037/a0029350

Lederman, J. (2012). Anti-bullying Ad campaign targets parents, Obama administration vows to a make it a 'national priority. http://www.huffingtonpost.com/2012/08/06/anti-bullying-adcampaign_ n_ 1749158.html?view=print&comm_ ref=false

Libbey, H. P. (2004). Measuring student relationships to school: Attachment, bonding, connectedness, and engagement. Journal of School Health, 74(7), 274–283. https://doi.org/10.1111/j.1746-1561.2004.tb08284.x

Limber, S. P. (2002, May). Addressing youth bullying behaviors. In Proceedings of the From the American Medical Association Educational Forum on Adolescent Health: Youth Bullying. Chicago, IL. American Medical Association.

Lindsey, R. B., Robins, K. N., Terrell, R. D., & Lindsey, D. B. (2019). Cultural proficiency: A manual for school leaders. Corwin Press, a Solid Action on Globalization and Environment Company.

Morrison, B. (2002). Bullying and victimisation in schools: A restorative justice approach, 219. Australian Institute of Criminology.

Motti-Stefanidi, F., Pavlopoulos, V., Obradović, J., & Masten, A. S. (2008). Acculturation and adaptation of immigrant adolescents in Greek urban schools. International Journal of Psychology, 43(1), 45–58. https://doi.org/10.1080/00207590701804412

Murie, C. (2004). Effects of communication on student learning. Kagan Publishing.

Nansel, T. R., Overpeck, M., Pilla, R. S., Ruan, W. J., Simons-Morton, B., & Scheidt, P. (2001). Bullying behaviors among US youth: Prevalence and association with psychosocial adjustment. JAMA, 285(16), 2094–2100. https://doi.org/10.1001/jama.285.16.2094

National Center for Education Statistics. (2017). Trends in High School Dropout and Completion Rates in the United States. Retrieved from https://nces.ed.gov/programs/dropout/ind_02.asp

Olivo, S. M. C. (2007). The effects of a culturally adapted social-emotional learning curriculum on social-emotional and academic outcomes of Latino immigrant high school students [Doctoral Dissertation]. University of Oregon.

—. (2000). Policy and research publications online reports. Final Report of the 21st Century Workforce Commission Released. https://wdr.doleta.gov/opr/fulltext/document.cfm?docn=6113. Employment & Training Administration. United States Department of Labor. (n.d.).

Reschly, A. L., Appleton, J. J., & Christenson, S. L. (2007). Student engagement at school and with learning: Theory and interventions. NASP Communiqué, 35(8).

Reschly, A. L., & Christenson, S. L. (2012). Jingle, jangle, and conceptual haziness: Evolution and future directions of the engagement construct. In Handbook of research on student engagement (pp. 3–19). Springer.

Robers, S., Zhang, J., Truman, J., & Snyder, T. D. (2012). Indicators of school crime and safety, 2011. Washington, DC. National Center for Education Statistics. United States Department of Education, and Bureau of Justice Statistics.

Rumberger, R. W., & Rotermund, S. (2012). The relationship between engagement and high school dropout. In Handbook of research on student engagement (pp. 491–513). Springer.

Shernoff, D. J., & Schmidt, J. A. (2008). Further Evidence of an Engagement–Achievement Paradox Among US High School Students. Journal of Youth and Adolescence, 37(5), 564–580. https://doi.org/10.1007/s10964-007-9241-z

Smith, P. K., Catalano, R., Junger-Tas, J. J., Slee, P. P., Morita, Y., & Olweus, D. (Eds.). (1999). The nature of school bullying: A cross-national perspective. Psychology Press.

Soriano, M., & Gerrard, B. (2013). School-based family counseling: An overview. In B. Gerrard & M. Soriano (Eds.), School-based family counseling: Transforming family-school relationships. Phoenix (pp. 2–15). Createspace.

Suárez-Orozco, M., & Suárez-Orozco, C. (2015). Children of immigration. Phi Delta Kappan, 97(4), 8–14. https://doi.org/10.1177/0031721715619911

Part 6

Community Prevention

19 The SBFC Practitioners' Role in Promoting Immigrant and Refugee Children's Social Participation in Community Life

Erwin D. Selimos

In addition to providing mental health and family support services, the school-based family counseling (SBFC) practitioner's key role is to assist immigrant and refugee children in expanding their social participation in the broader community. The chapter uses the SBFC case conceptualization approach to suggest why and how SBFC practitioners can help immigrant and refugee children connect to various programs and organizations.

Background

What Is Settlement?

Immigrant and refugee family settlement is defined as the process of establishing a new life in a new society of residence. Settlement involves the adaptation of immigrant and refugee families to the norms of their new host society and involves building attachments to various social institutions that comprise community life. The settlement process involves the concrete matters of finding housing, enrolling in school, securing employment, and building friendships with neighbors. Immigrant and refugee settlement involves the processes of entering the arenas of life that make up a community—that is, social participation (Drachman, 1992).

Canadian research demonstrates that immigrant and refugee families face significant challenges and barriers to their settlement in Canada. The degree of cultural similarity or difference between their country of origin and the receiving country may create stress that impacts their well-being (Drachman, 1992). Immigrant and refugee newcomers face barriers in finding adequate housing and accessing essential social, educational, and healthcare-related services. Many confront problems of underemployment and unemployment and difficulty in accessing social services. Concern and worry over family members living in conflict areas, refugee camps, or generally precarious life situations and problems associated with the accumulation of stress,

DOI: 10.4324/9781003097891-25

trauma, and violence further complicate building a life. Finally, xenophobia, discrimination, and racism limit refugees' access to essential domains of social participation and injure their sense of worth and dignity.

Canada, the context of my work as a sociologist, has a strong tradition in studying immigrant settlement in Canada. Within Canadian immigrant settlement research, scholarship has focused on various aspects of child and youth migration and settlement, emphasizing adolescents. This body of research explores the challenges young immigrants face in the new "host" countries and how these challenges are shaped by multiple variables, including race, social class, gender, pre-migration experience, and ethnic background (Dlamini et al., 2009).

Some of the problems identified in this literature include the difficulties young immigrants and refugees face learning English (Anisef & Murphy Kilbride, 2003), the psychosocial anxieties that accompany moving to a new society (James, 1997), the stressors young immigrants face as they negotiate changing family dynamics (Merali & Violato, 2002), peer victimization, violence, and bullying (McKenney et al., 2006), and barriers to their labor market participation or transitions to higher education (Lauer et al., 2012). Many Canadian studies focus on young migrants' experiences of schooling, especially their educational aspirations, needs, struggles, and the factors influencing their academic outcomes (Anisef & Murphy Kilbride, 2003; Garnett et al., 2008; Sweet et al., 2010; Wilkinson et al., 2013). A growing body of scholarly attention focuses on refugee children's mental health (see Guruge & Butt, 2015).

The Multi-faceted Role of the SBFC Practitioner

The SBFC meta-model assumes that immigrant and refugee children's wellbeing is shaped by an ecology of psychological, familial, and social factors, ranging from community life's unique arrangements to the interpersonal interactions between children and their peers and their teachers. The model sensitizes us to the contextual differences in which immigrant and refugee families settle: not all schools, peer groups, families, and communities are the same. In other words, SBFC practitioners have a complicated job. They have to attend to the problems and pressures children face that exist at multiple levels and consider at which level to intervene. Sometimes teaching children stress-reduction techniques within a clinical setting is required. Other times, addressing problematic norms undergirding peer relations, such as in a school with bullying issues, is needed.

Further, immigrant and refugee children experience social challenges, such as social isolation, which produces anxiety, frustration, and disappointment among many immigrant families and their children. As newcomers to society, immigrant children and their families require assistance in making attachments to various organizations, groups, and institutions. In some communities, specialized organizations exist to meet newcomer children and their families' settlement needs, and schools have developed robust educational supports for immigrant populations. But this is not the case everywhere. Regardless of the level of formal organizational support for immigrant family settlement, the SBFC practitioner occupies a vital position to assist immigrant children and their families in making these critical community connections. Through their work, SBFC practitioners gain intimate knowledge of their clients' lives in different ways from teachers and principals. Chapter 1 of this volume illustrates how immigrant families often consider their SBFC practitioner more than just therapists. They view the SBFC practitioner as friends, confidants, and knowledgeable community insiders who can help them solve some of the problems they face.

Gerrard and Soriano (2013, 2018) make a compelling case that SBFC practitioners do more than provide clinical services: they are mediators of solutions within their school and community. The authors make a persuasive case in their 2018 article "The Role of Community Intervention in School-based Family Counseling" that the SBFC practitioner plays an essential role in mobilizing community resources to improve their clients' lives. This chapter takes Gerrard and Soriano's arguments seriously and should be read as an extension of their theoretical and practical insights. The next section will draw on the SBFC case conceptualization method, as discussed in detail in Chapter 3 of this volume, to illustrate how SBFC practitioners can become an essential mediator of social engagement in community life. The procedures suggested here assume that immigrant children's positive social engagements filter back into the family to help with its overall functioning. As such, an SBFC practitioner's vital role involves assisting clients with enhancing their overall social engagement in the community.

Procedures

Step 1: Develop a SBFC Case Conceptualization as Outlined in Chapter 3 in This Volume

Gerrard specifies an approach to understanding the ecology of a young person's life and the potential source of their issues and problems. The goal here is to gain a clear and detailed picture of their lives and the variety of social relationships they have developed in the community. Your inquiry, as Gerrard specifies, should address some of the following questions:

- How is their relationship with their family?
- Do they have friends? How is that going?
- How about school? Are they doing well? Are they meeting their academic expectations and their families'?
- Are they working? If so, what do they do, and how is that going?

- How do they feel about their neighborhood?
- What sort of things are they doing for leisure? Do they have specific interests in music, art, or athletics? Are they finding an outlet to express those interests?

The importance of developing a detailed and rigorous case conceptualization cannot be overstated. To help someone, you need a holistic view of their life that emphasizes both the client's current struggles and their strengths and interests. By employing the SBFC case conceptualization approach, you will gain precisely this holistic view.

Step 2: Analyze Your Case Conceptualization and Discuss It in Collaboration With Your Clients

What are the sources of their suffering, anxiety, frustration, or disappointment? Young people will speak about conflicts or disagreements with their parents, "drama" among their friends, difficulty securing friendships, conflict with specific teachers, and longing for family living in other countries. They may also speak of being bored and not having adequate avenues to express their energies. I hypothesize that many problems young immigrants and refugees express will relate to their lack of social participation within the larger community.

Once you have conceptualized your case share your analysis with your clients and ask them for their thoughts. Here, I would say to the client,

> I have been thinking about your family quite a bit, and I would like to offer you some thoughts on your current situation. After listening to your story over the last few sessions, it sounds like these are three of the biggest issues you face: [List the issues]. Would you agree with me, or am I missing something?

The hope is to open up a conversation that would refine your analysis in dialogue with your clients. The goal is that collectively you would have a refined list of challenges upon which to focus. Then, ask the clients upon what issue they would like to focus.

Step 2: Get to Know the Community's Resources and Consider How Linking the Children and Their Families With Those Resources May Alleviate the Problems They Face

Take some time to get to know the community's resources focused on young people more generally. I suggest creating a document that includes a list of organizations that provide after-school programs, cultural immersion programs, extracurricular activities, and leisure pursuits for young people. I also suggest including a name of a point person and their contact information. The goal is to have a ready-made list to which you can easily refer. You may wish to use a chart format to organize this information (the names on this chart are fictitious):

Name of organizations or program	Activities offered	Contact person
Boundless Youth	Variety of after-school enrichment programs Tutoring	Joan Doe
Newcomers Thriving	Variety of programs targeting immigrants and refugees, including housing support, English as a Second Language, and youth groups	Cassy Devoy
Learn to Skate	Low-cost learn how to skate program	George Selimos
. . .	. . .	. . .
. . .	. . .	. . .

It is paramount that practitioners get to know people in these organizations through community events, or even just calling to introduce yourself is crucial. You will learn about many potential activities you can link your client to only through word of mouth. Young people's participation in interest-driven activities improves their social inclusion and social engagement, provides them with enjoyable activities, connects them to caring relationships, and enhances their opportunities for socialization and skill development (Ben-Eliyahi et al., 2014). It may also increase parents' social participation in community life and improve their prospects for socialization and building connections in the community. The impact of expanding relationships like this can be quite powerful.

Step 3: Consider If Enhancing Social Participation Is a Crucial Ingredient of Your Treatment Plan

The problems that immigrant and refugee children and families face can be quite multifaceted. Degni et al. (2006) discuss in their work with Somali migrant families in Finland how multiple factors, including parental unemployment and new cultural norms in the host society regarding gender relations, produce disorganization within the family. In such cases, interventions would involve assisting these families in securing employment, negotiating expectations in parenting, and resolving negative interactional dynamics among family members. Their work illustrates that some issues will need interventions at the therapeutic level. You will need to help in negotiating their relationship with family members or peers. This volume identifies excellent approaches to dealing with issues related to parenting and parent-child relationships. I suggest consulting those chapters for thoughts on how to address these sorts of problems.

In some cases, your analysis may point to having to assist the parents with their struggles. Perhaps the negative interactions and relationships between father and son are due to the father's inability to find work. Can you, as the SBFC practitioner, assist in connecting the father to available employment services?

In many cases, the "treatment" may be finding opportunities for young people and their families to expand their social participation within the community. Through this participation, young immigrants will meet new people, develop new skills, and gain knowledge. Here are some questions to ask yourself when determining to what extent assisting in expanding social engagements in community life might be a helpful intervention strategy:

- Does the child have a particular interest—in athletics, art, science—that is not being cultivated? Are there programs in the school or community that you can help tap into to satisfy these interests?
- Are the parents working long hours and concerned that their children are not getting adequate supervision? Are there after-school programs that the child could be enrolled in that would also provide an opportunity for the child to meet new people who share similar interests?
- Is the child having difficulty forming friends in school? Are there after-school youth groups, run through religious or voluntary organizations, that the child can participate in and that would allow building new friendships?
- Are the parents concerned that their child is "losing" their culture and absorbing too much of the new host society? Is the child amiable to attending activities to practice their native language? Are there programs to do this?
- Is the child having difficulty in school? Are there tutoring services available through the school or in the community that you can tap?

Step 4: Discuss Your Analysis With the Young Person and Present Them With Options for Social Engagement

Present to the parents and child some of the potential engagement opportunities that you think would benefit them. For example, perhaps you have a child who has always been interested in music and is, in fact, an excellent singer and traditional drummer. You also know that this particular young person has difficulty meeting friends at school, making her feel sad and distracting her from learning. Luckily, you also know of an after-school music program. Could you be the person who makes those connections for her?

An Example of the Power of Expanding Social Participation

While conducting my dissertation research on immigrant and refugee youth settlement, I met a young refugee from eastern Africa named Moti. A case study of his early settlement experiences is published in Chen et al. (2017).

In short, Moti viewed Canada, the national context of my study, as a place of opportunity and was grateful to the Canadian government for accepting his family as refugees. However, since moving to Canada, Moti had become increasingly sensitive to a growing xenophobic atmosphere amplified by experiences of everyday racism in his community and the extensive media coverage of ISIS. In response, Moti told me that he intentionally distanced himself from making friends with White Canadian peers in fear that "if something happens," his White Canadian friends would reject him. He told me in quite stirring words that "[t]o respect my reputation . . . I get away from people who are not from my race or my religion." His logic made sense to me. Why risk the chance of being rejected? In my estimate, his fears were legitimate and expressed his desire to protect himself from interpersonal rejection. So, when I concluded my study, Moti only hung out with other African immigrants.

In 2019, about 2 years after my research study, I learned from a friend who worked in a local voluntary organization that served new immigrants to Canada that Moti's life had changed significantly. Through her organization, Moti participated in a theatre play about the struggles and resiliency of young refugees. From that experience, he fell in love with all aspects of the performing arts. To follow his passion, he transferred schools, away from a school that served many new immigrants to the city and his existing peer group's comfort, to one known for its excellent theatre program, but a school with not many immigrant students. It was a bold move for this young man. She informed me that the school welcomed him with open arms and that he was now pursuing training in music and stage production, having become interested in the intricacies of lighting and sound.

Moti's participation in the refugee theatre group was significant to his settlement. It exposed him to an interest that drove his decision to change schools, despite his deep existential fears. While I do not wish to downplay the real negative consequences of discrimination and racism, Moti's choice to change schools helped cultivate his professional training and career and expand his community's social participation. Moti's story illustrates that critical point that children and youth who have the opportunity to expand their connections to people, places, and organizations help children develop their possibilities. The same is true for immigrant and refugee youth. SBFC practitioners can play a vital role in this essential component of youth development.

Multicultural Considerations

Immigrant and refugee children and families are diverse. These diversities include differing pre-migration lives, migration experiences and pathways, educational level, race and ethnicity, and cultural norms. All these factors play into how immigrant and refugee families cope with the stresses of settlement. When conducting case conceptualizations and associated intervention plans, SBFC practitioners must consider these varied forms of diversity. When an SBFC practitioner suggests organizations, programs, or extracurricular activities, they should do so by considering the family's sensitivities. Of course, all decisions should be left up to the child and family. The SBFC practitioner's role is to assist in negotiating the stressors of settlement in a supportive and collaborative manner.

Challenges and Solutions

Three significant barriers exist when attempting to connect young immigrants and refugees to programs and opportunities in the community:

1. **Time**. Some young immigrants and refugees have significant out-of-school responsibilities that might include working or caring for family members. In helping children and immigrants make these community connections, it is crucial to consider these time constraints. In some cases, a young person's participation in extracurricular activities might require renegotiating responsibilities and tasks within the family.
2. **Financial resources.** A significant factor that prevents people from expanding their connections in the community and getting involved in various extracurricular activities is cost. "Pay-to-Play" programming limits the extent to which low-income, including new immigrants and refugees, can participate. I understand that SBFC practitioners work in various institutional settings, so my only advice here would be to consider how you can develop a fund of some sort to help offset participation costs.
3. **Reluctance and fear.** Some parents may be particularly wary about allowing their children to participate in extracurricular activities. Families characterized by more traditional gender role socialization patterns may be particularly resistant to allowing their daughters to participate. The young person may also be worried about meeting new people and lack confidence in their language capacities. To address some of these situations, I would be sure to discuss why these programs would be helpful. If you have established yourself as a trusted mediator between the family and the larger society, presenting options that communicate how participation in these activities will help develop their children's skills might help combat parental resistance. Attending community programs and events can be scary, especially for immigrants and refugees who are new to a place and fearful that people may not be welcoming. In such cases, it is always helpful to be a point of support. Take them to the door, if you can! You would be surprised at how powerful such a gesture of encouragement can be!

Conclusion

In this chapter, I emphasized that the SBFC practitioners are mediators of solutions within school and community. My research with immigrants and refugees suggests that many of the psychological problems they face relate to the specific challenges of settlement and their difficulties in negotiating and navigating their social participation in community life. I take the ecological approach to the SBFC meta-model seriously. As such, a critical avenue of activity for SBFC practitioners is to consider how they can leverage their positions to enhance immigrant and refugee children's social engagement in community life. My suggestions in this chapter assume that expanding our connections to people, places, and institutions helps us develop and grow. As newcomers, immigrant and refugee children and families may need assistance in making these connections. SBFC practitioners are well placed to be mediators of connections between the immigrant children and the community, and they should consider how to facilitate these connections in their treatment plans.

Resources

Ben-Eliyahu, A., Rhodes, J. E., & Scales, P. (2014). The Interest-Driven Pursuits of 15 Year Olds: "Sparks" and Their Association With Caring Relationships and Developmental Outcomes. Applied Developmental Science, 18(2), 76–89. https://doi.org/10.1080/10888691.2014.894414

This article clarifies how connecting young people to various extracurricular activities improves positive developmental outcomes.

Degni, F., Pöntinen, S., & Mulki, M. (2006). Somali parents' experiences of bringing up children in Finland: Exploring social-cultural change within migrant households. Forum Qualitative Sozialforschung. Forum: Qualitative Social Research, 7(3), Art. 8. http://www.qualitative-research.net/index.php/fqs/article/view/139

This article provides fascinating insights into how migration impacts family relationships.

Gerrard, B. (2021). Chapter 3. Of this volume.

This chapter outlines how to develop an SBFC case conceptualization with immigrant and refugee clients. The case conceptualization represents the first step in assisting clients in addressing their problems. Without a detailed case conceptualization, appropriate interventions or therapies cannot be identified.

Gerrard, B., & Soriano, M. (2018). The role of community intervention in school-based family counseling. International Journal for School-Based Family Counseling. http://www.instituteschoolbasedfamilycounseling.com/journal.html, 10.

This article is a must-read as it provides a definitive statement on the SBFC practitioner's role in community intervention for the child's sake. It also offers excellent practical advice on how to conduct community interventions as an SBFC practitioner.

Hernandez, D. J., & Charney, E. (1998). Generation to generation: The health and wellbeing of children in immigrant families. http://www.ncbi.nlm.nih.gov/books/NBK230361/. National Academies Press.

While over 20 years old, this book, compiled by the National Research Institute and the Institute of Medicine Committee on the Health and Adjustment of Children in Immigrant Families, provides an important picture of immigrant children's developmental challenges.

Bridging refugee youth and children services. The website can be accessed here. https://brycs.org/
This website provides various resources on strengthening immigrant and refugee-serving and mainstream organizations in their efforts to support refugee and immigrant youth. The Promising Practices page allows you to search by region and program type. The Clearinghouse page offers a variety of additional resources.

Bibliography

Anisef, P., & Murphy Kilbride, K. (2003). Managing two worlds: The experiences and concerns of immigrant youth in Ontario. Canadian Scholars' Press.

Ben-Eliyahu, A., Rhodes, J. E., & Scales, P. (2014). The Interest-Driven Pursuits of 15 Year Olds: "Sparks" and Their Association With Caring Relationships and Developmental Outcomes. Applied Developmental Science, 18(2), 76–89. https://doi.org/10.1080/10888691.2014.894414

Chen, X., Raby, R., & Albanese, P. (2017). The sociology of childhood and youth in Canada. Canadian Scholars.

Degni, F., Pöntinen, S., & Mulki, M. (2006). Somali parents' experiences of bringing up children in Finland: Exploring social-cultural change within migrant households. Forum Qualitative Sozialforschung. Forum: Qualitative Social Research, 7(3), Art. 8.

Dlamini, N., Wolfe, B., Anucha, U., & Yan, M. C. (2009). Engaging the Canadian diaspora: Youth social identities in a Canadian border city. McGill Journal of Education, 44(3), 405–434.

Drachman, D. (1992). A stage-of-migration framework for services to immigrant populations. Social Work, 37(1), 68–72.

Garnett, B., Adamuti-Trache, M., & Ungerleider, C. (2008). The academic mobility of students for whom English is not a first language: The roles of ethnicity, language, and class. Alberta Journal of Educational Research, 54(3), 309–326.

Gerrard, B., & Soriano, M. (2013). School-based family counseling: An overview. In B. Gerrard & M. Soriano (Eds.), School-based family counseling: Transforming family-school relationships (pp. 2–15). San Francisco: Institute for School-Based Family Counseling.

Gerrard, B., & Soriano, M. (2018). The role of community intervention in school-based family counseling. International Journal for School-Based Family Counseling. http://www.instituteschoolbasedfamilycounseling.com/journal.html, 10.

Guruge, S., & Butt, H. (2015). A scoping review of mental health issues and concerns among immigrant and refugee youth in Canada: Looking back, moving forward. Canadian Journal of Public Health, 106(2), e72–e78. https://doi.org/10.17269/cjph.106.4588

James, D. C. (1997). Coping with a new society: The unique psychosocial problems of immigrant youth. Journal of School Health, 67(3), 98–102. https://doi.org/10.1111/j.1746-1561.1997.tb03422.x

Lauer, S., Wilkinson, L., Yan, M. C., Sin, R., & Tsang, A. K. T. (2012). Immigrant youth and employment: Lessons learned from the analysis of LSIC and 82 lived stories.

Journal of International Migration and Integration / Revue de l'Integration et de la Migration Internationale, 13, 1–19. https://doi.org/10.1007/s12134-011-0189-1

McKenney, K. S., Pepler, D., Craig, W., & Connolly, J. (2006). Peer victimization and psychosocial adjustment: The experiences of Canadian immigrant youth. Electronic Journal of Research in Educational Psychology, 4(2), 239–264.

Merali, N., & Violato, C. (2002). Relationships between demographic variables and immigrant parents' perceptions of assimilative adolescent behaviours. Journal of International Migration and Integration / Revue de l'Integration et de la Migration Internationale, 3(1), 65–81. https://doi.org/10.1007/s12134-002-1003-x

Selimos, E. D. (2021). The SBFC practitioner's role in promoting immigrant and refugee children's social participation in community life, A1.

Sweet, R., Anisef, P., & Walter, D. (2010). Immigrant parents' investments in their children's post-secondary education. Canadian Journal of Higher Education, 40(3), 59–80. https://doi.org/10.47678/cjhe.v40i3.2015

Wilkinson, L., Yan, M. C., Tsang, A. K. T., Sin, R., & Lauer, S. (2013). The school-to-work transitions of newcomer youth in Canada. Canadian Ethnic Studies, 44(3), 29–44. https://doi.org/10.1353/ces.2013.0000

Index

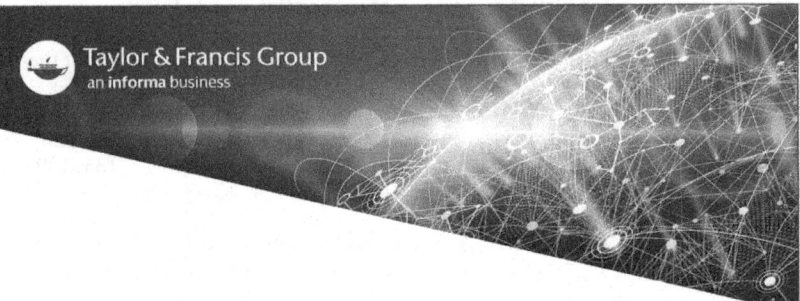
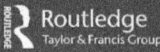
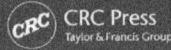